Immune Rebalancing

Immune Rebalancing
The Future of Immunosuppression

Diana Boraschi
Institute of Protein Biochemistry of the National Research Council,
Napoli, Italy

Giselle Penton-Rol
Center for Genetic Engineering and Biotechnology (CIGB), Havana, Cuba

ELSEVIER

AMSTERDAM • BOSTON • HEIDELBERG • LONDON
NEW YORK • OXFORD • PARIS • SAN DIEGO
SAN FRANCISCO • SINGAPORE • SYDNEY • TOKYO
Academic Press is an imprint of Elsevier

Academic Press is an imprint of Elsevier
125, London Wall, EC2Y 5AS.
525 B Street, Suite 1800, San Diego, CA 92101-4495, USA
50 Hampshire St. Cambridge, MA 02139, USA
The Boulevard, Langford Lane, Kidlington, Oxford OX5 1GB, UK

Notices
Knowledge and best practice in this field are constantly changing. As new research and experience broaden our understanding, changes in research methods, professional practices, or medical treatment may become necessary.

Practitioners and researchers must always rely on their own experience and knowledge in evaluating and using any information, methods, compounds, or experiments described herein. In using such information or methods they should be mindful of their own safety and the safety of others, including parties for whom they have a professional responsibility.

To the fullest extent of the law, neither the Publisher nor the authors, contributors, or editors, assume any liability for any injury and/or damage to persons or property as a matter of products liability, negligence or otherwise, or from any use or operation of any methods, products, instructions, or ideas contained in the material herein.

ISBN: 978-0-12-803302-9

Library of Congress Cataloging-in-Publication Data
A catalog record for this book is available from the Library of Congress.

British Library Cataloguing-in-Publication Data
A catalogue record for this book is available from the British Library.

For Information on all Academic Press publications
visit our website at http://store.elsevier.com/

  Working together
to grow libraries in
developing countries

ELSEVIER | Book Aid International

www.elsevier.com • www.bookaid.org

CONTENTS

List of Contributors... xi

Chapter 1 Pharmacological Strategies Using Biologics as
Immunomodulatory Agents...1
Diana Boraschi and Giselle Penton-Rol

1.1 Introduction..1
1.2 From Nonspecific to Targeted Immunosuppression....................2
1.3 From Immunosuppression to Immune Rebalancing..................6
1.4 Conclusions 8
Acknowledgments...9
References..9

PART I MECHANISMS OF IMMUNE-RELATED
PATHOLOGIES AND THEIR CURRENT
TREATMENT...13

Chapter 2 Advance in Therapies for Rheumatoid Arthritis:
New Perspectives..15
Flavio A. Amaral, Thiago H.C. Oliveira, Debora C. Calderaro,
Gilda A. Ferreira and Mauro M. Teixeira

2.1 Introduction..15
2.2 Rheumatoid Arthritis Management...................................16
2.3 New Alternatives for the Treatment of RA 24
2.4 Loss of Immune Tolerance as a Factor for
RA Development: A Possible Target..................................24
2.5 Resolution of Inflammation 25
2.6 Challenges 29
2.7 Concluding Remarks 31
References..31

Chapter 3 Immune Based Therapies for Inflammatory Bowel Disease **37**

Preetika Sinh, Claudio Fiocchi and Jean-Paul Achkar

3.1 Introduction...37
3.2 Immune Regulation in IBD...37
3.3 Current Immune Based Therapies in IBD 39
3.4 Immunomodulators 39
3.5 Biological Agents...42
3.6 Next Generation Immune Based Therapies in IBD.............49
3.7 Conclusion..54
References...54

Chapter 4 Multiple Sclerosis and Neurodegenerative Diseases **63**

Maira Gironi, Caterina Arnò, Giancarlo Comi, Giselle Penton-Rol and Roberto Furlan

4.1 Introduction...63
References...80

Chapter 5 Therapeutic Approaches in Allergic Diseases....................**85**

IlariaPuxeddu, Francesca Levi-Schaffer and Paola Migliorini

5.1 General Aspects of Allergic Diseases.................................85
5.2 Modulation of Allergen-Specific Responses 88
5.3 Targeting Th2 Cytokines: IL-5, IL-4, and IL-13 92
5.4 Targeting IgE and FcεRI..94
5.5 Targeting Mast Cells and Eosinophils................................96
5.6 Conclusions 99
References...99

Chapter 6 Immunotherapy for Transforming Advanced Cancer into a Chronic Disease: How Far Are We?......................**105**

Tania Crombet and Agustin Lage

6.1 Introduction: The Basic Biology of Chronic Diseases 105
6.2 The Evidence of a Transition to Chronicity 106
6.3 The Pharmacologic Consequence: Anticancer Drugs for Long-Term Use 109
6.4 The Expanding Role of Immunotherapy................................110
6.5 A Methodological Consequence: The Need of Novel Approaches to Clinical Trial Design and Evaluation 113

6.6   Immune Rebalancing: The Research Agenda for the
        Age of Chronicity 114
References 117

**PART II BIOLOGICS AS IMMUNOSUPPRESSIVE
              AGENTS** **121**

Chapter 7 Modulation of Macrophage Activation **123**
        Paola Italiani, Elfi Töpfer and Diana Boraschi
7.1   Introduction 123
7.2   An Overview on Macrophage Polarization/Activation 124
7.3   M1/M2 Skewing: Detrimental and Beneficial Consequences 128
7.4   Mechanisms of Macrophage Activation 132
7.5   Local Conditions and Cell–Cell Interactions:
        Other Cues in Macrophage Polarization 137
7.6   Therapeutic Applications Based on Modulation
        of Macrophage Polarization/Activation in the Tumor 140
7.7   Conclusions 141
Acknowledgments 143
Conflict of Interest 143
References 143

Chapter 8 Modulating Inflammatory Cytokines: IL-1 .... **151**
        Mark S. Gresnigt and Frank L. van de Veerdonk
8.1   Introduction 151
8.2   Biologicals Targeting IL-1 154
8.3   Blocking IL-1 in Disease 155
8.4   Conclusions 163
References 163

**Chapter 9 Systems Medicine of Autoimmune Diseases: From
              Understanding Complexity to Precision Treatments** **173**
        Julio Raúl Fernández Massó
9.1   Introduction 173
9.2   From Systems Biology to Systems Medicine 175
9.3   Systems Biology and the Emerging Technologies 175

9.4   Application of Emerging Technologies in Autoimmune
       Research 176
9.5   From Systems Medicine to Precision Medicine 183
References... 183

**Chapter 10 The Microbiota and Its Modulation in
            Immune-Mediated Disorders 191**
            *Meirav Pevsner-Fischer, Chagai Rot, Timur Tuganbaev
            and Eran Elinav*

10.1   Introduction.. 191
10.2   Development of the Gut Microbiota 192
10.3   Microbiota Effects on Immune Development....................... 193
10.4   Microbiota Modulation 197
10.5   Microbiota Involvement in Prevalence and Progression
        Immune-Related Disease 200
10.6   Summary and Conclusions 211
Acknowledgements 215
References... 215

**Chapter 11 Natural Products: Immuno-Rebalancing
            Therapeutic Approaches 229**
            Eduardo Penton-Arias and David D. Haines

11.1   Introduction.. 229
11.2   Modulation of Immune Responses for Disease Prevention
        and Treatment 231
11.3   Traditional Medicinal Preparations have Immunoactive
        Properties.. 233
11.4   Natural Products can Influence and Modify Intersystem
        Interactions and Infection Resistance 234
11.5   Immunosuppression is not the Abrogation but the
        Rebalancing of Immune Functions.................................... 236
11.6   The Oxidant versus Antioxidant Argument does not
        Provide Responses but Creates Uncertainty 238
11.7   Neuroprotection/Restoration is Achievable by Natural
        Products.. 240
11.8   C-Phycocyanin/Phycocyanobilin Properties, Mechanisms
        and Prospects... 241

11.9   Conclusions...243
References...245

Chapter 12 Nanomedicine...**251**
         Albert Duschl
12.1   Why Nanomaterials? 251
12.2   Products on the Market or in Development 253
12.3   Suppressing Immunity: Autoimmunity and Other Cases........255
12.4   Activating Immunity: The Future of Vaccines?......258
12.5   Cancer as an Immunological Disease 260
12.6   Allergy..262
12.7   What Are We Really Using?....................................264
12.8   Rebalancing Exciting New Prospects and
         Over-Optimistic Hype...266
12.9   Acknowledgements 267
References...267

Index...**275**

LIST OF CONTRIBUTORS

Jean-Paul Achkar
Department of Gastroenterology and Hepatology, Digestive Disease Institute, Cleveland Clinic, Cleveland, OH, USA; Department of Pathobiology, Lerner Research Institute, Cleveland Clinic, Cleveland, OH, USA

Flavio A. Amaral
Immunopharmacology, Department of Biochemistry and Immunology, Institute of Biological Science, Universidade Federal de Minas Gerais, Minas Gerais, Brazil

Caterina Arnò
Institute of Experimental Neurology, Division of Neuroscience, San Raffaele Scientific Institute, Milan, Italy

Diana Boraschi
Institute of Protein Biochemistry, National Research Council, Napoli, Italy

Debora C. Calderaro
Department of Rheumatology, Universidade Federal de Minas Gerais, Minas Gerais, Brazil

Giancarlo Comi
Institute of Experimental Neurology, Division of Neuroscience, San Raffaele Scientific Institute, Milan, Italy

Tania Crombet
Center of Molecular Immunology, Havana, Cuba

Albert Duschl
Department of Molecular Biology, University of Salzburg, Salzburg, Austria

Eran Elinav
Department of Immunology, Weizmann Institute of Science, Rehovot, Israel

Gilda A. Ferreira
Department of Locomotor System Medicine, Faculty of Medicine, Universidade Federal de Minas Gerais, Minas Gerais, Brazil

Claudio Fiocchi
Department of Gastroenterology and Hepatology, Digestive Disease Institute, Cleveland Clinic, Cleveland, OH, USA; Department of Pathobiology, Lerner Research Institute, Cleveland Clinic, Cleveland, OH, USA

Julio Raúl Fernández Massó
Department of Systems Biology, Center for Genetic Engineering and Biotechnology, Cubanacan, Havana, Cuba

Roberto Furlan
Institute of Experimental Neurology, Division of Neuroscience, San Raffaele Scientific Institute, Milan, Italy

Maira Gironi
Institute of Experimental Neurology, Division of Neuroscience, San Raffaele Scientific Institute, Milan, Italy

Mark S. Gresnigt
Department of Internal Medicine, Radboud University Medical Center, Nijmegen, The Netherlands

David D. Haines
University of Connecticut, Faculty of Pharmacy, Department of Pharmacology Health Science Center, University of Debrecen, Hungary

Paola Italiani
Institute of Protein Biochemistry, National Research Council, Napoli, Italy

Agustin Lage
Center of Molecular Immunology, Havana, Cuba

Francesca Levi-Schaffer
Pharmacology Unit, Faculty of Medicine, School of Pharmacy, Institute for Drug Research, Hebrew University of Jerusalem, Jerusalem, Israel

Paola Migliorini
Immuno-Allergology Unit, Department of Clinical and Experimental Medicine, Pisa University, Pisa, Italy

Thiago H.C. Oliveira
Immunopharmacology, Department of Biochemistry and Immunology, Institute of Biological Science, Universidade Federal de Minas Gerais, Minas Gerais, Brazil

Eduardo Penton-Arias
Latin American School of Medicine (ELAM) and Biomedical Research Direction of Center for Genetic Engineering and Biotechnology (CIGB), Havana, Cuba

Giselle Penton-Rol
Center for Genetic Engineering and Biotechnology, Havana, Cuba

Meirav Pevsner-Fischer
Department of Immunology, Weizmann Institute of Science, Rehovot, Israel

Ilaria Puxeddu
Immuno-Allergology Unit, Department of Clinical and Experimental Medicine, Pisa University, Pisa, Italy

Chagai Rot
Department of Immunology, Weizmann Institute of Science, Rehovot, Israel

Preetika Sinh
Department of Gastroenterology and Hepatology, Digestive Disease Institute, Cleveland Clinic, Cleveland, OH, USA

Mauro M. Teixeira
Immunopharmacology, Department of Biochemistry and Immunology, Institute of Biological Science, Universidade Federal de Minas Gerais, Minas Gerais, Brazil

Elfi Töpfer
Institute of Protein Biochemistry, National Research Council, Napoli, Italy

Timur Tuganbaev
Department of Immunology, Weizmann Institute of Science, Rehovot, Israel

Frank L. van de Veerdonk
Department of Internal Medicine, Radboud University Medical Center, Nijmegen, The Netherlands

CHAPTER 1

Pharmacological Strategies Using Biologics as Immunomodulatory Agents

Diana Boraschi[1] and Giselle Penton-Rol[2]

[1]Institute of Protein Biochemistry of the National Research Council, Napoli, Italy [2]Center for Genetic Engineering and Biotechnology (CIGB), Habana, Cuba

1.1 INTRODUCTION

Immunosuppression has been used by physicians for many decades for blocking the unwanted activities of the immune system. In the last century, the history of therapeutic immunosuppression has paralleled the history of immunology as studies on "transplantation immunity" have allowed us to gain a deeper understanding of the rules of activation and regulation of adaptive immunity.[1] The discovery of the major histocompatibility complex (MHC) dates back to 1967,[2] and since then we have understood the rules of antigen presentation and cross-presentation, cognate interaction, activation of the different T cell subsets, and antibody production. MHC typing has allowed us to better match organ donors with recipients, but has not avoided the need for immunosuppressive treatments to the recipient. Depending on the type of transplant (bone marrow or solid organs), immunosuppressive regimens could include whole body irradiation and immunosuppressive drugs, such as cytostatic molecules (azathioprine was first used as an immunosuppressive treatment in a kidney transplant in 1959), antimetabolites, corticosteroids, and antibodies against leukocytes and their products. The rough concept is that during an immune response against the allotransplant, the specific immune cells start proliferating and are metabolically active, thus they are better targets for drugs inhibiting metabolism and proliferation. The drawback is that several other cell types in the body are metabolically active and proliferating, for instance the epithelial cells of respiratory and gastrointestinal mucosae, hair follicles, and several others, including immune cells when combating an infection or a disease. Thus, life-long generalized immunosuppression may allow the allotransplant to survive in the host, but it can cause side effects that can become severe and life-threatening.

Immune Rebalancing. DOI: http://dx.doi.org/10.1016/B978-0-12-803302-9.00001-4

Table 1.1 Classical Immunosuppressive Regimens			
Drug/Treatment	**Application**	**Target**	**Side Effects**
Irradiation, antimetabolites, cytostatic drugs (eg, azathioprine, metothrexate)	Bone marrow transplantation, autoimmune diseases	Hematopoietic precursors in the BM, proliferating and activated leukocytes	Immunosuppression (increase of opportunistic infections), cytopenia, epithelial and mucosal damage (diarrhea, damage of endocrine organs, teeth, hair, skin)
Antilymphocyte and anticytokine antibodies, corticosteroids, calcineurin inhibitors (cyclosporine, tacrolimus, sirolimus)	Solid organ transplantation, Graft-versus-host disease, autoimmune diseases	Lymphocytes	Immunosuppression (increase of opportunistic infections), damage of the gastric mucosa, renal dysfunction and consequent hypertension, osteoporosis

Immunosuppressive strategies are used not only for transplanted patients but also, more widely, for treating asthma and allergies, and autoimmune and chronic inflammatory and degenerative diseases, that is, pathologies due to the deranged reaction of the immune system either to innocuous agents (eg, pollens), or to endogenous molecules and structures (autoreactivity), including cell membrane components, nuclei, DNA, and myelin. Most of these diseases have, in addition to the component of anomalous adaptive immune reactivity (for instance the production of autoantibodies), a strong inflammatory component. This includes all the mechanisms of innate immunity, with activation of leucocytes, production of inflammatory factors, and consequent tissue damage/destruction. The persistent inflammatory activation can also bring about the anomalous feed-back activation of repair mechanisms that may lead to nonfunctional neotissue apposition and pathological fibrosis, as in the case of systemic sclerosis. Immunosuppressive and anti-inflammatory treatments are in the vast majority of cases life-long treatments, since the immunosuppressive strategies basically address the damage-inducing immune activation caused by the disease, rather than the cause of the disease.

A summary of the classical immunosuppressive treatments that are being used is provided in Table 1.1.

1.2 FROM NONSPECIFIC TO TARGETED IMMUNOSUPPRESSION

Immunosuppressive approaches have experienced a wide development in more recent times, with the advent of two important technological advancements, that is, the recombinant DNA and the monoclonal antibody technologies. The use of recombinant proteins and of mono-specific antibodies has allowed the physician to direct the immunosuppressive drug to a single molecule/mechanism involved in the disease, in the attempt to achieve better efficacy and lower side effects.

Anticytokine antibodies and cytokine inhibitors are among the most important treatments for autoimmune/chronic inflammatory diseases.

In the list of the best-selling drugs in 2014 (Table 1.2), it is impressive that eight of the first 25 are immunosuppressive drugs, and of these five are biologics. This underlines the still open medical need for more efficient immunosuppressive treatments, and the current success of biologics.

Three anti-TNFα biologics are within the first five best-selling drugs: Humira (a human mAb recognizing the inflammatory cytokine TNFα) is the first in the list, with Remicade (humanized mAb) and Enbrel (chimeric receptor) at the third and fifth position, respectively. The anti-TNF treatments, usually after or in combination with DMARDs (disease modifying antirheumatic drugs) are active in autoimmune and chronic inflammatory diseases, in particular rheumatoid arthritis, osteoarthritis, juvenile idiopathic arthritis, psoriatic arthritis, plaque psoriasis, ankylosing spondilitis, Crohn's disease, and ulcerative colitis.[3] Another very successful immunosuppressive biological drug is Rituxan, a mouse/human chimeric mAb against CD20, an antigen preferentially expressed by activated B cells. Rituxan is used in a series of different diseases in which inhibition of B cell responses is beneficial (eg, autoimmune diseases, transplant rejection) and also for killing tumor cells in B cell lymphomas and leukemias.

The cost of therapies with biologics is significant. For instance, one-year treatment with anti-TNF therapy costs about US$20,000 for a single patient. The cost of Sovaldi (which however is not a biologic drug) peaks at US$84,000 for the full 12-week treatment course. These costs are excessive and necessarily limit the access to the cure. Also, a recent study has highlighted the fact that the success of many of these drugs is partial, with about 25% of treated US patients actually benefiting from anti-TNF therapy, while for other drugs the success is even lower (Table 1.2).[4] Thus, given the costs, predicting response and patients' stratification are a priority for the public health services. On the other hand, given the partial success of these treatments, it is obvious that new more effective approaches are required.[5]

Table 1.2 The 25 Best-selling Drugs in 2014

Name (Compound)	Company	Characteristics/Application	Sales 2014 (billion US$)	Success Rate (USA)
Humira (adalimumab)	AbbVie	Human mAb to TNFα/RA, plaque psoriasis, Crohn's disease, ulcerative colitis, ankylosing spondilitis, psoriatic arthritis, JIA	12.543	25%
Sovaldi (sofosbuvir)	Gilead Science	Small molecule, inhibitor of HCV RNA polymerase/eradication chronic HCV infection	10.283	
Remicade (infliximab)	Johnson & Johnson, Merck & Co.	Humanized mAb to TNFα/RA, Crohn's disease, ankylosing spondilitis, psoriatic arthritis, plaque psoriasis, ulcerative colitis	9.240	25%
Rituxan (rituximab, Mab Thera)	Roche (Genetech), Biogen Idec	Anti-CD20 antibody, kills activated B cells/lymphomas (NHL), leukemias (CLL), autoimmune diseases (RA), transplant rejection	8.678	
Enbrel (etanercept)	Amgen, Pfizer	Chimeric soluble TNFα receptor/RA, JIA, psoriasis	8.538	25%
Avastin (bevacizumab)	Roche	Humanized mAb to VEGF-A, inhibits tumor angiogenesis/carcinomas (colon, nonsmall cell lung, kidney), glioblastoma	6.957	
Herceptin (trastuzumab)	Roche	Humanized mAb to HER2, blocks HER2 signaling and shedding, mediates killing by ADCC/HER2-expressing tumors (breast, gastric, stomach)	6.793	
Lantus (insulin glargine)	Sanofi	Recombinant insulin, diabetes	6.557	
Advair/Seretide (fluticasone-salmeterol)	GSK	Corticosteroid + β_2 adrenergic receptor agonist/anti-inflammatory + bronchodilator; asthma, COPD	6.431	4%
Crestor (rosuvastatin calcium)	AstraZeneca, Shionogi	Small molecule (statin class); hypercholesterolemia	5.869	5%
Neulasta/ Neupogen (pegfilgrastim)	Amgen, Kyowa Hakko Kirin	PEGylated recombinant G-CSF/ chemotherapy-induced neutropenia	5.857	8%
Lyrica (pregabalin)	Pfizer	Small molecule, binds voltage-dependent calcium channels, anticonvulsant/ neuropathies	5.168	
Abilify (aripiprazole)	Otsuka Pharmaceutical, Bristol-Myers Squibb	Small molecule, partial agonist D_2 and $5HT_{1A}$ receptors/schizophrenia, bipolar I, depression	5.269	20%
Revlimid (lenalidomide)	Celgene	Lymphoma, myeloma	4.980	

(Continued)

Table 1.2 (Continued)				
Name (Compound)	**Company**	**Characteristics/Application**	**Sales 2014 (billion US$)**	**Success Rate (USA)**
Gleevec (imatinib mesylate)	Novartis	Small molecule, tyrosine kinase inhibitor; Ph + leukemias	4.746	
Prevnar	Pfizer	Vaccines against multiple *S. pneumoniae* strains (7 or 13), conjugates of streptococcal capsule polysaccharides with a recombinant carrier protein CRM197 of *C. diphteriae*/prevention pneumonia and otitis media in children and elderly	4.464	
Copaxone (glatiramer)	Teva Pharmaceutical Industries	Synthetic random peptide from myelin, acting as decoy for autoantibodies/ relapsing MS	4.237	6%
Zetia/Vytorin (ezetimibe)	Merck & Co.	Small molecules, inhibitor of intestinal absorption of cholesterol/ hypercholesterolemia	4.166	
Januvia (sitagliptin)	Merck & Co.	Small molecule, inhibitor dipeptidyldipeptidase 4, decreases blood sugar/type 2 diabetes mellitus	4.004	
Symbicort (budesonide and formoterol)	AstraZeneca	Cortocosteroid + β_2 adrenergic receptor agonist, anti-inflammatory+ bronchodilator/asthma, COPD, chronic bronchitis, emphysema	3.801	
Nexium (esomeprazole)	AstraZeneca	Small molecules, proton pump inhibitor/ *H. pylori* eradication, oesophageal reflux, gastric ulcers	3.655	4%
Atripla (efavirenz, emtricitabine, and tenofovir)	Gilead Sciences, Bristol-Myers Squibb	Cocktail antiretroviral small molecules/ HIV-1 infection	3.470	
Truvada (emtricitabine and tenofovir disoproxil fumarate)	Gilead Sciences	Cocktail antiretroviral small molecules/ HIV-1 infection	3.340	
Avonex	Biogen Idec	Recombinant interferon β-1A/relapsing MS	3.013	
Celebrex (celecoxib)	Pfizer	Small molecule, anti-inflammatory COX-2 inhibitor/RA, JIA, osteoarthritis	2.699	

In bold-italic: immunosuppressive/anti-inflammatory biologics; in italic: non-biologic immunosuppressive/ anti-inflammatory drugs; in bold: biologics not aiming at immune suppression.
mAb: monoclonal antibody; TNFα: tumor necrosis factor α; RA: rheumatoid arthritis; JIA: juvenile idiopathic arthritis; HCV: hepatitis C virus; CD20: cluster of differentiation 20 (surface molecule expressed by B cells); HL: non-Hodgkin's lymphoma; CLL: chronic lymphocytic leukemia; VEGF-A: vascular endothelial growth factor A; HER2 (human epidermal growth factor receptor 2); ADCC: antibody-dependent cellular cytotoxicity; COPD: chronic obstructive pulmonary disease; G-CSF: granulocyte colony stimulating factor; MS: multiple sclerosis; COX-2: cyclooxygenase 2.
Source: *Information taken from Genetic Engineering and Biotechnology News, February 23, 2015.*

1.3 FROM IMMUNOSUPPRESSION TO IMMUNE REBALANCING

The range of applications of immunosuppressive therapies has become increasingly wider as the mechanisms of disease initiation and progression are being clarified. Thus, it is now obvious that most diseases are based on anomalous immune regulation. In fact, it is known that the immune system needs to establish and maintain an effective balance between reaction to foreign possibly dangerous agents (such as invading microorganisms) and unresponsiveness to harmless agents (eg, the microbiota) and self-molecules. Disruption of the balance between response and tolerance, and the consequent immune dysregulation can cause pathologies such as cancer (in which inflammation and immunosuppression play an important role in allowing tumor growth), metabolic diseases (obesity, diabetes), degenerative diseases including Alzheimer, Parkinson, Amyotrophic Lateral Sclerosis, respiratory and cardiovascular diseases, in addition to the typical allergic and autoimmune diseases.

The new biologics and the single-target small molecules that have been developed in the last decades have allowed the design of better treatment protocols for some specific diseases (see for instance the case of the anti-CD20 mAb for B cell lymphomas and leukemias), but have also underlined the complexity of many diseases that in most cases cannot be treated by inhibiting a single target. Also, inhibition of single specific targets has given us a glimpse of the importance of such targets in the organism's homeostasis. This is the case of anti-TNF therapies, which have revealed to the medical community the importance of TNFα for protection against *Mycobacterium tuberculosis*. In fact, treated patients are more prone to get infected or to reactivate tuberculosis (if they are carriers). This limits the application of the anti-TNF therapy to people that are tuberculin negative, to limit the risk of reactivation.

Many other mAbs and biologics have been/are being developed for targeting immune cells, in particular in cancer therapy. Antibodies that disrupt the PD-1 receptor on activated T cells (pembrolizuman and nivolumab) essentially block their apoptosis thereby allowing immune recognition and destruction of the cancer cells. Ipilimumab, an antibody against CD152 (CTLA4, an inhibitory molecule of T cells), blocks the immunosuppression mediated by it and allows more efficient T cell activation and consequently a better response against cancer. These Immune Checkpoint Inhibitors (ICI) are the most promising new anti-cancer approach. Cancer disrupts the normal regulation of immune responses, by inhibiting most of them to increase its chances of successful growth, thus the new treatments that are being devised intend to reattain the normal defensive immune functions by eliminating the blocks that do not allow full antitumor activation. As an example, it is known that pathological events induce the so-called emergency hematopoiesis for increasing the number of immune cells, and that tumors can reprogram this process giving rise to immature immunosuppressive myeloid cells.[6] The identification of the switch molecule used by tumors for reprogramming such myelopoiesis, and the efficacy of its blockade in inhibiting tumor growth, open the way to a new immune rebalancing approach in anticancer therapy.[7]

Although biologics represent a major advance in the treatment of several diseases, notably rheumatoid arthritis, inflammatory bowel disease, and psoriasis, effective therapy for other autoimmune conditions, such as type 1 diabetes, remain elusive and will likely require targeting multiple immune components. Approaches of ex vivo immune cell "education" or combination therapies with different biologics and cells are being actively investigated, in the attempt to control autoimmune disease manifestations and restore the tolerant state.[8]

Restoration of tolerance is a medical issue of key importance that is gaining great attention. Knowledge of the role of regulatory T cells (Tregs) in the establishment and maintenance of immunological tolerance[9,10] opens the possibility of targeting the Treg suppressive functions as an effective way of controlling immune responses, Thus, Treg modulation may become an important therapeutic opportunity for the treatment of a number of important diseases. The importance of achieving an accurate balance, when attempting to modulate immune responses, was shown in several studies. As an example, exploiting Treg activity in haploidentical hematopoietic cell transplantation (a potential therapeutic strategy for patients with hematological malignancies[11,12]) would need a deeper understanding of how to modulate the T cell regulatory networks.[13] Indeed, if T cells are included in the donor graft, this would cause graft-versus-host disease (GVHD), while T cell depletion would avoid GVHD and considerably increase the risk of severe infections and tumor relapse.

The US Food and Drug Administration (FDA) has approved several agents for modulating Treg activity in anticancer trials. Cyclophosphamide, fludarabine, anti-CTLA4 antibodies, and PD-1 blockers have had considerable success in circumventing Treg activity through different mechanisms of action and, in turn, in enhancing killer cell activity.[14–18] Treg transfer is also a promising therapeutic option in controlling severe inflammatory diseases, as shown in experimental models of colitis.[19] There are also indications that the immunosuppressive and anti-inflammatory effects of corticosteroids may in part be via Treg activation.[20,21]

An important issue in the use of biologics for modulating immune responses is their immunogenicity, which could induce the host reaction and the production of antidrug antibodies (ADA) thereby hampering their efficacy. In the case of monoclonal or chimeric antibodies, ADA usually target foreign sequences that are not present in natural human antibodies. Replacement of foreign sequences with human sequences ("humanization") is the most common approach for decreasing antibody immunogenicity. However, even fully human mAbs can be immunogenic. In such cases, the introduction of T regulatory epitopes can be adopted, so that the biologic drug would induce tolerance rather than immunity.[22] The most recent document issued by FDA regarding the immunogenicity of biologics is the Draft Guidance for Industry "Immunogenicity Assessment for Therapeutic Protein Products" in August 2014.[23] The European Commission and EFPIA have started a Europe-wide project, in the context of the Innovative Medicine Initiative-Joint Undertaking (IMI-JU), to merge academic and industrial efforts in addressing the problem of immunization against biologics. The project ABIRISK (Anti-Biopharmaceutical Immunization: Prediction and Analysis of Clinical Relevance to Minimize the Risk) puts together nine companies and 25 academic institutions with the aim of solving the problem of biologics' immunogenicity to design new nonimmunogenic drugs, and also to generate tools for predicting the patients' response to the biological drugs.[24]

1.4 CONCLUSIONS

As detailed in this chapter, it is obvious that immune rebalancing is the future direction that immunosuppressive and immunotherapeutic strategies will take, with a particular focus on autoimmune, inflammatory, and degenerative diseases (such as rheumatoid arthritis, Crohn's disease and inflammatory bowel disease, multiple sclerosis and neuro-degenerative diseases, allergies) and cancer. The immune rebalancing strategy includes a series of approaches that need a concomitant harmonized development.

1. Precision medicine. Treatment should be tailored to the individual patient, like in the old concepts of Chinese traditional medicine, because there are no drugs that are good for everybody.[5] From this perspective, systems medicine, which exploits omics technologies for profiling the patient and its reactivity, may help to establish new medical concepts. Also, new valuable information will come from a better understanding of the "chimeric" state of human beings, who encompass 10 times more bacterial cells than human cells. Modulating the microbiota hosted in our body provides a precious strategy for modulating our immune responses.[25]

2. New drugs, new targets. Rediscovering natural products, both as a source of new molecules and as treatment procedures, could provide strategies of treatment that are more suited to precision medicine than the classical drugs.[26,27] New targets that are common to practically all patients could come from the knowledge of innate immune mechanisms (that are practically unaltered in living organisms), and could include mononuclear phagocytes and their products (eg, IL-1).[28]

3. New delivery approaches. A very promising technological advancement, ie, nanotechnology, has provided us with the possibility of using a practically endless array of novel carriers that can be built to form whatever kind of material, shape, size, surface characteristics, layers and tropism, we could wish.[29] Taking drugs specifically to their targets, without being eliminated by the body's defense mechanisms and without unwanted interaction with bystander cells could indeed be achieved by nanomedicine.[30]

ACKNOWLEDGMENTS

DB is supported by the EU projects HUMUNITY (FP7-PEOPLE-INT-2012 GA n. 316383) and BioCoG (FP7-HEALTH-2013-INNOVATION-1 GA n. 602461), and the Cluster project "Medintech" of the Italian Ministry of Education, University and Research.

REFERENCES

1. Chinen J, Buckley RH. Transplantation immunology: solid organ and bone marrow. *J Allergy Clin Immunol* 2010;**125**:S324−35.

2. Bach FH, Amos DB. Hu-1: major histocompatibility locus in man. *Science* 1967;**156**:1506−8.

3. Monaco C, Nanchahal J, Taylor P, Feldmann M. Anti-TNF therapy: past, present and future. *Int Immunol* 2015;**27**:55−62.

4. Schork NJ. Time for one-person trials. *Nature* 2015;**520**:609−11.

5. Bluestone JA, Tang Q. Immunotherapy: making the case for precision medicine. *Sci Transl Med* 2015;**7** 280ed3.

6. Ueha S, Shand FHW, Matsushima K. Myeloid cell population dynamics in healthy and tumor-brearing mice. *Int Immunopharmacol* 2011;**11**:783–8.

7. Strauss L, Sangaletti S, Consonni FM, Szebeni G, Morlacchi S, Totaro MG, et al. RORC1 regulates tumor-promoting "emergency" granulo-monocytopoiesis. *Cencer Cell* 2015;**28**: 253–69.

8. Smilek DE, Ehlers MR, Nepom GT. Restoring the balance: immunotherapeutic combinations for autoimmune disease. *Dis Model Mech* 2014;**7**:503–13.

9. Sakaguchi S, Wing K, Onishi Y, Prieto-Martin P, Yamaguchi T. Regulatory T cells: how do they suppress immune responses? *Int Immunol* 2009;**21**:1105–11.

10. Pandiyan P, Zheng L, Lenardo MJ. The molecular mechanisms of regulatory T cell immunosuppression. *Front Immunol* 2011;**2**:60.

11. Di Ianni M, Falzetti F, Carotti A, Terenzi A, Castellino F, Bonifacio E, et al. Tregs prevent GVHD and promote immune reconstitution in HLA-haploidentical transplantation. *Blood* 2011;**117**:3921–8.

12. Aversa F, Martelli MF. Transplantation of haploidentically mismatched stem cells for the treatment of malignant diseases. *Springer Semin Immunopathol* 2004;**26**:155–68.

13. Humblet-Baron S, Baron F, Liston A. Regulatory T cells fulfil their promise? *Immun Cell Biol* 2011;**89**:825–6.

14. Grosso J, Jure-Kunkel M. CTLA-4 blockade in tumor models: an overview of preclinical and translational research. *Cancer Immun* 2013;**13**:5–18.

15. Sharma RK, Yolcu ES, Shirwan H. The promise of PD-1 signaling pathway for cancer immunotherapy. *J Clin Cell Immunol* 2012;**3**:e110.

16. Berd D, Mastrangelo MJ. Effect of low dose cyclophosphamide on the immune system of cáncer patients: depletion of CD4 + , 2H4 + suppressor-inducer T-cells. *Cancer Res* 1988;**48**:1671–5.

17. Hegde U, Chhabra A, Chattopadhyay S, Das R, Ray S, Chakraborty NG. Presence of low dose of fludarabine in cultures blocks regulatory T cell expansion and maintains tumor-specific cytotoxic T lymphocyte activity generated with peripheral blood lymphocytes. *Pathobiology* 2008;**75**:200–8.

18. Karimi S, Chattopadhyay S, Chakraborty NG. Manipulation of regulatory T cells and antigen-specific cytotoxic T lymphocyte-based tumour immunotherapy. *Immunology* 2014; **144**:186–96.

19. Powrie F. Immune regulation in the intestine: a balancing act between effector and regulatory T cell responses. *Ann NY Acad Sci* 2004;**1029**:132–41.

20. Robinson DS. Regulatory T cells and asthma. *Clin Exp Allergy* 2009;**39**:1314–23.

21. de Paz B, Prado C, Alperi-Lopez M, Ballina-Garcia FJ, Rodriguez-Carrio J, Lopez P, et al. Effects of glucocorticoid treatment on CD25⁻FOXP3 + population and cytokine-producing cells in rheumatoid arthritis. *Rheumatology* 2012;**51**:1198–207.

22. De Groot AS, Terry F, Cousens L, Martin W. Beyond humanization and de-immunization: tolerization as a method for reducing the immunogenicity of biologics. *Expert Rev Clin Pharmacol* 2013;**6**:651–62.

23. U.S. Department of Health and Human Services, Food and Drug Administration Center for Drug Evaluation and Research (CDER), and Center for Biologics Evaluation and Research (CBER). Guidance for Industry: Immunogenicity Assessment for Therapeutic Protein Products. <www.fda.gov/downloads/Drugs/GuidanceComplianceRegulatoryInformation/Guidances/ UCM338856.pdf>; 2014.

24. ABIRISK. Anti-Biopharmaceutical Immunization: prediction and analysis of clinical relevance to minimize the RISK. Available from: <www.abirisk.eu>.

25. Palm NW, de Zoete MR, Flavell RA. Immune-microbiota interactions in health and disease. *Clin Immunol* 2015;**159**:122–7.

26. Banerjee P, Erehman J, Gohlke B-O, Wilhelm T, Preissner R, Dunkel M. Super Natural II – a database of natural products. *Nucleic Acids Res* 2015;**43**:D935–9.

27. Penton-Rol G, Martinez-Sanchez G, Cervantes-Llanos M, Lagumersindez-Denis N, Acosta-Medina EF, Falcon-Cama V, et al. C-phycocyanin ameliorates experimental autoimmune encephalomyelitis and induces regulatory T cells. *Int Immunopharmacol* 2011;**11**:29–38.

28. Bronte V, Murray PJ. Understanding local macrophage phenotypes in disease: modulating macrophage function to treat cancer. *Nat Med* 2015;**21**:117–19.

29. Smith DM, Simon JK, Baker JR. Applications of nanotechnology for immunology. *Nat Rev Immunol* 2013;**13**:592–605.

30. Stylianopoulos T, Jain RK. Design considerations for nanotherapeutics in oncology. *Nanomedicine* 2015. pii:S1549-9634(15)00158-6

Mechanisms of Immune-Related Pathologies and their Current Treatment

CHAPTER 2

Advance in Therapies for Rheumatoid Arthritis: New Perspectives

Flavio A. Amaral[1], Thiago H.C. Oliveira[1], Debora C. Calderaro[2], Gilda A. Ferreira[3] and Mauro M. Teixeira[1]

[1]Immunopharmacology, Department of Biochemistry and Immunology, Institute of Biological Science, Universidade Federal de Minas Gerais, Minas Gerais, Brazil [2]Department of Rheumatology, Universidade Federal de Minas Gerais, Minas Gerais, Brazil [3]Department of Locomotor System Medicine, Faculty of Medicine, Universidade Federal de Minas Gerais, Minas Gerais, Brazil

2.1 INTRODUCTION

Rheumatoid arthritis (RA) is a chronic inflammatory disease characterized by synovial inflammation and hyperplasia, autoantibody production, cartilage and bone destruction, and systemic features, including cardiovascular, pulmonary, and skeletal disorders, leading to severe disability, premature mortality, and socioeconomic costs.[1] It affects 1% of the population and is associated with significant morbidity and increased mortality in developed regions of the world.[2]

Environmental factors (smoking, microbial agents) and polymorphisms of specific genes that contribute to T-cell activation (*PTPN22*, *CTLA4*), production of autoantibodies (*HLA-DRB1, PADI4*), or impairment of cell signaling (*TNFAIP3*) are directly associated with the development of RA.[3] The production of the autoantibodies rheumatoid factor (RF—antibody against the Fc portion of autologous IgG) and anticitrullinated proteins antibodies (ACPA) indicate a breach of self-tolerance that often precedes the onset of RA by many years and are strongly correlated to more severe clinical disease and complications than seronegative patients.[4] The autoantibodies associate with self-antigens and form immune complexes, which can precipitate in synovial vessels and tissues that initiate and perpetuate local inflammation.[3]

Immune Rebalancing. DOI: http://dx.doi.org/10.1016/B978-0-12-803302-9.00002-6

Several cytokines, including TNF, IL-1β, IFN-γ, IL-17 and IL-6, chemokines, metalloproteinases, and prostanoids coordinate the constant and intense recruitment and activation of leukocytes to the synovium and stimulate osteoclastogenesis and osteoclast activity, leading to tissue damage and articular pain.[3] Furthermore, damaged cells release endogenous molecules (alarmins) that also activate neighbor cells and amplify joint inflammation.[5] In the joint, antigen present cells, T cells, and B cells can accumulate in a coordinated manner in the synovium, creating a tertiary lymphoid organ, which contributes to continuous local cell activation and perpetuation of inflammation.[6] All cellular types and molecules mentioned previously are targets for the treatment of RA. Here we explore the benefits and disadvantages of the current therapies and discuss novel possibilities for the treatment of RA.

2.2 RHEUMATOID ARTHRITIS MANAGEMENT

At present, the management of patients with RA is based on early methotrexate and other disease-modifying antirheumatic drugs (DMARDs). Biological agents are indicated for incomplete responders to DMARDs. Low-dose oral glucocorticoids used as bridging add on to DMARD therapy should be considered in the initial disease management. This regimen allows rapid control of disease activity in terms of clinical and subclinical reduction of the inflammatory process, thus ensuring long-standing structural benefits.[7,8] The benefits and risks of the main treatments used to control inflammation in RA patients are presented below and in Table 2.1.

2.2.1 Glucococorticoids

The discovery of the anti-inflammatory actions of glucocorticoids (GCs) was a major breakthrough for the treatment of inflammatory disorders.[9] GC therapy was first introduced by Dr. Philip Hench in the 1940s for the treatment of RA.[10] Since then, it has been used to treat inflammatory and autoimmune diseases.[9] Twelve clinical trials have documented that long-term low-dose prednisone or prednisolone (10 mg/day or less) is efficacious to improve function, maintain status, and/or slow radiographic progression in patients with RA. Gaps in knowledge about the optimal duration of therapy and the best method to taper and possibly discontinue GC treatment remain.[11] Despite their therapeutic benefits, GC use is associated with severe side effects,

Table 2.1 Current Therapies for Rheumatoid Arthritis: Mechanisms of Action and Clinical Outcomes

Drug	Benefits	Major Adverse Events
Glucococorticoids • Induction of apoptosis of leukocytes • Macrophage cytokine production modulation (inhibiting p38 MAPK) • Expression of IL-1β, MCP-1, MIP-2 and IFN-γ-inducible protein 10 regulation in neutrophils and macrophages	• Improvement of RA activity, slow radiographic progression, maintains function	• Osteoporosis, Diabetes, hypertension, dyslipidemia, glaucoma, growth retardation, infection
Methotrexate • Dihydrofolate reductase inhibition (Inhibits purine and pyrimidine synthesis) • Polyamines generation ⇒ toxic products (eg, ammonia, hydrogen peroxide) ⇒ T cells inhibition • Catabolism of adenosine and adenine nucleotides reduction	• Improvement of RA activity, physical function, quality of life, reduction of radiographic progression • Protection against development of atherosclerotic heart disease	• Hepatotoxicity (hepatic fibrosis or cirrhosis), bone marrow suppression, alopecia, stomatitis, induction of nodules, pulmonary fibrosis, somnolence, infection
Leflunomide • Inhibits dihydroorotate dehydrogenase (inhibits pyrimidine)	• Improvement of RA activity, physical function, quality of life, reduction of radiographic progression	• Hepatotoxicity alopecia, diarrhea, allergic reactions, infection
Sulfasalazine – Unknown – Antimicrobial properties, immunosuppressant effects of 5-aminosalicylic acid, inhibition of folate-dependent enzymes leading to impaired lymphocytes function	• Improvement of RA activity, reduction of radiographic progression	• Dyspepsia, nausea, vomiting, loss of appetite, diarrhea, skin rash and pruritus, headache, dizziness, oligospermia, neutropenia, aplasticor hemolytic anemia, bone marrow depression, hepatotoxicity
Cyclosporine A • Calcineurin inhibition	• Improvement of RA activity, physical function, reduction of radiographic progression, protection against development of atherosclerotic heart disease	• Renal toxicity (reversible or irreversible), hypertension, tremor, increased infections and malignancies
Azathioprine • Purine synthesis inhibition	• Improvement of RA activity, reserved to extra-articular severe of RA	• Bone marrow suppression, hepatotoxicity, nausea and vomiting
Cyclophophamide • Alkylating antiproliferative agent	• Improvement of RA activity • Reserved to extra-articular severe manifestations of RA	• Hemorrhagic cystitis, bladder cancer, nausea, vomiting, bone marrow suppression alopecia, infertility, amenorrhea, malignant neoplasias and infections

(Continued)

Table 2.1 (Continued)

Drug	Benefits	Major Adverse Events
Antimalarials (Hydroxichloroquine or Chloroquine Diphosphate) • Not well understood • Raises pH of intracellular lysosomes and other cytoplasmic vesicles, alters protein processing, leading to a reduction in autoantibody formation, T-cell activation and to the inhibition of TLR3/7/9	• Improvement of RA activity	• Excellent safety profile • Epigastric burning, nausea, bloating, diarrhea, skin rashes, alopecia • Ocular toxicity
TNF-inhibitor • **Etanercept:** Fusion protein TNF receptor inhibitor • **Infliximab:** Anti-TNF monoclonal chimeric antibody • **Adalimumab:** Fully anti-TNF human monoclonal antibody • **Golimumab:** Anti-TNF human monoclonal antibody • **CertolizumabPegol:** Pegylated humanized anti-TNF antibody	• Improvement of RA activity, physical function, quality of life, reduction of radiographic progression	• Headache, abdominal pain, diarrhea, vomiting, rash, injection site reaction, bleeding, bruising, itching, infections, positive anti-double-stranded DNA antibodies, positive antinuclear antibodies, reactivation of latent tuberculosis (TB), reactivation of virus B hepatitis, *Listeria* infections, nontuberculous mycobacterial infections, neutropenia, demyelinating disease, cutaneous psoriasis • Increased risk of pulmonary fibrosis and malignancies
Abatacept • T-cell costimulation modulator • Soluble fusion protein	• Improvement of RA activity, physical function, quality of life, reduction of radiographic progression	• Infections, headache, nausea, nasopharyngitis, antibody formation may exacerbate COPD
Rituximab • Monoclonal antibody anti-CD20 antigen (B-cells)	• Improvement of RA activity, physical function, quality of life, reduction of radiographic progression	• Infusion related reactions, infections, TB reactivation, increased risk of progressive multifocal leukoencephalopathy
Anakinra • IL-1 Receptor antagonist	• Improvement of RA activity, physical function, quality of life, reduction of radiographic progression	• Site reactions to daily subcutaneous injections infections
Tocilizumab • IL-6 receptor antagonist (monoclonal antibody that inhibits IL-6 receptors)	• Improvement of RA activity, physical function, quality of life, reduction of radiographic progression	• Infection, transient elevations of hepatic transaminases, neutropenia, TB reactivation, increases in total cholesterol and triglyceride levels, gastrointestinal perforation
Tofacitinib • JAK (1,2,3 and TYK2) inhibitor	• Improvement of RA activity, physical function, quality of life	• Increased risk for TB, serious infections, lymphoma and other malignancies and elevated cholesterol, long-term safety issues are not well known yet

including osteoporosis, diabetes, hypertension, dyslipidemia, glaucoma, muscle atrophy and growth retardation, and others, depending on the dose and duration of treatment.[12]

2.2.2 Methotrexate

Methotrexate (MTX) is currently considered, among DMARDs, the "anchor-drug" and is among the most commonly prescribed drug in the treatment of RA. Its low cost, associated with good long-term efficacy and safety profile, justifies the recommendation for its use as the first disease-modifying drug for treating RA.[7,8,13] MTX is a folic acid antagonist that inhibits the synthesis of deoxyribonucleic acid (DNA), ribonucleic acid (RNA), and proteins by binding to dihydrofolate reductase. Polyglutamates, important MTX metabolites are potent inhibitors of the enzyme aminoimidazole carboxamide ribonucleotide, leading to the accumulation of this enzyme and its metabolites, which inhibit adenosine deaminase and AMP deaminase. By reducing the catabolism of adenosine and adenosine nucleotides, adenosine levels increase, leading to a variety of anti-inflammatory effects.[14]

It is efficacious and safe when used in monotherapy or combined therapy with other DMARDs or biologic agents.[7,8,13] In parallel design clinical trials including RA patients with no prior exposure to either drug, MTX results in similar outcomes to biological agents. Superiority of biologics over MTX on the treatment of RA was only demonstrated in a parallel clinical trial including patients with prior incomplete response to MTX, in a step-up design (adding a biologic agent to MTX).[15]

MTX adverse events are attributed to its antimetabolite and antiproliferative effects, and include bone marrow suppression, alopecia, and stomatitis. Increased levels of adenosine have been associated to MTX-induced hepatotoxicity, characterized by hepatic fibrosis and cirrhosis, that may be worsened by ethanol ingestion, and to somnolence that some patients taking MTX experience.[14,15]

2.2.3 Leflunomide

Leflunomide is a DMARD with immunomodulating, immnosuppressive, and antiproliferative properties. Its active metabolite (A771726) blocks the enzyme dihydrorotate deydrogenase, thus, inhibiting the synthesis of pyrimidines. Leflunomide relieves symptoms and signs of RA with good effectiveness. It is efficacious and safe when used in monotherapy or combined therapy with other nonbiologic or biologic DMARDs. Frequent adverse events attributed to leflunomide are hepatotoxicity, alopecia, diarrhea, allergic reactions, and infections.[16]

2.2.4 Sulfasalazine

Sulfasalazine (SSZ) is a sulfapyridine and 5-aminosalicylic acid and is absorbed either as intact SSZ or as sulfapyridine, and both appear to be active in RA. The specific mode of action of SSZ has yet to be identified. It exerts effects on the gut microbiota, on inflammatory cell function, cytokine and antibody production, inhibition of folate-dependent enzymes, inhibition of synovial neovascularization, and an increase in free radical scavenging activity.[17] Placebo-controlled studies have demonstrated the efficacy of SSZ as a DMARD in RA. It improves swollen and tender joint counts, pain and grip strength, patient's assessment, morning stiffness, erythrocyte sedimentation rate, and slows radiographic progression of RA. It is safe and efficacious when used in monotherapy or combined therapy with other DMARDs or biologic agents. However, some studies have suggested that SSZ is less effective than other DMARDs. Monotherapy with SSZ has been recommended for patients with contraindications to other DMARDs, mild forms of RA or women who desire to become pregnant.[7,8,13,15]

Adverse events of SSZ include relatively common minor gastrointestinal (eg, dyspepsia, nausea, vomiting, loss of appetite, diarrhea) and neurological (headache, dizziness, depression) abnormalities and skin rash and pruritus, and uncommon serious hematological events, such as bone marrow suppression.[17]

2.2.5 Cyclosporin A

Cyclosporin A is a calcineurin inhibitor, leading to inhibition of the transcription and production of IL-2 and other inflammatory cytokines triggered by T-cell activation. It is indicated for the treatment of severe, active RA unresponsive or inadequately responsive to MTX, in monotherapy or in combination with MTX. Though effective in improving RA activity and slowing radiographic progression, it is a third-line DMARD in the treatment of RA, because of its frequent side effects and drug interactions.[18] Side effects include renal toxicity (reversible or irreversible), hypertension, tremor, increased infections, and malignancies. Drug interactions are frequent, leading to the increase or decrease of cyclosporin A levels, affecting toxicity and effectiveness.[18]

2.2.6 Azathioprine

The active metabolite of azathioprine is 6-mercaptopurine that blocks purine synthesis and DNA repair, inhibiting cell proliferation, particularly of rapidly dividing cells, such as lymphocytes and hematopoietic cells. Azathioprine is effective for active RA treatment, however, its efficacy was found to be inferior to that of MTX and its use in RA has become third line or as therapy for severe extra-articular RA manifestations, such as pneumonitis and cutaneous vasculitis. The most common side effects of azathioprine are bone marrow suppression, hepatotoxicity, nausea, and vomiting.[18,19]

2.2.7 Cyclophosphamide

Cyclophosphamide is an alkylating agent with antiproliferative effects. Although its therapeutic effects on RA articular activity, bone marrow and bladder toxicity, and the potential for late malignancy have restricted its use to refractory and life-threatening conditions such as severe vasculitis and interstitial lung disease secondary RA. Toxicities include bone marrow suppression, loss of fertility, bladder toxicity, cancer, and infections.[18,20]

2.2.8 Antimalarials

Antimalarials interfere with antigen presentation and the activation of the immune response by increasing pH within macrophage phagolysosomes. They have efficacy in mild to moderate RA and are primarily used in combination with other DMARDs, but may be used in monotherapy in patients with mildly active RA without poor prognostic features.[21] The antimalarials have an excellent safety profile. Common side effects include epigastric burning, nausea, bloating, diarrhea, skin rashes, and alopecia. Patients may develop hyperpigmentation in sun exposed areas. Retinal toxicity with macular damage and corneal deposits are infrequent, however, ophthalmological monitoring is recommended during antimalarial treatment.[21]

2.2.9 Biologics

Biologics are purified, modified and/or reconstructed proteins derived from the genetic sequences of living cells, which are used to modify a patient's immune response. In RA, they are indicated to suppress active and destructive inflammatory responses by specifically targeting key mediators, such as cytokines, cells, or cellular interactions.[22] Biologics developed for the treatment of RA currently available include different tumor necrosis factor inhibitors (anti-TNF), IL-1 and IL-6 inhibitors, and B and T lymphocytes targeting biologic agents.[7,8,13,18,22]

2.2.10 Tumor Necrosis Factor Inhibitors

Tumor necrosis factor α (TNFα, referred to here simply as TNF) is a cytokine involved in systemic inflammation which is abundant in the serum and synovial fluid of RA patients and plays a major role in the pathogenesis of RA.[18] Five anti-TNF are currently approved for RA treatment: etanercept (recombinant human soluble fusion protein), infliximab (chimeric murine-human IgG1 monoclonal antibody), adalimumab (fully human monoclonal antibody), golimumab (human monoclonal antibody), and certolizumabpegol (Fc free humanized pegylated anti-TNF Fab fragment). All of them are effective in controlling RA activity, keeping function, and slowing radiographic progression.[7,8,13,18,21,22] When combined with MTX or others DMARDs, they are more effective than when used in monotherapy.[22] Common side effects include headache, abdominal pain, diarrhea, vomiting, rash, injection site reaction, bruising, itching, infections (including serious and/or opportunistic), antinuclear antibodies formation, reactivation of latent tuberculosis (TB), reactivation of virus B hepatitis, *Listeria* infections, nontuberculous mycobacterial infections, neutropenia, demyelinating disease, and cutaneous psoriasis. TB screening before initiating anti-TNF therapy is recommended. Patients with latent TB must be treated first for at least one month prior to starting anti-TNF therapy.[7,8,13,18,21,22]

2.2.11 T-Lymphocyte Costimulation Blocker: Abatacept

Abatacept is a selective costimulation modulator that inhibits T-cell activation by binding to CD80 and CD86 on antigen-presenting cells (APCs) and, thus, blocking the required CD28 interaction between APCs and T-cells. It is effective in patients with active RA that failed at least one DMARD or have not adequately responded to the combination of MTX with an anti-TNF. It may be given in monotherapy, although its efficacy is enhanced when give concomitantly with DMARDs. Side effects include a higher frequency of chronic obstructive pulmonary disease adverse reactions, headache, nausea, nasopharyngitis, infections and antibody formation.[21,22]

2.2.12 Anti-B-Cell Therapy: Rituximab

Rituximab is currently the only licensed anti-B cell therapy in RA. It targets the CD20 antigen on B-lymphocytes, resulting in a depletion of B cells and the reduction of autoantibodies and T-cell/B-cell interactions, potentially suppressing both humoral and cellular autoimmunity.[18,21,22] The combination of Rituximab and MTX or leflunomide resulted in good response in RA patients resistant to DMARDS alone or in combination with anti-TNF. It is recommended as a second-line therapy, after anti-TNF failure. Adverse events include infusion related reactions, infections, and an increased risk of progressive multifocal leukoencephalopathy and of TB reactivation.[18,21,22]

2.2.13 Anakinra

Anakinra is a recombinant human IL-1 receptor antagonist. In recent years, it has been shown to be less effective than anti-TNF and other biologics. Hence, because of the cumbersome daily administration by subcutaneous injection and its very short half-life, this compound has a minor role in the routine clinical care of RA patients.[18,21,22] Site reactions to daily subcutaneous injections and, less frequently, infections, are potential side effects.[22] Novel inhibitors of IL-1β function, such as antibodies, may redefine the use of IL-1β-based strategies in the context of RA.

2.2.14 Tocilizumab

Tocilizumab is a humanized monoclonal antibody that targets soluble and membrane-bound IL-6. IL-6 is a pro-inflammatory cytokine produced by T and B lymphocytes, monocytes, and fibroblasts, whose effects include the induction of synovial neovascularization, osteoclast activation, and the upregulation of metalloproteinases and C-reactive protein. It also promotes the differentiation of pro-inflammatory Th17 cells.[18,21,22] Tocilizumab reduces synovitis and radiographic progression of RA and improves systemic features of inflammation, including anemia, anorexia, fever, and fatigue. It is approved to be used as a first-line therapy after inadequate response to one or more DMARDs, or after anti-TNF therapy failure. It can be used in monotherapy or in combination with DMARDs.[7,8,13,18,21,22] Side effects of tocilizumab include infection, transient elevations of hepatic transaminases, neutropenia, TB reactivation, and increases in total cholesterol and triglyceride levels. Rare events of gastrointestinal perforation have also been reported.[18,21,22]

2.2.15 Protein Kinase Inhibitors

Protein kinases are small intracellular enzymes that modify the function of other proteins by attaching phosphate groups to them. Janus kinase (JAK) is a tyrosine kinase. Four kinds of JAKs have been described: JAK1, JAK2, JAK3, and tyrosine kinase 2 (TYK2). JAKs mediate the signaling of cytokine and growth factors responsible for hematopoiesis and immune function. JAK mediated signaling involves recruitment of signal transducers and activators of transcription (STATs) to cytokine receptors which leads to the modulation of gene expression.[18,21]

Tofacitinib is the first JAK inhibitor approved for use in RA patients. It inhibits primarily JAK 1 and JAK 3 and, to a lesser extent, JAK 2 and TYK2 and can be taken orally. Tofacitinib can be used as monotherapy or in combination with MTX or other DMARDs, after inadequate response to at least one DMARD. Patients treated with tofacitinib are at increased risk for TB, infections, lymphoma and other malignancies, and elevated cholesterol. Long-term safety issues are not known at present.[13,18,21]

2.3 NEW ALTERNATIVES FOR THE TREATMENT OF RA

As described early, RA is a chronic inflammatory disease with a significant and continuous migration of leukocytes to the joint that contribute to cartilage and bone destruction, causing intense articular pain and dysfunction. There is also significant systemic inflammation and related comorbidities.[3] The causes for the chronification in RA are still unclear, but the loss of immunological tolerance and the impairment of the resolution of inflammation are thought to contribute to chronic inflammation.

2.4 LOSS OF IMMUNE TOLERANCE AS A FACTOR FOR RA DEVELOPMENT: A POSSIBLE TARGET

It is thought that RA arises from a breakdown of immunological self-tolerance leading to aberrant immune responses to autoantigens.[23] Defects in the number or function of T regulatory (Treg) cells potentially allow effector T cells to escape from suppression leading to the production of pro-inflammatory cytokines.[24-26] Treg cells express high levels of CD25 (α chain of IL-2 receptor) and the master transcription factor forkhead box P3 (Foxp3), which are essential for their activity.[27] The mechanisms used by Treg cells to suppress inflammation can be broadly divided into those that target T cells (suppressor cytokines, IL-2 consumption, cytolysis) and those that primarily target antigen-presenting cells (decreased costimulation or decreased antigen presentation).[28] A recent study demonstrated that RA patients unresponsive to methotrexate present reduced expression of CD39 on Treg cells. CD39 is an ectonucleoside that, together with CD73, converts ATP to adenosine, a molecule that suppress the pro-inflammatory actions of effector T cells.[29]

Komatsu and colleagues showed that under arthritic conditions, CD25[lo]Foxp3 + CD4 + T cells lose the expression of Foxp3, and undergo transdifferentiation into Th17 cells.[30] Interestingly, the treatment with a TNF-specific antibody restored Treg cells function in subjects with RA, and was associated with increased Foxp3 phosphorylation in Treg cells.[31] Similarly, patients with RA treated with tocilizumab showed a decrease in the percentage of Th17 and an increase in the percentage of Treg cells.[32] Furthermore, peripheral blood mononuclear cells obtained from RA patients and treated in vitro with methotrexate alone or in combination with methylprednisolone showed an increase in the population of Th17 cells that expressed IL-10 and Treg cells.[33] Thus, the reestablishment of Treg population and function in RA and other autoimmune diseases could be a strategy to prevent disease progression. Two ongoing clinical trials aim to investigate the potential use of recombinant IL-2 for the treatment of RA patients in order to reestablish the population of Treg cells and control the RA progression (Clinicaltrials.gov identifier: NCT02467504 and NCT01988506).

2.5 RESOLUTION OF INFLAMMATION

The current therapies for RA are based on the concept that targeting the influx activation and migration of leukocytes prevents disease progression. This has been a useful concept that has led to the development of the current available strategies. Another potential approach to controlling inflammation is the termination of inflammation by inducing its resolution. It is now clear that the resolution of inflammation is a very active process that associates with the prevention of the progression of inflammation to a persistent and chronic state.[34] The underlying idea is that active induction of the resolution of inflammation during chronic inflammatory diseases may lead to decreased tissue injury and restoration of tissue homeostasis. Here, we will briefly describe the contribution of some molecules to the resolution of inflammation and their actions in experimental and clinical arthritis.

2.5.1 Lipid Mediators

Eicosanoids (prostaglandins, leukotrienes) are lipid mediators originating from essential fatty acid omega-6 arachidonic acid and classically promote acute inflammation. However, several other lipid mediators that originate from either arachidonic acid (lipoxin A4—LXA4) or mainly from the omega-3 polyunsaturated fatty acid eicosapentaenoic acid and docosahexaenoic acid (resolvins, protectins and maresins) have been described as potent promoters of the resolution of inflammation.[35] The description of these proresolving lipid mediators has heralded the new era of inflammation resolution and its potential for the development of novel anti-inflammatory drugs. In experimental models of spontaneously resolving inflammation, the metabololipidomic analyzes of exudate by liquid chromatography with tandem mass spectrometry (LC-MS/MS) showed a lipid class switch along the time course of the inflammation and revealed different bioactive forms of these so called specialized proresolving mediators (SPMs).[36] Clinically, the LC-MS/MS analysis in synovial fluid from RA patients identified the presence of LXA4, Resolvin D5, and Maresin 1.[37] Although descriptive, this study could be used in the future to identify the state of severity of the disease and direct an appropriate treatment of RA patients. In this sense, epidemiological studies indicated that a diet enriched with omega-3 fatty acid improves clinical signs and symptoms of RA patients.[38,39]

The impairment or blockade of the recruitment of leukocytes, and the induction of apoptosis of pro-inflammatory cells are key features during the resolution of inflammation. All of these actions are regulated by the SPMs.[40–42] Furthermore, the clearance of apoptotic cells (efferocytosis) and the return of nonapoptotic cells to vasculature or lymphatics limit inflammation.[43] In an experimental model of arthritis, the induction of apoptosis of migrated neutrophils into the knee increases their efferocytosis by macrophages and anticipates the resolution of inflammation, decreasing tissue damage.[44] Importantly, efferocytosis changes the pro-inflammatory phenotype of macrophages to alternatively anti-inflammatory and proresolutive macrophages. This increases the synthesis of proresolutive molecules, decreases the production of pro-inflammatory molecules and promotes the recruitment of nonphlogistic mononuclear cells, leading to tissue homeostasis.[34] Thus, triggering the resolution machinery gradually tends to restore the function of tissue.

LXA4 is product of arachidonic acid metabolism by the 5/12/15-lipoxygenase enzymes. Furthermore, the acetylation of cyclooxygenase-2 (COX2) by aspirin lead to the production of 15-epimeric lipoxin A4, named aspirin-triggered 15-epi-lipoxin A4 (ATL).[45] A descriptive study showed that LXA4 and its receptor FPR2/ALX are present in synovial fluid and synovial tissue, respectively, of patients with RA and there was a positive correlation between LXA4 and PGE2 or LTB4 in synovial fluid.[46] In fact, the synthesis of LXA4 is dependent on the first wave of PGE2. The blockade of COX2 decreased the production of LXA4 and perpetuated arthritis in mice. In that study, administration of PGE2 restored the production of LXA4 and consequently controlled joint inflammation.[47] Mechanistically, LXA4 decreased the production of the metalloproteinases MMP-1 and MMP-3 in human synovial fibroblasts stimulated with IL-1.[48] In mice, the treatment with LXA4 reduced edema and neutrophil migration to the joint in a model of zymosan-induced arthritis.[49] In a model of inflammation of the temporomandibular joint, rabbits overexpressing 15-LO exhibited markedly reduced bone loss and local inflammation in a mechanism dependent on the synthesis of LXA4.[50] In addition, the administration of microparticles obtained from human neutrophils and enriched with an analog of LXA4 or aspirin triggered-resolvin D1 limited the number of neutrophils and enhanced the joint wound healing.[51]

Besides a direct role on leukocytes, different studies demonstrated that resolvin E1 (RvE1), RvE2, protectin 1 (PD1) and maresin 1 are potent molecules that decrease the perception of different types of pain, including neuropathic and articular inflammatory pain.[52–55] Furthermore, the administration of RvE1 in rabbit completely restored bone loss and decreased the production of the cytokine IL-1β in a model of periodontitis.[56] A possible mechanism could be a direct effect of RvE1 on osteoclast activity, since RvE1 is able to inhibit the osteoclast differentiation *in vitro*.[57]

The immunosuppression caused by the current treatments for RA is a significant problem among RA patients due to the risk of opportunistic infections and malignancies.[58] However, the beneficial effects of SPMs for the control of inflammation also extend to better control of certain infections. Indeed, RvE5 and PD1 were found in self-resolving *Escherichia coli* exudates. These molecules enhanced the phagocytosis of *E. coli*, reduced the bacterial titers and increased the survival of infected mice. Furthermore, RvD1 enhanced the therapeutic actions of ciprofloxacin.[59] In another study, human macrophages incubated with RvE2 increased the phagocytosis of *E. coli* and the efferocytosis of apoptotic neutrophils. Experimentally, RvE2 enhanced the clearance of *E. coli* and *Staphylococcus aureus* in infected mice and accelerated the resolution of inflammation by the binding of RvE2 on the GPR18 receptor.[60] In a different mechanism, LXA4 increased the survival of rats submitted to sepsis (cecal ligation and puncture model) by stimulating the recruitment of macrophages to the peritoneal cavity (focus of infection) without interfering with their phagocytic ability, yet reducing systemic inflammation.[61] Altogether, SPMs could be an alternative strategy to promote the resolution of inflammation without compromising the capacity of immune cells to deal with infections.

2.5.2 Annexin A1

Annexin A1, a 37 KDa glucocorticoid induced protein and its active derived peptide Ac2-26 share the same receptor of LXA4, FPR2/ALX.[62] Activation of this receptor triggers a range of proresolutive actions, including the decrease of leukocyte interaction with endothelial cells,[63] increase of neutrophil apoptosis,[64] and enhancement of efferocytosis.[65,66] Furthermore, using a humanized model of arthritis, the overexpression of Annexin A1 in the monocytic cell line U937 reduced their capacity to migrate towards RA synovial tissue implanted in severe combined immunodeficient mice.[40] Thus, annexin A1 is a molecule that actively influences leukocyte biology and could be a target to control inflammation in clinical conditions.

The presence of anti-annexin A1 antibody has been reported in the serum of RA patients treated with hydrocortisone.[67] Also, RA fibroblast-like synoviocytes had reduced binding sites for annexin A1.[68] These studies could provide an explanation for certain cases of glucocorticoid resistance in RA patients. Several preclinical studies have suggested that annexin A1 has a very important role in the control of inflammation in the context of experimental arthritis. In rats, the administration of anti-annexin A1 antibody reversed the beneficial effects of dexamethasone on antigen-induced arthritis, including an increase in TNF and PGE2 production in synovial tissue.[69] These data were corroborated using Annexin A1-deficient (AnxA1$^{-/-}$) mice. Although there was no difference in arthritis intensity between AnxA1$^{-/-}$ and wild type mice, the treatment with dexamethasone was impaired in AnxA1$^{-/-}$ mice.[70] Therefore, as seen for LXA4 and Annexin A1, the use of agonists for FPR2/ALX could be an alternative therapy for RA and other chronic inflammatory diseases.

2.6 CHALLENGES

There are now several therapies that provide control of inflammation in RA patients including therapies that block pro-inflammatory and intracellular signaling molecules and lymphocytic activity (Table 2.1 and Figure 2.1). However, several of these strategies lead to secondary immunosuppression that increase the risk of infection and tumor development. Furthermore, a portion of RA patients are still unresponsive or intolerant to currently available treatment. Thus, efforts to develop novel therapies are still necessary and the search for new targets and approaches must be taken into account for this growing challenge. The activation of the resolution of inflammation may be an interesting concept for the development of novel therapies for inflammatory disorders.[71] There is now a lot of data demonstrating the effectiveness of proresolving strategies in preclinical models but these need to be translated into patients. In addition, there is a great need to understand the mechanisms underlying resolution of chronic inflammation. Indeed, although efficient in the control of acute inflammation, very few studies have demonstrated the beneficial actions of proresolutive molecules in chronic conditions, especially those associated with significant tissue fibrosis.[72]

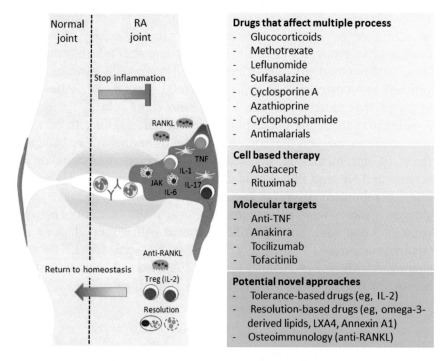

*Figure 2.1 **Current and potential novel approaches for the treatment of RA.** Scheme showing normal and RA joints, including the main inflammatory mediators associated to joint inflammation and damage. The current therapies for RA target cells and mediators involved in RA pathology. Alternatively, potential novel approaches could reduce local inflammation that lead to a homeostatic status.*

Another concept that should be considered in the search for new therapies for RA relies on the close relationship between the bone and the immune system, an area of research referred to as osteoimmunology. Bone damage is a hallmark of severe RA but is usually detected in patients with the end stage of joint destruction. However, bone remodeling appears to occur much earlier and appears to cross-talk with the various leukocytes in the joint.[73] The fine-tuning of bone metabolism is regulated by the actions of osteoblasts (responsible for bone formation) and osteoclasts (responsible for bone degradation). The upregulation of osteoclasts activation depends on the increase in expression of the so-called receptor activator of nuclear factor κB ligand (RANKL) relative to osteoprotegerin (OPG).[74,75] T cells, specially Th17 cells, and synovial cells present in the joints of patients with RA release pro-inflammatory molecules, such as TNF, IL-6, IL-1, and IL-17, that drive the production of RANKL.[76–78] On the other hand, degraded bone can modify the function of the immune system. Osteoblasts, osteoclasts and osteocytes regulate hematopoiesis and, consequently, the composition of the immune system.[79,80] Thus, the modification of joint homeostasis may generate global impairment in the inflamed joint. There are several interesting reviews in the literature deepening the role of osteoimmunology in chronic inflammatory diseases, including RA.[81–83] There is a clinical trial exploring the potential benefits of Denosumab, an antibody against RANKL, in RA (ClinicalTrials.gov Identifier: NCT01973569).

2.7 CONCLUDING REMARKS

In conclusion, there have been many exciting developments in the treatment of RA in the last few years. Novel treatments alone or in association with older therapies, especially methotrexate, have revolutionized the way we treat RA and other chronic inflammatory diseases. There is still room for improvement and the cost of medication is a very major issue for individual patients and in developing countries. Because most treatments have been around only for a decade or less, we still need to assess the long-term safety of these treatments. An interesting issue relates to the cost of developing new therapies in addition to the existing ones. New trials will need to show benefits in addition to currently available therapies, which are not cheap, and may take many years to complete. Finally, it is now time for us to fully consider the safety, real cost, and impact of biogenerics, antibodies developed from existing effective therapies.

REFERENCES

1. Firestein GS. Evolving concepts of rheumatoid arthritis. *Nature* 2003;**423**:356–61.

2. Carbonell J, Cobo T, Balsa A, Descalzo MA, Carmona L, Group SS. The incidence of rheumatoid arthritis in Spain: results from a nationwide primary care registry. *Rheumatology (Oxford)* 2008;**47**:1088–92.

3. McInnes IB, Schett G. The pathogenesis of rheumatoid arthritis. *N Engl J Med* 2011; **365**:2205–19.

4. Nielen MM, van Schaardenburg D, Reesink HW, van de Stadt RJ, van der Horst-Bruinsma IE, de Koning MH, et al. Specific autoantibodies precede the symptoms of rheumatoid arthritis: a study of serial measurements in blood donors. *Arthritis Rheum* 2004;**50**:380–6.

5. Jiang W, Pisetsky DS. Mechanisms of disease: the role of high-mobility group protein 1 in the pathogenesis of inflammatory arthritis. *Nat Clin Pract Rheumatol* 2007;**3**:52–8.

6. Manzo A, Bugatti S, Caporali R, Prevo R, Jackson DG, Uguccioni M, et al. CCL21 expression pattern of human secondary lymphoid organ stroma is conserved in inflammatory lesions with lymphoid neogenesis. *Am J Pathol* 2007;**171**:1549–62.

7. da Mota LM, Cruz BA, Brenol CV, Pereira IA, Rezende-Fronza LS, Bertolo MB, et al. 2012 Brazilian Society of Rheumatology Consensus for the treatment of rheumatoid arthritis. *Rev Bras Reumatol* 2012;**52**:152–74.

8. Singh JA, Furst DE, Bharat A, Curtis JR, Kavanaugh AF, Kremer JM, et al. 2012 update of the 2008 American College of Rheumatology recommendations for the use of disease-modifying antirheumatic drugs and biologic agents in the treatment of rheumatoid arthritis. *Arthritis Care Res (Hoboken)* 2012;**64**:625–39.

9. Rhen T, Cidlowski JA. Antiinflammatory action of glucocorticoids – new mechanisms for old drugs. *N Engl J Med* 2005;**353**:1711–23.

10. Hench PS, Kendall EC, Slocumb CH, Polley HF. The effect of a hormone of the adrenal cortex (17-hydroxy-11-dehydrocorticosterone: compound E) and of pituitary adrenocortical hormone in arthritis: preliminary report. *Ann Rheum Dis* 1949;**8**:97–104.

11. Pincus T, Cutolo M. Clinical trials documenting the efficacy of low-dose glucocorticoids in rheumatoid arthritis. *Neuroimmunomodulation* 2015;**22**:46–50.

12. Nussinovitch U, de Carvalho JF, Pereira RM, Shoenfeld Y. Glucocorticoids and the cardiovascular system: state of the art. *Curr Pharm Des* 2010;**16**:3574–85.

13. Smolen JS, Breedveld FC, Burmester GR, Bykerk V, Dougados M, Emery P, et al. Treating rheumatoid arthritis to target: 2014 update of the recommendations of an international task force. *Ann Rheum Dis* 2015.

14. Chan ES, Cronstein BN. Mechanisms of action of methotrexate. *Bull Hosp Jt Dis (2013)* 2013;(71 Suppl. 1):S5–8.

15. Lopez-Olivo MA, Siddhanamatha HR, Shea B, Tugwell P, Wells GA, Suarez-Almazor ME. Methotrexate for treating rheumatoid arthritis. *Cochrane Database Syst Rev* 2014;**6**: CD000957.

16. Golicki D, Newada M, Lis J, Pol K, Hermanowski T, Tlustochowicz M. Leflunomide in monotherapy of rheumatoid arthritis: meta-analysis of randomized trials. *Pol Arch Med Wewn* 2012;**122**:22–32.

17. Weinblatt ME, Reda D, Henderson W, Giobbie-Hurder A, Williams D, Diani A, et al. Sulfasalazine treatment for rheumatoid arthritis: a metaanalysis of 15 randomized trials. *J Rheumatol* 1999;**26**:2123–30.

18. Miller AV, Ranatunga SK. Immunotherapies in rheumatologic disorders. *Med Clin North Am* 2012;**96**:475–96 ix–x.

19. Suarez-Almazor ME, Spooner C, Belseck E. Azathioprine for treating rheumatoid arthritis. *Cochrane Database Syst Rev* 2000;CD001461.

20. Suarez-Almazor ME, Belseck E, Shea B, Wells G, Tugwell P. Cyclophosphamide for treating rheumatoid arthritis. *Cochrane Database Syst Rev* 2000;CD001157.

21. Kumar P, Banik S. Pharmacotherapy options in rheumatoid arthritis. *Clin Med Insights Arthritis Musculoskelet Disord* 2013;**6**:35–43.

22. Meier FM, Frerix M, Hermann W, Muller-Ladner U. Current immunotherapy in rheumatoid arthritis. *Immunotherapy* 2013;**5**:955–74.

23. Cooles FA, Isaacs JD, Anderson AE. Treg cells in rheumatoid arthritis: an update. *Curr Rheumatol Rep* 2013;**15**:352.

24. Viglietta V, Baecher-Allan C, Weiner HL, Hafler DA. Loss of functional suppression by CD4 + CD25 + regulatory T cells in patients with multiple sclerosis. *J Exp Med* 2004;**199**:971–9.

25. Ehrenstein MR, Evans JG, Singh A, Moore S, Warnes G, Isenberg DA, et al. Compromised function of regulatory T cells in rheumatoid arthritis and reversal by anti-TNFalpha therapy. *J Exp Med* 2004;**200**:277–85.

26. Lindley S, Dayan CM, Bishop A, Roep BO, Peakman M, Tree TI. Defective suppressor function in CD4(+)CD25(+) T-cells from patients with type 1 diabetes. *Diabetes* 2005;**54**:92–9.

27. Fontenot JD, Rasmussen JP, Williams LM, Dooley JL, Farr AG, Rudensky AY. Regulatory T cell lineage specification by the forkhead transcription factor foxp3. *Immunity* 2005;**22**:329–41.

28. Shevach EM. Mechanisms of foxp3 + T regulatory cell-mediated suppression. *Immunity* 2009;**30**:636–45.

29. Peres RS, Liew FY, Talbot J, Carregaro V, Oliveira RD, Almeida SL, et al. Low expression of CD39 on regulatory T cells as a biomarker for resistance to methotrexate therapy in rheumatoid arthritis. *Proc Natl Acad Sci USA* 2015;**112**:2509–14.

30. Komatsu N, Okamoto K, Sawa S, Nakashima T, Oh-hora M, Kodama T, et al. Pathogenic conversion of Foxp3 + T cells into TH17 cells in autoimmune arthritis. *Nat Med* 2014;**20**:62–8.

31. Nie H, Zheng Y, Li R, Guo TB, He D, Fang L, et al. Phosphorylation of FOXP3 controls regulatory T cell function and is inhibited by TNF-alpha in rheumatoid arthritis. *Nat Med* 2013;**19**:322–8.

32. Samson M, Audia S, Janikashvili N, Ciudad M, Trad M, Fraszczak J, et al. Brief report: inhibition of interleukin-6 function corrects Th17/Treg cell imbalance in patients with rheumatoid arthritis. *Arthritis Rheum* 2012;**64**:2499–503.

33. Guggino G, Giardina A, Ferrante A, Giardina G, Schinocca C, Sireci G, et al. The in vitro addition of methotrexate and/or methylprednisolone determines peripheral reduction in Th17 and expansion of conventional Treg and of IL-10 producing Th17 lymphocytes in patients with early rheumatoid arthritis. *Rheumatol Int* 2015;**35**:171–5.

34. Buckley CD, Gilroy DW, Serhan CN. Proresolving lipid mediators and mechanisms in the resolution of acute inflammation. *Immunity* 2014;**40**:315–27.

35. Headland SE, Norling LV. The resolution of inflammation: principles and challenges. *Semin Immunol* 2015;**27**:149–60.

36. Levy BD, Clish CB, Schmidt B, Gronert K, Serhan CN. Lipid mediator class switching during acute inflammation: signals in resolution. *Nat Immunol* 2001;**2**:612–19.

37. Giera M, Ioan-Facsinay A, Toes R, Gao F, Dalli J, Deelder AM, et al. Lipid and lipid mediator profiling of human synovial fluid in rheumatoid arthritis patients by means of LC-MS/MS. *Biochim Biophys Acta* 2012;**1821**:1415–24.

38. Geusens P, Wouters C, Nijs J, Jiang Y, Dequeker J. Long-term effect of omega-3 fatty acid supplementation in active rheumatoid arthritis. A 12-month, double-blind, controlled study. *Arthritis Rheum* 1994;**37**:824–9.

39. Goldberg RJ, Katz J. A meta-analysis of the analgesic effects of omega-3 polyunsaturated fatty acid supplementation for inflammatory joint pain. *Pain* 2007;**129**:210–23.

40. Perretti M, Ingegnoli F, Wheller SK, Blades MC, Solito E, Pitzalis C. Annexin 1 modulates monocyte-endothelial cell interaction in vitro and cell migration in vivo in the human SCID mouse transplantation model. *J Immunol* 2002;**169**:2085–92.

41. Spite M, Norling LV, Summers L, Yang R, Cooper D, Petasis NA, et al. Resolvin D2 is a potent regulator of leukocytes and controls microbial sepsis. *Nature* 2009;**461**:1287–91.

42. Oh SF, Dona M, Fredman G, Krishnamoorthy S, Irimia D, Serhan CN. Resolvin E2 formation and impact in inflammation resolution. *J Immunol* 2012;**188**:4527–34.

43. Serhan CN, Savill J. Resolution of inflammation: the beginning programs the end. *Nat Immunol* 2005;**6**:1191–7.

44. Lopes F, Coelho FM, Costa VV, Vieira EL, Sousa LP, Silva TA, et al. Resolution of neutrophilic inflammation by H2O2 in antigen-induced arthritis. *Arthritis Rheum* 2011;**63**:2651–60.

45. Chiang N, Takano T, Clish CB, Petasis NA, Tai HH, Serhan CN. Aspirin-triggered 15-epi-lipoxin A4 (ATL) generation by human leukocytes and murine peritonitis exudates: development of a specific 15-epi-LXA4 ELISA. *J Pharmacol Exp Ther* 1998;**287**:779−90.

46. Hashimoto A, Hayashi I, Murakami Y, Sato Y, Kitasato H, Matsushita R, et al. Antiinflammatory mediator lipoxin A4 and its receptor in synovitis of patients with rheumatoid arthritis. *J Rheumatol* 2007;**34**:2144−53.

47. Chan MM, Moore AR. Resolution of inflammation in murine autoimmune arthritis is disrupted by cyclooxygenase-2 inhibition and restored by prostaglandin E2-mediated lipoxin A4 production. *J Immunol* 2010;**184**:6418−26.

48. Sodin-Semrl S, Spagnolo A, Barbaro B, Varga J, Fiore S. Lipoxin A4 counteracts synergistic activation of human fibroblast-like synoviocytes. *Int J Immunopathol Pharmacol* 2004;**17**:15−25.

49. Conte FP, Menezes-de-Lima Jr. O, Verri Jr. WA, Cunha FQ, Penido C, Henriques MG, et al. (4) attenuates zymosan-induced arthritis by modulating endothelin-1 and its effects. *Br J Pharmacol* 2010;**161**:911−24.

50. Serhan CN, Jain A, Marleau S, Clish C, Kantarci A, Behbehani B, et al. Reduced inflammation and tissue damage in transgenic rabbits overexpressing 15-lipoxygenase and endogenous anti-inflammatory lipid mediators. *J Immunol* 2003;**171**:6856−65.

51. Norling LV, Spite M, Yang R, Flower RJ, Perretti M, Serhan CN. Cutting edge: humanized nano-proresolving medicines mimic inflammation-resolution and enhance wound healing. *J Immunol* 2011;**186**:5543−7.

52. Park CK, Xu ZZ, Liu T, Lu N, Serhan CN, Ji RR. Resolvin D2 is a potent endogenous inhibitor for transient receptor potential subtype V1/A1, inflammatory pain, and spinal cord synaptic plasticity in mice: distinct roles of resolvin D1, D2, and E1. *J Neurosci* 2011;**31**:18433−8.

53. Serhan CN, Dalli J, Karamnov S, Choi A, Park CK, Xu ZZ, et al. Macrophage proresolving mediator maresin 1 stimulates tissue regeneration and controls pain. *FASEB J* 2012;**26**:1755−65.

54. Xu ZZ, Liu XJ, Berta T, Park CK, Lu N, Serhan CN, et al. Neuroprotectin/protectin D1 protects against neuropathic pain in mice after nerve trauma. *Ann Neurol* 2013;**74**:490−5.

55. Klein CP, Sperotto ND, Maciel IS, Leite CE, Souza AH, Campos MM. Effects of D-series resolvins on behavioral and neurochemical changes in a fibromyalgia-like model in mice. *Neuropharmacology* 2014;**86**:57−66.

56. Hasturk H, Kantarci A, Goguet-Surmenian E, Blackwood A, Andry C, Serhan CN, et al. Resolvin E1 regulates inflammation at the cellular and tissue level and restores tissue homeostasis in vivo. *J Immunol* 2007;**179**:7021−9.

57. Herrera BS, Ohira T, Gao L, Omori K, Yang R, Zhu M, et al. An endogenous regulator of inflammation, resolvin E1, modulates osteoclast differentiation and bone resorption. *Br J Pharmacol* 2008;**155**:1214−23.

58. Ramiro S, Gaujoux-Viala C, Nam JL, Smolen JS, Buch M, Gossec L, et al. Safety of synthetic and biological DMARDs: a systematic literature review informing the 2013 update of the EULAR recommendations for management of rheumatoid arthritis. *Ann Rheum Dis* 2014;**73**:529−35.

59. Chiang N, Fredman G, Backhed F, Oh SF, Vickery T, Schmidt BA, et al. Infection regulates pro-resolving mediators that lower antibiotic requirements. *Nature* 2012;**484**:524−8.

60. Chiang N, Dalli J, Colas RA, Serhan CN. Identification of resolvin D2 receptor mediating resolution of infections and organ protection. *J Exp Med* 2015;**212**:1203−17.

61. Walker J, Dichter E, Lacorte G, Kerner D, Spur B, Rodriguez A, et al. Lipoxin a4 increases survival by decreasing systemic inflammation and bacterial load in sepsis. *Shock* 2011;**36**:410−16.

62. Perretti M, D'Acquisto F. Annexin A1 and glucocorticoids as effectors of the resolution of inflammation. *Nat Rev Immunol* 2009;**9**:62−70.

63. Lim LH, Solito E, Russo-Marie F, Flower RJ, Perretti M. Promoting detachment of neutrophils adherent to murine postcapillary venules to control inflammation: effect of lipocortin 1. *Proc Natl Acad Sci USA* 1998;**95**:14535−9.

64. Vago JP, Nogueira CR, Tavares LP, Soriani FM, Lopes F, Russo RC, et al. Annexin A1 modulates natural and glucocorticoid-induced resolution of inflammation by enhancing neutrophil apoptosis. *J Leukoc Biol* 2012;**92**:249−58.

65. Maderna P, Yona S, Perretti M, Godson C. Modulation of phagocytosis of apoptotic neutrophils by supernatant from dexamethasone-treated macrophages and annexin-derived peptide Ac(2-26). *J Immunol* 2005;**174**:3727−33.

66. Dalli J, Jones CP, Cavalcanti DM, Farsky SH, Perretti M, Rankin SM. Annexin A1 regulates neutrophil clearance by macrophages in the mouse bone marrow. *FASEB J* 2012;**26**:387−96.

67. Podgorski MR, Goulding NJ, Hall ND, Flower RJ, Maddison PJ. Autoantibodies to lipocortin-1 are associated with impaired glucocorticoid responsiveness in rheumatoid arthritis. *J Rheumatol* 1992;**19**:1668−71.

68. Sampey AV, Hutchinson P, Morand EF. Annexin I surface binding sites and their regulation on human fibroblast-like synoviocytes. *Arthritis Rheum* 2000;**43**:2537−42.

69. Yang Y, Hutchinson P, Morand EF. Inhibitory effect of annexin I on synovial inflammation in rat adjuvant arthritis. *Arthritis Rheum* 1999;**42**:1538−44.

70. Patel HB, Kornerup KN, Sampaio AL, D'Acquisto F, Seed MP, Girol AP, et al. The impact of endogenous annexin A1 on glucocorticoid control of inflammatory arthritis. *Ann Rheum Dis* 2012;**71**:1872−80.

71. Serhan CN. Pro-resolving lipid mediators are leads for resolution physiology. *Nature* 2014;**510**:92−101.

72. Qu X, Zhang X, Yao J, Song J, Nikolic-Paterson DJ, Li J. Resolvins E1 and D1 inhibit interstitial fibrosis in the obstructed kidney via inhibition of local fibroblast proliferation. *J Pathol* 2012;**228**:506−19.

73. Tanaka S. Regulation of bone destruction in rheumatoid arthritis through RANKL-RANK pathways. *World J Orthop* 2013;**4**:1−6.

74. Takahashi N, Akatsu T, Udagawa N, Sasaki T, Yamaguchi A, Moseley JM, et al. Osteoblastic cells are involved in osteoclast formation. *Endocrinology* 1988;**123**:2600−2.

75. Gravallese EM, Manning C, Tsay A, Naito A, Pan C, Amento E, et al. Synovial tissue in rheumatoid arthritis is a source of osteoclast differentiation factor. *Arthritis Rheum* 2000;**43**:250−8.

76. Moon YM, Yoon BY, Her YM, Oh HJ, Lee JS, Kim KW, et al. IL-32 and IL-17 interact and have the potential to aggravate osteoclastogenesis in rheumatoid arthritis. *Arthritis Res Ther* 2012;**14**:R246.

77. Nakashima T, Kobayashi Y, Yamasaki S, Kawakami A, Eguchi K, Sasaki H, et al. Protein expression and functional difference of membrane-bound and soluble receptor activator of NF-kappaB ligand: modulation of the expression by osteotropic factors and cytokines. *Biochem Biophys Res Commun* 2000;**275**:768−75.

78. Sato K, Suematsu A, Okamoto K, Yamaguchi A, Morishita Y, Kadono Y, et al. Th17 functions as an osteoclastogenic helper T cell subset that links T cell activation and bone destruction. *J Exp Med* 2006;**203**:2673−82.

79. Sato M, Asada N, Kawano Y, Wakahashi K, Minagawa K, Kawano H, et al. Osteocytes regulate primary lymphoid organs and fat metabolism. *Cell Metab* 2013;**18**:749−58.

80. Sesler CL, Zayzafoon M. NFAT signaling in osteoblasts regulates the hematopoietic niche in the bone microenvironment. *Clin Dev Immunol* 2013;**2013**:107321.

81. Crotti TN, Dharmapatni AA, Alias E, Haynes DR. Osteoimmunology: Major and Costimulatory Pathway Expression Associated with Chronic Inflammatory Induced Bone Loss. *J Immunol Res* 2015;**2015**:281287.

82. Takayanagi H. Osteoimmunology: shared mechanisms and crosstalk between the immune and bone systems. *Nat Rev Immunol* 2007;**7**:292–304.

83. Vis M, Guler-Yuksel M, Lems WF. Can bone loss in rheumatoid arthritis be prevented? *Osteoporos Int* 2013;**24**:2541–53.

CHAPTER 3

Immune Based Therapies for Inflammatory Bowel Disease

Preetika Sinh[1], Claudio Fiocchi[1,2] and Jean-Paul Achkar[1,2]

[1]Department of Gastroenterology and Hepatology, Digestive Disease Institute, Cleveland Clinic, Cleveland, OH, USA [2]Department of Pathobiology, Lerner Research Institute, Cleveland Clinic, Cleveland, OH, USA

3.1 INTRODUCTION

The two major forms of inflammatory bowel diseases (IBD), ulcerative colitis (UC) and Crohn's disease (CD), are chronic relapsing diseases of the gastrointestinal tract with increasing incidence and prevalence throughout the world.[1] The etiology of IBD is unclear but there is an interplay of genetic, environmental, microbial, and immunological factors that results in persistent inflammation and gut damage.[2] Immune dysregulation is pivotal in IBD pathogenesis and extensive research has highlighted the key role of the adaptive and innate immune systems of the gut. However, with our expanding knowledge, comes the realization that immune dysfunction does not completely explain the mechanisms that lead to inflammatory response in the gut. The interplay of immune system (immunome), environmental factors (exposome), gut microbiota (microbiome), and genetic factors (genome) need to be considered and better defined. Recent strides in research have narrowed our knowledge gap and led to the development of medical therapies that are currently in use and newer therapies that are awaiting bench-to-bedside application.[2,3]

3.2 IMMUNE REGULATION IN IBD

Immune dysregulation plays a central role in IBD pathogenesis and both innate and adaptive immune systems mediate an aggressive response against environmental factors and gut microbiota in genetically

Immune Rebalancing. DOI: http://dx.doi.org/10.1016/B978-0-12-803302-9.00003-8

susceptible hosts. In the last few decades greater emphasis has been placed on the innate immune system and the role of epithelial cells, dendritic cells, macrophages, and natural killer cells in the pathogenesis of IBD. In addition, other cells like platelets, mesenchymal cells, and endothelial cells have been recognized to play an active role in the inflammatory response.[4]

The antigens that trigger an inflammatory process are taken up by antigen presenting cells, primarily dendritic cells, and undergo intracellular degradation in the proteasomes exposing the epitope, the antigenic moiety, which triggers a T cell mediated immune response along with a costimulatory signal.[5] The immune response in UC is different from that of CD.[6] CD is considered a T helper (Th) 1 and Th17 cell response, while UC is considered an atypical Th2 immune response. In CD, Th1 and Th17 cells primarily produce cytokines like interferon (IFN)γ, interleukin (IL)-17, and tumor necrosis factor (TNF)α in response to IL-12, 18, and 23. The cytokines in turn stimulate other immune and nonimmune cells to produce TNFα, IL-1, 6, 8, 12, and 18, all of which contribute to amplify and perpetuate the inflammatory damage.[3,7] On the other hand in UC the Th2 immune response is mediated primarily by IL-5, and IL-13 and low IL-4[3,4,8] (Fig. 3.1).

Signaling molecules like Janus kinases (JAK), that act downstream of cytokine-mediated lymphocyte activation, also have an important role in the immune response.[9] By using JAK inhibitors, signal transduction through the common gamma receptors of multiple cytokines including IL-2, 4, 7, 9, 15, and 21 can be blocked by small molecules that are being explored as a treatment option for IBD patients.[9,10]

In addition to this immune response, adhesion molecules expressed on endothelial cells, and integrin and chemokine receptors expressed on the leukocytes are critical in trafficking additional leukocytes into the mucosa and amplifying the immune response.[11]

With this understanding of the immune system in IBD, numerous cytokine and chemokine inhibitors, T cell function blocking drugs, and leukocyte trafficking inhibitors have been tested in clinical trials. However, less than half have shown promising results highlighting the reality that our current knowledge of IBD pathogenesis remains incomplete[3,4] (Fig. 3.2).

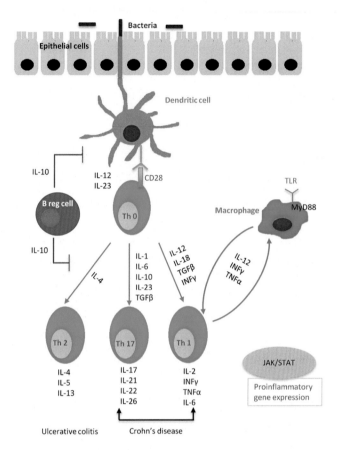

Figure 3.1 Innate and adaptive immune system in IBD. B reg, B regulatory; IL, interleukin; INF, interferon; JAK, Janus kinases; MyD, myeloid differentiation primary response gene; Th, T helper; TLR, toll like receptor; TNF, tumor necrosis factor; TGF, transforming growth factor.

3.3 CURRENT IMMUNE BASED THERAPIES IN IBD

Currently available therapies in IBD that target various aspects of the immune system include immunomodulators, anti-TNF agents and newer anti-integrin antibodies (Table 3.1).

3.4 IMMUNOMODULATORS

Several immunomodulating agents are used for treatment of IBD including corticosteroids, thiopurines, methotrexate (Mtx), cyclosporine, and tacrolimus. We highlight a few of the drugs in this section.

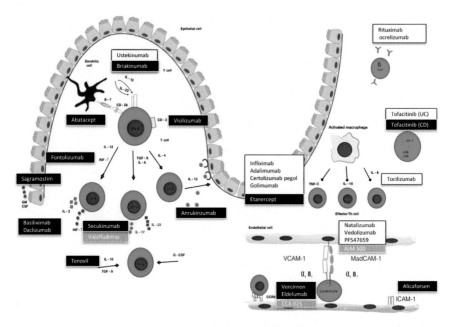

Figure 3.2 Successful and unsuccessful therapeutic programs in IBD. White boxes: Treatments with a positive out-come. Gray boxes: Potentially effective or ongoing treatments. Black boxes: Treatments failed. ICAM, intracellu-lar cell adhesion molecule; IL, interleukin; INF, interferon; MAdCAM, mucosal addressin cell adhesion molecule; TGF, transforming growth factor; Th, T helper; TNF, tumor necrosis factor; VCAM, vascular cell adhesion mole-cule. Adapted with permission from Danese (Gut 2012;61:918–932).

Table 3.1 Current Therapies in IBD					
Medication		**Induction**		**Maintenance**	
Drug Class	**Drug Name**	**UC**	**CD**	**UC**	**CD**
5-Aminosalicylic acid	Multiple agents	+	−	+	−
Steroids	Prednisone	+	+	−	−
	Budesonide	+	+	−	−
Immunonodulators	Thiopurines	−	−	+	+
	Mtx	−	+	+ / −	+
	Cyclosporine	+	−	−	−
	Tacrolimus	+	+	−	+ / −
Anti-TNF antibodies	Infliximab	+	+	+	+
	Adalimumab	+	+	+	+
	Certolizumab	−	+	−	+
	Golimumab	+	−	+	−
Anti-integrin antibodies	Natalizumab	−	+	−	+
	Vedolizumab	+	+	+	+

3.4.1 Thiopurines

Azathioprine (AZA) is a prodrug and an imidazole derivative of mercaptopurine that is converted nonenzymatically in tissue and red blood cells by sulphydryl-containing compounds to 6-mercaptopurine (6MP) and then enzymatically by thiopurine-S-methytransferase (TPMT), xanthine oxidase, and hypoxanthine phosphoribosyltransferase to 6-methylmercatopurine, 6-thiouric acid, and 6-thioguanine nucleotides (6TGN), respectively.[12] The active metabolite 6TGN is a purine analog that is incorporated in replicating DNA and blocks *de novo* purine synthesis. However, the effect on DNA replication does not completely explain the immunosuppressive effect of AZA and 6MP. T cell function is dependent on activation of both T cell receptor (TCR) ligand and a second costimulatory signal.[13] TCR stimulation without a costimulatory signal can result in T cell unresponsiveness or in some instances apoptosis.[14] 6TGN inhibits CD28 costimulatory signaling through Rac1 leading to T cell apoptosis and immunosuppression.[15]

The target dosing for therapy with these agents is weight-based: 2−2.5 mg/kg/day for AZA and 1−1.5 mg/kg/day for 6MP. Dose adjustments are based on baseline TPMT levels, measurement of metabolite levels, and development of leukopenia.

AZA and 6MP have generally been used in moderate to severe CD for maintenance of remission.[16] However, recent data from two randomized trials of AZA monotherapy for early moderate to severe CD for induction of remission have been discouraging.[17,18] Despite this, thiopurine analogs still have a place in management of postoperative CD and as combination therapy with biologics.[19−21] A meta-analysis of four clinical trials with 433 patients showed that purine analogs have a modest effect in preventing clinical and endoscopic postoperative recurrence at 1 year [number needed to treat (NNT) = 7 and NNT = 4, respectively].[19] The strongest indication of use of thiopurines in CD may be as part of combination therapy with anti-TNF agents.[21,22] In UC, AZA is more effective than 5-aminosalicylic acid in inducing clinical and endoscopic remission in steroid dependent cases[23] but, evidence is weaker as compared to CD for maintenance of remission.[24]

3.4.2 Methotrexate

Mtx is a folate analog that is metabolized intracellularly to polyglutamate metabolites and inhibits dihydroflate reductase. Mtx has high affinity for enzymes that require folate cofactors like thymidylatesynthetase (TS) and

5-aminoimidazole-4-carboxamide ribonucleotide (AICAR) transformylase. By binding to TS it inhibits DNA synthesis leading to its cytotoxic effect.[25] In addition, the effect of Mtx on AICAR enzyme causes an increase in extracellular adenosine concentration that has been shown to mediate anti-inflammatory effects by altering cytokine and eicosanoid synthesis.[25,26]

High dose Mtx, 25 mg once per week as subcutaneous or intramuscular injection, is effective in inducing remission in steroid refractory or steroid dependent CD patients as compared to placebo.[27] For maintenance of remission in CD, Mtx at 15 mg once per week by intramuscular injection is superior to placebo.[28]

In UC, there is no good evidence-based data for the use of Mtx although the number of randomized clinical trials is limited.[29,30] Recent trials have further evaluated the use of Mtx in UC. The multicenter European double blind placebo controlled METEOR trial did not show a benefit of Mtx in induction of remission in UC patients at week 16 (32% vs 20%, $P = 0.15$).[31] There is an ongoing US multicenter placebo controlled trial, Methotrexate Response In Treatment of UC, which showed positive results in an interim report.

The teratogenic potential of Mtx is restrictive for females who wish to conceive. Other potential adverse events associated with Mtx include bone marrow suppression, nausea, vomiting, hepatic fibrosis, and hypersensitivity pneumonitis.[32]

3.5 BIOLOGICAL AGENTS

There are several potential cytokine targets in IBD. These include inflammatory cytokines like TNFα, IFNγ, IL-1, 18, 22, 32, 35; immunoregulatory cytokines like IL-2, 4, 5, 6, 10, 12, 23, 27; cell adhesions molecules like intracellular cell adhesion molecule (ICAM)-1, mucosal addressin cell adhesion molecule (MAdCAM)-1, integrin α4β7; growth factors like platelet activating factor, keratinocyte growth factor, transforming growth factor β (TGF)β; neuropeptides like substance P; reactive oxygen species like nitric oxide; and chemokines like CXCL-10 and CCR-9. From this wide array of potential targets, several biological agents have been developed and investigated in animal colitis models and in clinical trials. Among these, only the anti-TNFα and anti-integrin inhibitors are currently approved for treatment of IBD while several others are in the pipeline at various stages of development (Table 3.2, Fig. 3.2).

Table 3.2 Next Generation Immune Based Therapies in IBD

Class	Target Molecule	Name	CD	UC	Trial Phase	Outcome
Cytokine pathway	IL-12/23	Ustekinumab	+	+	Phase 3	Underway
	IL-12/23	Briakunumab[1,2]	+	−	Phase 2	Failed
	IL-13	Anrukinzumab[3]	−	+	Phase 2	Failed
	IL-17A	Secukinumab[4]	+	−	Phase 2	Failed
	IL-17/IL-17R	Vidofludimus[a 5]	+	+	Phase 2	Success
	IL-17R	Brodalumab	+	−	Phase 2	Failed
	IL-21	PF05230900	+	−	Phase 1	Failed
	IL-6R	Tocilizumab[6]	+	−	Phase 1	Response
	IL-6/soluble gp130	sgp130Fc	−	−	Preclinical	Response
	IL-6	C326	+	−	Phase 1	Underway
		PF04236921	+	−	Phase 2	Completed
	IRAK4/ TRAF4/MyD88	RDP58[a 7]	+	+	Phase 2	Underway
	JAK/STAT	Tofacitinib[a]	−	++	Phase 2	Underway
	TGFβ/SMAD7	Mongersen[a]	+	−	Phase 2	Response
	Syk	Fostamatinib	−	−	Preclinical	Response
	MAPKs	Semapimod[8]	+	−	Phase 2	Modest response
	GM-CSF	Sagramostim	+	−	Phase 3	Failed
	Anti-TNF	AVX-470 (Avaxia)[a]	−	+	Phase 1	Completed
		Etanercept	+	+	Phase 2	Failed
	IFNϒ	Fontolizumab	+	−	Phase 2	Failed
	CD3 chain of TCR	Visilizumab	+	+	Phase 1/2	Adverse events
	CTLA4/T cell costimulation	Abatacept	+	+	Phase 3	Failed
Chemokines	CCR-9	CCX-282B (Vercirnon)	+	−	Phase 3	Failed
		Biarylsulfinamide	−	−	Preclinical	Response
		CCX-025	+	−	Phase 1	Underway
	CXCL-10	Eldelumab	−	+	Phase 2	Failed
Integrins	α4β7	AMG 181	+	+	Phase 2	Suspended[b]
	β7 (α4β7, αEβ7)	Etrolizumab	−	+	Phase 3	Failed
	α4 (α4β7, α4β1)	AJM 300[a]	−	+	Phase 2	Successful
Adhesion molecules	MAdCAM	PF00547659	+	+	Phase 2	Underway
	ICAM1	Alicaforsen	+	+	Phase 2	Failed[c]

(*Continued*)

Table 3.2 (Continued)						
Class	Target Molecule	Name	CD	UC	Trial Phase	Outcome
T and B cell trafficking	S1P1receptor	RPC1063[a][9]	–	+	Phase 3	Successful
Purine receptor	P2X$_7$	AZD9056[a][10]	+	–	Phase 2	Modest response
Stem cells	Mesenchymal	MSCs	+	+	Phase 2	Successful
	Human placenta derived	PDA-001	+	–	Phase 2	Underway
Immunomodulators	IL-17, T cell migration	Laquinimod[a]	+	–	Phase 2	Successful
	Antibiotics	Rifaximin	+	–	Phase 3	Underway
		RHB141[d]	+	–	Phase 3	Underway

Note: CTLA, cytotoxic T-lymphocyte antigen; IFN, interferon; IL, interleukin; IRAK, interleukin-1 receptor associated kinase; JAK, Janus kinase; MAPKs, mitogen-activated protein kinases; MSCs, mesenchymal stem cells; MyD, myeloid differentiation primary response gene; TRAF, TNF receptor associated factor; TCR, T cell receptor; TNF, tumor necrosis factor; TGFβ, transforming growth factor β; S1P, sphingosine-1-phosphate; Syk, spleen tyrosine kinase.
[a]Orally active.
[b]Phase 2 trials suspended due to inaccuracy in study documentation.
[c]Phase 2 with IV trials for CD failed. Rectal administration in UC proctitis showed response.
[d]Clarithromycin, rifabutin, clofazimine.

3.5.1 Anti-TNF Agents

Infliximab was the first anti-TNFα agent approved by the United States Food and Drug Administration (FDA) for treatment of CD in 1998 and then for moderate to severe UC in 2005. Subsequently three other anti-TNFα agents were FDA approved for treatment of IBD: adalimumab (ADA) for both CD (2007) and UC (2012), certolizumab pegol for CD (2008), and golimumab for UC (2013). Evidence from large population based studies, retrospective and *post-hoc* analyses of clinical trials showed that thiopurines or biologics given for a prolonged period or earlier during the disease alter the disease course and decrease the need for surgery.[33−38]

Infliximab is a chimeric (75% human and 25% murine) monoclonal IgG-1 antibody against TNFα that is administered intravenously.

Infliximab monotherapy and infliximab combined with AZA regimens are more effective in treating moderate to severe CD as compared to AZA monotherapy in patients who are anti-TNFα and immunosuppressant naïve and who have failed steroids or mesalamine.[21]

In addition, infliximab has shown good results in the treatment of perianal CD.[39] Infliximab has also been evaluated for its ability to reduce postoperative CD recurrence in high-risk patients (smokers, younger age, penetrating disease, shorter disease duration).[40] Initial studies with small number of patients showed promise but a recent large multicenter placebo controlled trial presented in abstract form failed to show similar results.[41] Infliximab is used for induction and maintenance of remission[42] and in combination therapy with AZA for inducing steroid free remission in moderate to severe UC.[22] It is also efficacious and safe as a rescue therapy in patients with severe or moderately severe UC refractory to intravenous steroids and can reduce the rate of colectomy.[43]

Infliximab is generally well tolerated, but side effects include acute and delayed hypersensitivity infusion reactions.[32] The incidence of infusion reactions is higher in patients with antibody to infliximab (ATI).[44] There is evidence that ATI formation is associated with poor clinical outcomes in patients with CD.[45] Patients who are on concomitant immunomodulator therapy have a lower level of ATI.[21,44] Hence, it is intuitive to think that combination therapy would be associated with better sustained infliximab response and clinical remission rates. Although the rationale is compelling, long-term prospective studies are needed.[46−48] Other adverse events associated with infliximab are risk of serious and opportunistic infections, drug induced lupus, liver enzyme abnormality, lymphoma, skin cancer, and the more controversial risks of solid organ malignancy and heart failure.[49−53] The risk of lymphoma and skin cancers seems to be higher in patients with past or current use of thiopurines.

ADA is a fully humanized recombinant monoclonal antibody to TNFα. It is administered as a subcutaneous injection providing the patients the flexibility of self-administration.

ADA is used for induction and maintenance of remission in CD and UC patients.[54−57] Several randomized controlled trials in CD have established ADA as an alternative for patients with loss of response to infliximab treatment.[55,58,59] Subgroup analysis from CHARM study and two open labeled studies showed efficacy of ADA in fistula closure in anti-TNF naïve and experienced patients.[55,60,61] In terms of the efficacy of ADA in prevention of postoperative CD, a randomized trial showed that step up therapy with either thiopurines and/or ADA based on clinical risk factors and early endoscopic recurrence was better than conventional therapy for prevention of CD recurrence (67% vs 49%, $P = 0.003$ intention to treat analysis).[20]

The side effect profile of ADA is similar to infliximab, although the pooled analysis of clinical trials did not find an increased risk of cancer in patients treated with ADA.[62] With respect to immunogenicity, the rate of antibody formation seems to be lower in ADA (2.6% in CLASSIC II trial).[63] However, patients who are switched from infliximab to ADA due to infliximab antibody formation are more likely to develop anti-ADA antibodies, which in turn is associated with increased risk of treatment failure with ADA.[64]

Certolizumab pegol is a humanized monoclonal antibody that neutralizes soluble and membrane-bound TNFα activity. It lacks the Fc portion of the antibody and hence does not cause complement activation or increased apoptosis in in vitro assays.[65] The Fab fragment is linked to polyethylene glycol, which increases its plasma half-life and possibly reduces immunogenicity. Like ADA, this agent is administered subcutaneously.

Certolizumab is approved for induction and maintenance of remission in moderate to severe CD.[66,67] Open labeled trials have evaluated the efficacy of certolizumab in patients who have lost response or are intolerant to infliximab (secondary failures) and showed good rates of clinical and endoscopic remission.[68,69]

The safety profile of certolizumab is similar to that of other anti-TNF agents. Certolizumab has decreased transferability across the blood-placenta barrier compared to the other anti-TNF agents and hence might be considered as the anti-TNF drug of preference if a pregnant patient needs to start a biologic agent for moderate to severe CD.

Golimumab is the newest anti-TNF drug and is approved only for treatment of moderate to severe UC. It is a fully human monoclonal IgG-1 antibody to TNFα and is administered subcutaneously.[70,71] An in vitro and mouse model study showed that golimumab has higher affinity for soluble TNFα compared to infliximab and ADA (2.4 fold and 7.1 fold, respectively) and has more capacity to neutralize TNF.[70]

Golimumab is initiated with an induction phase of 200 mg at week 0 and 100 mg at week 2 followed by maintenance therapy of 100 mg every 4 weeks.[72,73] Of note, in the clinical trials, patients with prior anti-TNF exposure were excluded and hence the efficacy of golimumab in those with loss of response to other anti-TNF agents is unclear. The safety profile of golimumab in the drug trials was similar to other anti-TNF medications.[73]

3.5.2 Anti-Integrin Antibody Agents

Leukocyte recruitment to the intestinal mucosa plays an important role in the pathogenesis of IBD. Integrin molecules like α4β1/α4β7 are found on T lymphocytes and bind to adhesion molecules like vascular cell adhesion molecule (VCAM)-1/MAdCAM-1 that are expressed on the endothelium and upregulated in areas of active inflammation.[74] Hence blocking leukocyte trafficking can decrease inflammation in the intestinal mucosa (Fig. 3.3).

Several monoclonal antibodies that block integrins have been developed, like natalizumab, which is specific for the α4 integrin subunit, vedolizumab which is directed against an epitope comprising the α4β7 heterodimer, and etrolizumab directed against the β7 subunit.[75]

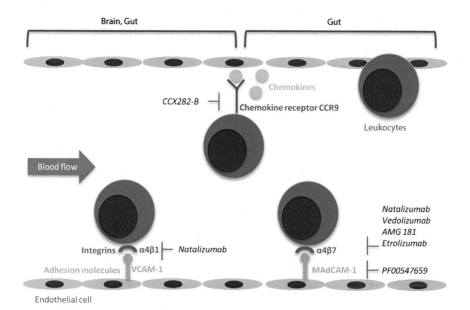

Figure 3.3 Role of chemokines and, adhesion (VCAM, MAdCAM) and integrin (α4β1, α4β7) molecules in leukocyte trafficking in various organs and their therapeutic drug targets in IBD. MAdCAM, mucosal vascular addressin cell adhesion molecule; VCAM, vascular cell adhesion molecule.

Natalizumab is a humanized IgG-4 molecule[76,77] that inhibits α4β1 and α4β7 interaction with adhesion molecules VCAM and MAdCAM-1, respectively. It is FDA approved for the treatment of CD patients who have lost response or are intolerant to anti-TNF agents. The inhibition of α4β1-VCAM interaction affects T cell mediated immune surveillance against John Cunningham (JC) virus infection, thus leading to an increased incidence of progressive multifocal encephalopathy (PML) of the central nervous system. Because of this adverse effect, natalizumab has had limited use in CD especially after vedolizumab became available.

Vedolizumab is a monoclonal IgG-1 antibody specific to gut leukocyte trafficking by selectively inhibiting α4β7/MAdCAM. It was FDA approved for the treatment of both UC and CD at 300 mg (week 0, 2, 6 induction followed by every 8 weeks maintenance) dose in June 2014.

The results of vedolizumab induction therapy for treatment of moderate to severe CD have not been very robust (14.5% clinical remission rate at week 6 compared to 6.8% in the placebo group, $P = 0.02$).[78] However, at week 52 the results were more promising with 39% clinical remission rates as compared to placebo (21.6%). There seems to be a delay in clinical effect of the drug in CD and the clinical response and remission rates become more prominent after 28 weeks of therapy. A possible explanation for this finding is that the transmural nature of CD may require a longer time for the drug to become effective. Another possible explanation could be the significant disease burden in the clinical trial. The study population included 37% patients with a history of fistulizing disease, 42% with at least one prior surgery, and 50% with primary or secondary loss of response to prior therapy.[78] Although the studies did not show remarkable efficacy of vedolizumab for induction of remission it is a good option for patients who have failed prior anti-TNF therapy and have complex and severe CD.

In UC the efficacy of vedolizumab was more impressive as compared to placebo (clinical response rate of 47.1% vs 25.5%, $P<0.001$ at week 6 and 41.8% vs 15.9% at week 52).[79]

The α4β7 receptors are also present in bronchial tissue and thus there was concern for increased risk of nasopharyngitis in CD patients who were part of treatment arm. However, there was no increase in the incidence of severe infections in the study population and current recommendations do not require screening of patients for tuberculosis or hepatitis B prior to initiation of the drug.

The theoretical advantage of gut selective inhibition of leukocyte trafficking is supported by the data that there have been no reported cases of PML with vedolizumab treatment in over 3000 patients in clinical trials. In the natalizumab treated patients, factors associated with increased incidence of PML were prior use of immunosuppressive agent, positive JC virus antibody, and duration of therapy.[80] In a review of risk of malignancy associated with biologics in IBD, there was one B cell lymphoma, three nonmelanoma skin cancers, and two melanomas among 3129 patients with 3097 patient years from three vedolizumab drug trials (two CD and one UC).[50] Even though the safety profile of vedolizumab regarding infections and malignancy is reassuring, long-term data are needed.

3.6 NEXT GENERATION IMMUNE BASED THERAPIES IN IBD

The current immune based therapies in IBD have variable clinical efficacy ranging from 15% to 60%. The long-term efficacy of these drugs is limited by development of antibodies, loss of response, and serious adverse events like opportunistic infections and cancers. Considering these aspects, numerous other targets in immune regulatory pathways of IBD are being explored. We review a few that have shown favorable efficacy in early phase human trials (Table 3.2, Fig. 3.2).

3.6.1 Blockage of Leukocyte Trafficking

In addition to natalizumab and vedolizumab, there are other anti-integrins and anti-adhesion molecules being investigated. These include AMG 181 (anti-$\alpha 4\beta 7$ antibody), etrolizumab (anti-$\beta 7$ subunit antibody), PF00547649 (anti-MAdCAM-1 antibody) and AJM 300 (anti-$\alpha 4$ antibody, orally administered). Antagonists to chemokines that mediate integrin activation are also being evaluated (anti-CXCL-10—eldelumab, anti-CCR-9—CCX282-B).[81] (Fig. 3.3).

AMG 181 is an IgG2 monoclonal antibody similar to vedolizumab that blocks $\alpha 4\beta 7$ interaction with MAdCAM-1. A trial evaluating the efficacy and safety of the drug in healthy subjects ($n = 68$) and four UC patients showed that the pharmacokinetic and pharmacodynamic profile was safe and suitable for further testing in IBD patients.[82] No treatment related serious adverse events were observed. Phase 2 trials for AMG 181 in UC (NCT01694485) and CD patients (NCT01696396) have been suspended due to issues with study documentation that required correction.[81,83]

Etrolizumab is a monoclonal antibody specific to β7 subunit of the integrin molecule that blocks α4β7 mediated T cell migration into the gut and αEβ7-E-cadherin interaction antagonizing the retention of lymphocytes in the mucosa. A phase 1 study showed that etrolizumab was safe and well tolerated.[84] The phase 2 EUCALYPTUS trial showed clinical efficacy for induction of remission at week 10 in moderate to severe UC.[85] A phase 3 double blind trial for induction and maintenance of remission in patients with moderate to severe UC who are refractory or intolerant to anti-TNF drugs is underway (NCT02100696).

PF00547659 is a highly specific fully humanized IgG2 antibody to MAdCAM.[86] MAdCAM, in contrast to VCAM is gut specific and is not found in the endothelium of the brain thus making it a good therapeutic option for treatment of IBD.[87] The first human trial of PF00547659 with 80 active UC patients showed a delayed clinical response at week 12. There were no obvious drug related side effects, although the number of patients who were exposed to the full dose was small. There was no evidence of immunogenic response during the study period or 1 month after last injection.[88] Larger phase 2 clinical trials are underway to determine its efficacy in CD (NCT01276509) and UC (NCT01620255) patients.

AJM 300 is an α4 integrin antagonist that inhibits the binding of α4β1 and α4β7 to VCAM-1 and MAdCAM-1, respectively. It is an orally active small molecule with targets similar to natalizumab.[76,77] A phase 2a multicenter Japanese trial in moderately active UC patients ($n = 102$) treated at doses of 960 mg three times a day showed clinical response in 62.7% patients as compared to 25.5% in the placebo group at week 8 ($P = 0.002$). No serious adverse events were reported.[89]

3.6.1.1 Chemokine Inhibitors

The two chemokine inhibitors CCX-282B (*Vercirnon*), which is an orally active molecule that blocks CCR-9 receptors, and *Eldelumab*, which targets IFNγ-inducible protein 10 (IP-10 or CXCL-10), failed to show significant efficacy in phase 2 and phase 3 clinical trials, respectively (Feagan B et al., abstract presentation CCFA 2013).[90-93]

In summary, the antileukocyte trafficking molecules bring a new array of therapeutic options for patients with IBD, especially those who are refractory to anti-TNF treatment. As more phase 2 and phase 3 trials are done, better safety and efficacy data will emerge. It is also important to recognize that other aspects of treatment will need to be answered, including the immunogenic potential of these agents and whether there is a role for concomitant treatment with anti-adhesion and anti-TNF drugs.

3.6.2 JAK-Stat Pathway Inhibitor (Tofacitinib)

JAKs regulate cellular proliferation, differentiation, and immune cell function.[94] Tofacitinib is an oral JAK-1, 2, and 3 inhibitor that acts by competing with adenosine triphosphate (ATP) for the ATP binding site in JAK enzymes.[95] In vitro specificity of tofacitinib for inhibition of JAK 1 and 3 blocks the signaling of cytokines like IL-2, 4, 7, 9, 15, and 21 that share the gamma-chain containing receptors. JAK-1 inhibition also results in blockage of IL-6 and IFNγ.[96]

Phase 2 trials of tofacitinib for moderate to severe UC showed good results in achieving clinical response and remission rates at week 8.[9] In contrast, the phase 2 trial in CD patients did not show significant differences in clinical response or remission rates after 4 weeks of treatment compared to placebo, but of note the placebo rates were unexpectedly high (47% response and 21% remission rates).[10] A reduction in fecal calprotectin and C-reactive protein levels were seen in 15 mg twice-daily tofacitinib dosing indicating biological activity. A current tofacitinib trial for CD is underway that has stricter inclusion criteria (requires demonstration of terminal ileum or colonic ulcers by endoscopy) and a long-term treatment option (NCT01393626). Increases in low and high-density lipoprotein cholesterol were observed in patients in both trials, especially those receiving higher doses.

3.6.3 TGFβ/SMAD7 Pathway Inhibitor (Mongersen)

TGFβ1 inhibits T cell proliferation and differentiation and reduces macrophage activation and dendritic cell maturation. Mice lacking TGFβ1 die soon after birth due to severe colitis, pulmonary and systemic inflammation.[97] In CD, high levels of SMAD7 protein block TGFβ signaling. The oral antisense oligonucleotide of SMAD7 causes degradation of SMAD7 messenger RNA and restores the TGFβ signaling and reduces inflammation.[97]

A phase 2 double blind, placebo controlled study evaluating the efficacy of an oral SMAD7 inhibitor (mongersen) in moderate to severe CD patients showed exciting clinical remission rates at day 15 after 2 weeks of treatment with mongersen at 10, 40, or 160 mg doses (12%, 55%, and 65%, respectively, as compared to 10% in placebo group).[98] Of note, the inclusion criteria were based on a clinical disease activity index and 39% of patients did not have elevated CRP levels with an overall low median CRP of 4–5 mg/liter at the time of induction. Interestingly, the clinical remission was sustained for 3 months even though the treatment was only given for 2 weeks. These results will need to be further evaluated in larger studies but they bring up the possibility of change in T cell homeostasis after unblocking TGFβ1 signaling for a short duration.[97]

3.6.4 Laquinimod

Laquinimod is an oral immunomodulator that has shown favorable efficacy and safety profile in multiple sclerosis.[99] It is a novel synthetic compound with high bioavailability that has a direct inhibitory effect on antigen presenting cells and T cells, resulting in downregulation of pro-inflammatory cytokines.[100] A phase 2 multicenter, double blind, sequential cohort, randomized controlled trial with 117 patients in laquinimod group (0.5, 1, 1.5, or 2 mg/day) and 63 patients in placebo group evaluated clinical remission and clinical response rates at week 8 with 4 week follow up and found efficacy with the 0.5 mg/day dose. The treatment was safe and well tolerated with overall rates of adverse events similar to placebo.[101]

3.6.5 IL-12/23 Pathway Inhibitor (Ustekinumab)

The IL-12/23 inflammatory pathway is linked with the pathogenesis of CD. There is overexpression of the IL-12 p35 and IL-12/23 p40 subunits in CD.[102,103] Data from human genetic and genome-wide association studies have shown polymorphism of IL-12/23 p40 genes in CD patients.[104,105]

Ustekinumab is an IL-12/23 inhibitor that blocks the p40 subunit common to both IL-12 and 23. Three trials reported modest effects of ustekinumab in CD patients.[106–108] The phase 2B induction and maintenance trial evaluated 526 patients with moderate to severe CD with anti-TNF failure who were randomized to ustekinumab (1, 3, or 6 mg/kg IV dose) or placebo during induction phase. Patients who had response to drug treatment at week 6 were enrolled and randomized to the maintenance phase with 90 mg/kg ustekinumab or placebo at weeks 8 and 16. The primary end point of clinical response at 6 weeks was achieved with statistical significance with the 6 mg/kg dose (39.7% vs 23.5%, $P = 0.005$). In the maintenance phase there were significant increases in clinical response (69.4% vs 42.5%, $P<0.001$) and remission rates (41.7% vs 27.4%, $P = 0.03$) in the treatment group as compared to placebo.[108] Serious infections occurred in 6 patients in treatment and 1 patient in the placebo group during the induction phase and in 11 patients (4 receiving ustekinumab) in the maintenance phase. There was one reported case of basal cell skin cancer in the treatment group.[108]

Ustekinumab is currently FDA approved for treatment of severe plaque psoriasis. In patients with moderate to severe CD refractory to anti-TNF medications, especially in those with psoriasis, it provides a viable off-label treatment option.

3.6.6 Stem Cell Therapy

Stem cells can be classified as embryonic (ESCs) or adult-derived. Some ESCs are retained as adult-derived stem cells. These can be hematopoietic stem cells (HSCs), intestinal stem cells, or mesenchymal stem cells (MSCs). The HSCs derived from bone marrow or blood differentiate into hematopoietic cells[109] and have been studied as a potential therapeutic modality in IBD patients, but systemic side effects may limit their use.[110–112] The intestinal stem cells are located at the base of the intestinal crypt at the leucine-rich repeat containing G protein coupled receptor 5 location and lead to renewal of intestinal epithelium.[113] The MSCs are present at various mesoderm-derived locations like adipocytes and have limited differentiation potential. However, they have immunomodulating capability in the gut and hence have been explored as potential treatment for fistulizing CD and luminal IBD.[112]

The results of treatment of refractory perianal and fistulizing disease with local MSCs therapy have been particularly favorable.[112,114–117] Treatment with systemic infusion of allogenic and umbilical cord derived MSCs has been evaluated in randomized trials with limited number of patients.[118–120] A meta-analysis of all studies with systemic stem cell treatment showed that 40.5% achieved remission after infusion of MSCs.[112] Most commonly reported adverse events with systemic MSCs were headache, diarrhea, mild transfusion reaction, and taste and smell disturbances, all of which were self limiting.[112]

MSC therapy has emerged as a safe and effective treatment option for refractory IBD, but is still in its early stages limited by cost and lack of data from larger randomized trials.

3.7 CONCLUSION

Immune dysregulation plays a key role in the pathogenesis of IBD, but the immune pathways are complex and not completely understood. The fact that current therapies are at best 60% effective and have the potential to lose efficacy over time has led to the development of several molecules targeting various aspects of the innate and adaptive immune system. A significant number of drugs failed to prove efficacious in early phases of clinical trials, which emphasizes the importance of interaction of the immunome with the exposome, genome, and the microbiome in the pathogenesis of IBD. However, there are a few potential therapeutic targets of the immune system (like SMAD7 and MAdCAM inhibitors) with acceptable side effect profiles that show promise. This will expand the horizon of IBD treatment in the coming years and hopefully provide better outcomes for patients with this chronic illness.

REFERENCES

1. Molodecky NA, Soon IS, Rabi DM, Ghali WA, Ferris M, Chernoff G, et al. Increasing incidence and prevalence of the inflammatory bowel diseases with time, based on systematic review. *Gastroenterology* 2012;**142**:46−54 e42; quiz e30.

2. Fiocchi C. Genes and 'in-vironment': how will our concepts on the pathophysiology of inflammatory bowel disease develop in the future? *Dig Dis* 2012;**30**(Suppl. 3):2−11.

3. Danese S. New therapies for inflammatory bowel disease: from the bench to the bedside. *Gut* 2012;**61**:918−32.

4. de Souza HSP, Fiocchi C. Immunopathogenesis of IBD: current state of the art. *Nat Rev Gastroenterol Hepatol* 2016 (in press).

5. Bruce E. Sands CAS. Crohn's disease. In: Feldman M, Friedman LS, Brandt LJ, eds. *Sleisenger and Fordtran's Gastrointestinal and Liver Disease*, vol. 2. 9th ed. Philadelphia PA: Elsevier; 2010.

6. Fonseca-Camarillo G, Yamamoto-Furusho JK. Immunoregulatory pathways involved in inflammatory bowel disease. *Inflamm Bowel Dis* 2015;**21**(9):2188−93.

7. MacDonald TT, Monteleone I, Fantini MC, Monteleone G. Regulation of homeostasis and inflammation in the intestine. *Gastroenterology* 2011;**140**:1768−75.

8. Fuss IJ, Heller F, Boirivant M, Leon F, Yoshida M, Fichtner-Feigl S, et al. Nonclassical CD1d-restricted NK T cells that produce IL-13 characterize an atypical Th2 response in ulcerative colitis. *J Clin Invest* 2004;**113**:1490−7.

9. Sandborn WJ, Ghosh S, Panes J, Vranic I, Su C, Rousell S, et al. Tofacitinib, an oral Janus kinase inhibitor, in active ulcerative colitis. *N Engl J Med* 2012;**367**:616−24.

10. Sandborn WJ, Ghosh S, Panes J, Vranic I, Wang W, Niezychowski W. A phase 2 study of tofacitinib, an oral Janus kinase inhibitor, in patients with Crohn's disease. *Clin Gastroenterol Hepatol* 2014;**12**:1485—93, e1482.

11. Bevilacqua MP. Endothelial-leukocyte adhesion molecules. *Annu Rev Immunol* 1993;**11**: 767—804.

12. Elion GB. The george hitchings and gertrude elion lecture. The pharmacology of azathioprine. *Ann NY Acad Sci* 1993;**685**:400—7.

13. Maltzman JS, Koretzky GA. Azathioprine: old drug, new actions. *J Clin Invest* 2003;**111**: 1122—4.

14. Rathmell JC, Thompson CB. Pathways of apoptosis in lymphocyte development, homeostasis, and disease. *Cell* 2002;**109**(Suppl):S97—107.

15. Tiede I, Fritz G, Strand S, Poppe D, Dvorsky R, Strand D, et al. CD28-dependent Rac1 activation is the molecular target of azathioprine in primary human CD4+ T lymphocytes. *J Clin Invest* 2003;**111**:1133—45.

16. Chande N, Tsoulis DJ, MacDonald JK. Azathioprine or 6-mercaptopurine for induction of remission in Crohn's disease. *Cochrane Database Syst Rev* 2013;4 CD000545.

17. Panes J, Lopez-Sanroman A, Bermejo F, Garcia-Sanchez V, Esteve M, Torres Y, et al. Early azathioprine therapy is no more effective than placebo for newly diagnosed Crohn's disease. *Gastroenterology* 2013;**145**:766—74, e761.

18. Cosnes J, Bourrier A, Laharie D, Nahon S, Bouhnik Y, Carbonnel F, et al. Early administration of azathioprine vs conventional management of Crohn's disease: a randomized controlled trial. *Gastroenterology* 2013;**145**:758—65 e752; quiz e714—755.

19. Peyrin-Biroulet L, Deltenre P, Ardizzone S, D'Haens G, Hanauer SB, Herfarth H, et al. Azathioprine and 6-mercaptopurine for the prevention of postoperative recurrence in Crohn's disease: a meta-analysis. *Am J Gastroenterol* 2009;**104**:2089—96.

20. De Cruz P, Kamm MA, Hamilton AL, Ritchie KJ, Krejany EO, Gorelik A, et al. Crohn's disease management after intestinal resection: a randomised trial. *Lancet* 2015;**385**:1406—17.

21. Colombel JF, Sandborn WJ, Reinisch W, Mantzaris GJ, Kornbluth A, Rachmilewitz D, et al. Infliximab, azathioprine, or combination therapy for Crohn's disease. *N Engl J Med* 2010;**362**:1383—95.

22. Panaccione R, Ghosh S, Middleton S, Marquez JR, Scott BB, Flint L, et al. Combination therapy with infliximab and azathioprine is superior to monotherapy with either agent in ulcerative colitis. *Gastroenterology* 2014;**146**:392—400, e393.

23. Ardizzone S, Maconi G, Russo A, Imbesi V, Colombo E, Bianchi Porro G. Randomised controlled trial of azathioprine and 5-aminosalicylic acid for treatment of steroid dependent ulcerative colitis. *Gut* 2006;**55**:47—53.

24. Timmer A, McDonald JW, Tsoulis DJ, Macdonald JK. Azathioprine and 6-mercaptopurine for maintenance of remission in ulcerative colitis. *Cochrane Database Syst Rev* 2012;9 CD000478.

25. Cutolo M, Sulli A, Pizzorni C, Seriolo B, Straub RH. Anti-inflammatory mechanisms of methotrexate in rheumatoid arthritis. *Ann Rheum Dis* 2001;**60**:729—35.

26. Morabito L, Montesinos MC, Schreibman DM, Balter L, Thompson LF, Resta R, et al. Methotrexate and sulfasalazine promote adenosine release by a mechanism that requires ecto-5′-nucleotidase-mediated conversion of adenine nucleotides. *J Clin Invest* 1998;**101**:295—300.

27. Feagan BG, Rochon J, Fedorak RN, Irvine EJ, Wild G, Sutherland L, et al. Methotrexate for the treatment of Crohn's disease. The North American Crohn's Study Group Investigators. *N Engl J Med* 1995;**332**:292—7.

28. Patel V, Wang Y, MacDonald JK, McDonald JW, Chande N. Methotrexate for mainte-nance of remission in Crohn's disease. *Cochrane Database Syst Rev* 2014;**8**:CD006884.

29. Chande N, Wang Y, MacDonald JK, McDonald JW. Methotrexate for induction of remis-sion in ulcerative colitis. *Cochrane Database Syst Rev* 2014;**8**:CD006618.

30. Oren R, Arber N, Odes S, Moshkowitz M, Keter D, Pomeranz I, et al. Methotrexate in chronic active ulcerative colitis: a double-blind, randomized, Israeli multicenter trial. *Gastroenterology* 1996;**110**:1416–21.

31. Carbonnel F, Colombel J-F, Filippi J, Katsanos K, Peyrin-Biroulet L, Allez M. et al. Methotrexate for corticosteroid-dependent ulcerative colitis: results of a placebo randomized controlled trial, *Gastroenterology* 2015;**148**:S-140.

32. Lichtenstein GR, Hanauer SB, Sandborn WJ. Management of Crohn's disease in adults. *Am J Gastroenterol* 2009;**104**:465–83; quiz 464, 484.

33. Crombe V, Salleron J, Savoye G, Dupas JL, Vernier-Massouille G, Lerebours E, et al. Long-term outcome of treatment with infliximab in pediatric-onset Crohn's disease: a population-based study. *Inflamm Bowel Dis* 2011;**17**:2144–52.

34. Peyrin-Biroulet L, Oussalah A, Williet N, Pillot C, Bresler L, Bigard MA. Impact of azathio-prine and tumour necrosis factor antagonists on the need for surgery in newly diagnosed Crohn's disease. *Gut* 2011;**60**:930–6.

35. Ramadas AV, Gunesh S, Thomas GA, Williams GT, Hawthorne AB. Natural history of Crohn's disease in a population-based cohort from Cardiff (1986–2003): a study of changes in medical treatment and surgical resection rates. *Gut* 2010;**59**:1200–6.

36. Lakatos PL, Golovics PA, David G, Pandur T, Erdelyi Z, Horvath A, et al. Has there been a change in the natural history of Crohn's disease? Surgical rates and medical management in a population-based inception cohort from Western Hungary between 1977–2009. *Am J Gastroenterol* 2012;**107**:579–88.

37. Lichtenstein GR, Yan S, Bala M, Hanauer S. Remission in patients with Crohn's disease is associated with improvement in employment and quality of life and a decrease in hospitaliza-tions and surgeries. *Am J Gastroenterol* 2004;**99**:91–6.

38. Chatu S, Subramanian V, Saxena S, Pollok RC. The role of thiopurines in reducing the need for surgical resection in Crohn's disease: a systematic review and meta-analysis. *Am J Gastroenterol* 2014;**109**:23–34; quiz 35.

39. Sands BE, Blank MA, Patel K, van Deventer SJ. Long-term treatment of rectovaginal fistu-las in Crohn's disease: response to infliximab in the ACCENT II Study. *Clin Gastroenterol Hepatol* 2004;**2**:912–20.

40. Regueiro M, Schraut W, Baidoo L, Kip KE, Sepulveda AR, Pesci M, et al. Infliximab prevents Crohn's disease recurrence after ileal resection. *Gastroenterology* 2009;**136**:441–50 e441; quiz 716.

41. Regueiro M, Feagan BG, Zou B, Johanns J, Blank M, Chevrier M. et al. Infliximab for prevention of recurrence of post-surgical Crohn's disease following ileocolonic resection: a randomized, Placebo-Controlled study. *Gastroenterology* 2015;**148**:S-141.

42. Rutgeerts P, Sandborn WJ, Feagan BG, Reinisch W, Olson A, Johanns J, et al. Infliximab for induction and maintenance therapy for ulcerative colitis. *N Engl J Med* 2005;**353**: 2462–76.

43. Jarnerot G, Hertervig E, Friis-Liby I, Blomquist L, Karlen P, Granno C, et al. Infliximab as rescue therapy in severe to moderately severe ulcerative colitis: a randomized, placebo-controlled study. *Gastroenterology* 2005;**128**:1805–11.

44. Baert F, Noman M, Vermeire S, Van Assche G, D'Haens G, Carbonez A, et al. Influence of immunogenicity on the long-term efficacy of infliximab in Crohn's disease. *N Engl J Med* 2003;**348**:601–8.

45. Vande Casteele N, Khanna R, Levesque BG, Stitt L, Zou GY, Singh S, et al. The relationship between infliximab concentrations, antibodies to infliximab and disease activity in Crohn's disease. *Gut* 2014;**64**(10):1539−45.

46. Jones JL, Kaplan GG, Peyrin-Biroulet L, Baidoo L, Devlin S, Melmed GY, et al. Effects of concomitant immunomodulator therapy on efficacy and safety of Anti-TNF therapy for Crohn's disease: a meta-analysis of placebo-controlled trials. *Clin Gastroenterol Hepatol* 2015;**13**(13):2233−40.e2.

47. Grossi V, Lerer T, Griffiths A, LeLeiko N, Cabrera J, Otley A, et al. Concomitant use of immunomodulators affects the durability of infliximab therapy in children with Crohn's disease. *Clin Gastroenterol Hepatol* 2015;**13**(10):1748−56.

48. Christophorou D, Funakoshi N, Duny Y, Valats JC, Bismuth M, Pineton De Chambrun G, et al. Systematic review with meta-analysis: infliximab and immunosuppressant therapy vs. infliximab alone for active ulcerative colitis. *Aliment Pharmacol Ther* 2015;**41**:603−12.

49. Lichtenstein GR, Feagan BG, Cohen RD, Salzberg BA, Diamond RH, Price S, et al. Serious infection and mortality in patients with Crohn's disease: more than 5 years of follow-up in the TREAT registry. *Am J Gastroenterol* 2012;**107**:1409−22.

50. Dulai PS, Siegel CA. The risk of malignancy associated with the use of biological agents in patients with inflammatory bowel disease. *Gastroenterol Clin North Am* 2014;**43**: 525−41.

51. Williams CJ, Peyrin-Biroulet L, Ford AC. Systematic review with meta-analysis: malignancies with anti-tumour necrosis factor-alpha therapy in inflammatory bowel disease. *Aliment Pharmacol Ther* 2014;**39**:447−58.

52. Diaz JC, Vallejo S, Canas CA. Drug-induced lupus in anti-TNF-alpha therapy and its treatment with rituximab. *Rheumatol Int* 2012;**32**:3315−17.

53. Bjornsson ES, Gunnarsson BI, Grondal G, Jonasson JG, Einarsdottir R, Ludviksson BR, et al. Risk of drug-induced liver injury from tumor necrosis factor antagonists. *Clin Gastroenterol Hepatol* 2015;**13**:602−8.

54. Hanauer SB, Sandborn WJ, Rutgeerts P, Fedorak RN, Lukas M, MacIntosh D, et al. Human anti-tumor necrosis factor monoclonal antibody (adalimumab) in Crohn's disease: the CLASSIC-I trial. *Gastroenterology* 2006;**130**:323−33; quiz 591.

55. Colombel JF, Sandborn WJ, Rutgeerts P, Enns R, Hanauer SB, Panaccione R, et al. Adalimumab for maintenance of clinical response and remission in patients with Crohn's disease: the CHARM trial. *Gastroenterology* 2007;**132**:52−65.

56. Sandborn WJ, van Assche G, Reinisch W, Colombel JF, D'Haens G, Wolf DC, et al. Adalimumab induces and maintains clinical remission in patients with moderate-to-severe ulcerative colitis. *Gastroenterology* 2012;**142**:257−65, e251−253.

57. Reinisch W, Sandborn WJ, Hommes DW, D'Haens G, Hanauer S, Schreiber S, et al. Adalimumab for induction of clinical remission in moderately to severely active ulcerative colitis: results of a randomised controlled trial. *Gut* 2011;**60**:780−7.

58. Sandborn WJ, Rutgeerts P, Enns R, Hanauer SB, Colombel JF, Panaccione R, et al. Adalimumab induction therapy for Crohn disease previously treated with infliximab: a randomized trial. *Ann Intern Med* 2007;**146**:829−38.

59. Rutgeerts P, Van Assche G, Sandborn WJ, Wolf DC, Geboes K, Colombel JF, et al. Adalimumab induces and maintains mucosal healing in patients with Crohn's disease: data from the EXTEND trial. *Gastroenterology* 2012;**142**:1102−11, e1102.

60. Panaccione R, Loftus Jr. EV, Binion D, McHugh K, Alam S, Chen N, et al. Efficacy and safety of adalimumab in Canadian patients with moderate to severe Crohn's disease: results of the Adalimumab in Canadian SubjeCts with ModErate to Severe Crohn's DiseaSe (ACCESS) trial. *Can J Gastroenterol* 2011;**25**:419−25.

61. Lofberg R, Louis EV, Reinisch W, Robinson AM, Kron M, Camez A, et al. Adalimumab produces clinical remission and reduces extraintestinal manifestations in Crohn's disease: results from CARE. *Inflamm Bowel Dis* 2012;**18**:1−9.

62. Osterman MT, Sandborn WJ, Colombel J-F, Robinson AM, Lau W, Huang B, et al. Increased risk of malignancy with adalimumab combination therapy, compared with monotherapy, for Crohn's disease. *Gastroenterology* 2014;**146**:941−9, e942.

63. Sandborn WJ, Hanauer SB, Rutgeerts P, Fedorak RN, Lukas M, MacIntosh DG, et al. Adalimumab for maintenance treatment of Crohn's disease: results of the CLASSIC II trial. *Gut* 2007;**56**:1232−9.

64. Frederiksen MT, Ainsworth MA, Brynskov J, Thomsen OO, Bendtzen K, Steenholdt C. Antibodies against infliximab are associated with de novo development of antibodies to adalimumab and therapeutic failure in infliximab-to-adalimumab switchers with IBD. *Inflamm Bowel Dis* 2014;**20**:1714−21.

65. Nesbitt A, Fossati G, Bergin M, Stephens P, Stephens S, Foulkes R, et al. Mechanism of action of certolizumab pegol (CDP870): in vitro comparison with other anti-tumor necrosis factor alpha agents. *Inflamm Bowel Dis* 2007;**13**:1323−32.

66. Sandborn WJ, Feagan BG, Stoinov S, Honiball PJ, Rutgeerts P, Mason D, et al. Certolizumab pegol for the treatment of Crohn's disease. *N Engl J Med* 2007;**357**:228−38.

67. Schreiber S, Khaliq-Kareemi M, Lawrance IC, Thomsen OO, Hanauer SB, McColm J, et al. Maintenance therapy with certolizumab pegol for Crohn's disease. *N Engl J Med* 2007;**357**:239−50.

68. Sandborn WJ, Abreu MT, D'Haens G, Colombel JF, Vermeire S, Mitchev K, et al. Certolizumab pegol in patients with moderate to severe Crohn's disease and secondary failure to infliximab. *Clin Gastroenterol Hepatol* 2010;**8**:688−95, e682.

69. Hebuterne X, Lemann M, Bouhnik Y, Dewit O, Dupas JL, Mross M, et al. Endoscopic improvement of mucosal lesions in patients with moderate to severe ileocolonic Crohn's disease following treatment with certolizumab pegol. *Gut* 2013;**62**:201−8.

70. Shealy DJ, Cai A, Staquet K, Baker A, Lacy ER, Johns L, et al. Characterization of golimumab, a human monoclonal antibody specific for human tumor necrosis factor alpha. *MAbs* 2010;**2**:428−39.

71. Weiner LM. Fully human therapeutic monoclonal antibodies. *J Immunother* 2006;**29**:1−9.

72. Sandborn WJ, Feagan BG, Marano C, Zhang H, Strauss R, Johanns J, et al. Subcutaneous golimumab induces clinical response and remission in patients with moderate-to-severe ulcerative colitis. *Gastroenterology* 2014;**146**:85−95; quiz e14−85.

73. Sandborn WJ, Feagan BG, Marano C, Zhang H, Strauss R, Johanns J, et al. Subcutaneous golimumab maintains clinical response in patients with moderate-to-severe ulcerative colitis. *Gastroenterology* 2014;**146**:96−109, e101.

74. Berlin C, Berg EL, Briskin MJ, Andrew DP, Kilshaw PJ, Holzmann B, et al. Alpha 4 beta 7 integrin mediates lymphocyte binding to the mucosal vascular addressin MAdCAM-1. *Cell* 1993;**74**:185−95.

75. Lin L, Liu X, Wang D, Zheng C. Efficacy and safety of antiintegrin antibody for inflammatory bowel disease: a systematic review and meta-analysis. *Medicine (Baltimore)* 2015;**94**, e556.

76. Targan SR, Feagan BG, Fedorak RN, Lashner BA, Panaccione R, Present DH, et al. Natalizumab for the treatment of active Crohn's disease: results of the ENCORE Trial. *Gastroenterology* 2007;**132**:1672−83.

77. Sandborn WJ, Colombel JF, Enns R, Feagan BG, Hanauer SB, Lawrance IC, et al. Natalizumab induction and maintenance therapy for Crohn's disease. *N Engl J Med* 2005;**353**:1912−25.

78. Sandborn WJ, Feagan BG, Rutgeerts P, Hanauer S, Colombel JF, Sands BE, et al. Vedolizumab as induction and maintenance therapy for Crohn's disease. *N Engl J Med* 2013;**369**:711–21.

79. Feagan BG, Rutgeerts P, Sands BE, Hanauer S, Colombel JF, Sandborn WJ, et al. Vedolizumab as induction and maintenance therapy for ulcerative colitis. *N Engl J Med* 2013;**369**:699–710.

80. Bloomgren G, Richman S, Hotermans C, Subramanyam M, Goelz S, Natarajan A, et al. Risk of natalizumab-associated progressive multifocal leukoencephalopathy. *N Engl J Med* 2012;**366**:1870–80.

81. Danese S, Panes J. Development of drugs to target interactions between leukocytes and endothelial cells and treatment algorithms for inflammatory bowel diseases. *Gastroenterology* 2014;**147**:981–9.

82. Pan W-J, Köck K, Rees WA, Sullivan BA, Evangelista CM, Yen M, et al. Clinical pharmacology of AMG 181, a gut-specific human anti-α4β7 monoclonal antibody, for treating inflammatory bowel diseases. *Br J Clin Pharmacol* 2014;**78**:1315–33.

83. Lobatón T, Vermeire S, Van Assche G, Rutgeerts P. Review article: anti-adhesion therapies for inflammatory bowel disease. *Aliment Pharmacol Ther* 2014;**39**:579–94.

84. Rutgeerts PJ, Fedorak RN, Hommes DW, Sturm A, Baumgart DC, Bressler B, et al. A randomised phase I study of etrolizumab (rhuMAb beta7) in moderate to severe ulcerative colitis. *Gut* 2013;**62**:1122–30.

85. Vermeire S, O'Byrne S, Keir M, Williams M, Lu TT, Mansfield JC, et al. Etrolizumab as induction therapy for ulcerative colitis: a randomised, controlled, phase 2 trial. *Lancet* 2014;**384**:309–18.

86. Pullen N, Molloy E, Carter D, Syntin P, Clemo F, Finco-Kent D, et al. Pharmacological characterization of PF-00547659, an anti-human MAdCAM monoclonal antibody. *Br J Pharmacol* 2009;**157**:281–93.

87. Allavena R, Noy S, Andrews M, Pullen N. CNS elevation of vascular and not mucosal addressin cell adhesion molecules in patients with multiple sclerosis. *Am J Pathol* 2010;**176**:556–62.

88. Vermeire S, Ghosh S, Panes J, Dahlerup JF, Luegering A, Sirotiakova J, et al. The mucosal addressin cell adhesion molecule antibody PF-00547,659 in ulcerative colitis: a randomised study. *Gut* 2011;**60**:1068–75.

89. Watanabe M, Yoshimura N, Motoya S, Tominaga K, Iwakiri R, Watanabe K, et al. 370 AJM300, an oral α4 integrin antagonist, for active ulcerative colitis: a multicenter, randomized, double-blind, placebo-controlled phase 2A study. *Gastroenterology* 2014;**146**:S-82.

90. Keshav S, Vanasek T, Niv Y, Petryka R, Howaldt S, Bafutto M, et al. A randomized controlled trial of the efficacy and safety of CCX282-B, an orally-administered blocker of chemokine receptor CCR9, for patients with Crohn's disease. *PLoS One* 2013;**8**:e60094.

91. An active treatment study to induce clinical response and/or remission with GSK1605786A in subjects with Crohn's disease (SHIELD-4). NCT01536418, <https://clinicaltrials.gov/ct2/show/NCT01536418>; 2015.

92. Mayer L, Sandborn WJ, Stepanov Y, Geboes K, Hardi R, Yellin M, et al. Anti-IP-10 antibody (BMS-936557) for ulcerative colitis: a phase II randomised study. *Gut* 2014;**63**:442–50.

93. Sandborn WJ, Colombel J-F, Ghosh S, Sands BE, Xu L-A, Luo A. 865 Phase IIB, randomized, placebo-controlled evaluation of the efficacy and safety of induction therapy with Eldelumab (Anti-IP-10 Antibody; BMS-936557) in patients with active ulcerative colitis. *Gastroenterology* 2014;**146**:S-150.

94. Lowenberg M, D'Haens G. Next-generation therapeutics for IBD. *Curr Gastroenterol Rep* 2015;**17**:21.

95. Karaman MW, Herrgard S, Treiber DK, Gallant P, Atteridge CE, Campbell BT, et al. A quantitative analysis of kinase inhibitor selectivity. *Nat Biotechnol* 2008;**26**:127−32.

96. Meyer DM, Jesson MI, Li X, Elrick MM, Funckes-Shippy CL, Warner JD, et al. Anti-inflammatory activity and neutrophil reductions mediated by the JAK1/JAK3 inhibitor, CP-690,550, in rat adjuvant-induced arthritis. *J Inflamm (Lond)* 2010;**7**:41.

97. Vermeire S. Oral SMAD7 antisense drug for Crohn's disease. *N Engl J Med* 2015;**372**: 1166−7.

98. Monteleone G, Neurath MF, Ardizzone S, Di Sabatino A, Fantini MC, Castiglione F, et al. Mongersen, an oral SMAD7 antisense oligonucleotide, and Crohn's disease. *N Engl J Med* 2015;**372**:1104−13.

99. Comi G, Jeffery D, Kappos L, Montalban X, Boyko A, Rocca MA, et al. Placebo-controlled trial of oral laquinimod for multiple sclerosis. *N Engl J Med* 2012;**366**:1000−9.

100. Yang JS, Xu LY, Xiao BG, Hedlund G, Link H. Laquinimod (ABR-215062) suppresses the development of experimental autoimmune encephalomyelitis, modulates the Th1/Th2 balance and induces the Th3 cytokine TGF-beta in Lewis rats. *J Neuroimmunol* 2004;**156**:3−9.

101. D'Haens G, Sandborn WJ, Colombel JF, Rutgeerts P, Brown K, Barkay H, et al. A phase II study of laquinimod in Crohn's disease. *Gut* 2015;**64**:1227−35.

102. Neurath MF. IL-23: a master regulator in Crohn disease. *Nat Med* 2007;**13**:26−8.

103. Strober W, Zhang F, Kitani A, Fuss I, Fichtner-Feigl S. Proinflammatory cytokines underlying the inflammation of Crohn's disease. *Curr Opin Gastroenterol* 2010;**26**:310−17.

104. Wang K, Zhang H, Kugathasan S, Annese V, Bradfield JP, Russell RK, et al. Diverse genome-wide association studies associate the IL12/IL23 pathway with Crohn disease. *Am J Hum Genet* 2009;**84**:399−405.

105. Duerr RH, Taylor KD, Brant SR, Rioux JD, Silverberg MS, Daly MJ, et al. A genome-wide association study identifies IL23R as an inflammatory bowel disease gene. *Science* 2006;**314**:1461−3.

106. Sandborn WJ, Feagan BG, Fedorak RN, Scherl E, Fleisher MR, Katz S, et al. A randomized trial of Ustekinumab, a human interleukin-12/23 monoclonal antibody, in patients with moderate-to-severe Crohn's disease. *Gastroenterology* 2008;**135**:1130−41.

107. Toedter GP, Blank M, Lang Y, Chen D, Sandborn WJ, de Villiers WJ. Relationship of C-reactive protein with clinical response after therapy with ustekinumab in Crohn's disease. *Am J Gastroenterol* 2009;**104**:2768−73.

108. Sandborn WJ, Gasink C, Gao LL, Blank MA, Johanns J, Guzzo C, et al. Ustekinumab induction and maintenance therapy in refractory Crohn's disease. *N Engl J Med* 2012;**367**: 1519−28.

109. Wilson A, Trumpp A. Bone-marrow haematopoietic-stem-cell niches. *Nat Rev Immunol* 2006;**6**:93−106.

110. Copelan EA. Hematopoietic stem-cell transplantation. *N Engl J Med* 2006;**354**:1813−26.

111. Garcia-Bosch O, Ricart E, Panes J. Review article: stem cell therapies for inflammatory bowel disease—efficacy and safety. *Aliment Pharmacol Ther* 2010;**32**:939−52.

112. Dave M, Mehta K, Luther J, Baruah A, Dietz AB, Faubion Jr. WA. Mesenchymal stem cell therapy for inflammatory bowel disease: a systematic review and meta-analysis. *Inflamm Bowel Dis* 2015;**21**(11):2696−707.

113. Koo BK, Clevers H. Stem cells marked by the R-spondin receptor LGR5. *Gastroenterology* 2014;**147**:289−302.

114. Garcia-Olmo D, Garcia-Arranz M, Garcia LG, Cuellar ES, Blanco IF, Prianes LA, et al. Autologous stem cell transplantation for treatment of rectovaginal fistula in perianal Crohn's disease: a new cell-based therapy. *Int J Colorectal Dis* 2003;**18**:451–4.

115. Ciccocioppo R, Bernardo ME, Sgarella A, Maccario R, Avanzini MA, Ubezio C, et al. Autologous bone marrow-derived mesenchymal stromal cells in the treatment of fistulising Crohn's disease. *Gut* 2011;**60**:788–98.

116. de la Portilla F, Alba F, Garcia-Olmo D, Herrerias JM, Gonzalez FX, Galindo A. Expanded allogeneic adipose-derived stem cells (eASCs) for the treatment of complex perianal fistula in Crohn's disease: results from a multicenter phase I/IIa clinical trial. *Int J Colorectal Dis* 2013;**28**:313–23.

117. Cho YB, Lee WY, Park KJ, Kim M, Yoo HW, Yu CS. Autologous adipose tissue-derived stem cells for the treatment of Crohn's fistula: a phase I clinical study. *Cell Transplant* 2013;**22**:279–85.

118. Liang J, Zhang H, Wang D, Feng X, Wang H, Hua B, et al. Allogeneic mesenchymal stem cell transplantation in seven patients with refractory inflammatory bowel disease. *Gut* 2012;**61**:468–9.

119. Forbes GM, Sturm MJ, Leong RW, Sparrow MP, Segarajasingam D, Cummins AG, et al. A phase 2 study of allogeneic mesenchymal stromal cells for luminal Crohn's disease refractory to biologic therapy. *Clin Gastroenterol Hepatol* 2014;**12**:64–71.

120. Duijvestein M, Vos AC, Roelofs H, Wildenberg ME, Wendrich BB, Verspaget HW, et al. Autologous bone marrow-derived mesenchymal stromal cell treatment for refractory luminal Crohn's disease: results of a phase I study. *Gut* 2010;**59**:1662–9.

CHAPTER 4

Multiple Sclerosis and Neurodegenerative Diseases

Maira Gironi[1], Caterina Arnò[1], Giancarlo Comi[1], Giselle Penton-Rol[2] and Roberto Furlan[1]

[1]Institute of Experimental Neurology, Division of Neuroscience, San Raffaele Scientific Institute, Milan, Italy [2]Center for Genetic Engineering and Biotechnology, Havana, Cuba

4.1 INTRODUCTION

Multiple sclerosis (MS) is a chronic immune-mediated inflammatory disease of the central nervous system (CNS) leading to demyelination and neuronal loss. It affects 2.5 million individuals worldwide, and represents the leading cause of nontraumatic disability in young and middle-aged people in the developed world. MS is present in all regions of the world, but its occurrence varies considerably, being very high in North America and Europe (108–140 per 100,000) and lower in Sub-Saharan Africa and East Asia (2–2.2 per 100,000).[1] MS is a very complex disease and no single factor has been shown to confer MS susceptibility.[2] MS shares with many other autoimmune diseases the fact that females have a greater risk of developing the disease than males. MS has a profound social impact, the cost of care dramatically increasing with the progression of disability. The effort made to guarantee education or employment to patients is necessary and beneficial; some studies demonstrated that people who were not employed and social active have a greater cognitive impairment.[3]

Healthy related quality of life (HRQoL) is a well-studied concept in MS and explains how many aspects of daily life are influenced by health status from the patient's point of view. The impact of a new treatment on HRQoL is now considered as a secondary/tertiary endpoint of efficacy during a clinical trial.[4]

4.1.1 Etiology

The real cause of MS is still unknown. Epidemiological data indicates that both genetic and environmental factors are important. The contribution

Immune Rebalancing. DOI: http://dx.doi.org/10.1016/B978-0-12-803302-9.00004-X

of genetic factors in MS development results from many studies of populations, geography, familial aggregation, and genome-wide association studies.[5] In the general population the risk is about 0.1%, while in first-degree relatives this risk is about 3% and in second or third-degree relatives is 1%.[6] The largest effect of the genetic contribution to developing MS is located in the human leukocyte antigen class II locus.[7] One third of the identified genetic loci were associated with at least one other autoimmune disease, thus underlying the indication that different autoimmune disorders probably share similar genetic features.

Environmental factors emerge from different studies, and the strongest associations with MS are infections, smoking, latitude, and vitamin D levels.[8] An involvement of Epstein Barr virus (EBV) infection is still debated. EBV affects about the 94% of general population, so it is difficult to identify a causal role within MS. It has been shown that people with high titers of anti-EBV antibodies have a greater risk than people with lower titers, but the reason is unknown.

4.1.2 Clinical Features

A significant number of people diagnosed with MS report earlier symptoms that could be attributed to a first demyelinating event. First symptoms at onset are extremely variable and include sensory disturbances, unilateral optic neuritis, diplopia, Lhermitte's sign, limb weakness, gait ataxia, neurogenic bladder and bowel symptoms, fatigue, and an increase in body temperature, depression, emotional liability, pain, sexual dysfunction, cognitive impairment, and other manifestation of CNS dysfunction.[9]

4.1.3 Disease Forms

In 2013 MS phenotypes were redefined to take into account clinical, imaging, and biomarker advances. According to this revision MS is divided into four clinical subtypes: clinically isolated syndrome (CIS), relapsing–remitting MS (RR-MS), secondary progressive MS (SP-MS), and primary progressive MS (PP-MS):

- CIS is the first clinical presentation of MS, suggestive of an inflammatory demyelination. This syndrome is isolated in time and generally the lesions of the white matter in magnetic resonance imaging (MRI) appear to be monofocal.[10]

- Relapsing–remitting MS: about 85% of people have RR-MS. It is characterized by recurrent acute relapse episodes followed by partial or total recovery. Between relapses the patient is in a relatively quiet neurological condition.
- Primary progressive MS: accounts for 10% of cases. Patients with PP-MS do not experience attacks but a progressive and steady decline of neurological functions from the onset.
- Secondary progressive MS: represents the clinical evolution of RR-MS. Transition between the two forms is gradual and patients experience a steady decline unassociated with relapses.
- Benign and malign MS: they are not MS phenotype descriptors per se, because they can apply to any MS phenotype. Benign refers to a disease course in which patient has minimal or no disability at least 15 years after disease onset. Malign refers to disease with a fast progressive course leading to strong disability or death in a short time after disease onset.

4.1.4 Pathology and Neuroradiology

MS is considered the prototype immune-mediated demyelinating disease of the CNS. The immune system, in fact, starts to see CNS myelin components as foreign and destroys myelin sheets, thus contributing to disease pathogenesis. The therapeutic efficacy of immunosuppressive drugs and of monoclonal antibodies interfering with leukocyte migration from the blood-stream to the brain is the strongest evidence that MS is primarily immune-mediated. Exacerbation of the disease after administration of altered myelin antigens, on the other hand, clearly suggests MS to be autoimmune.[11] This concept is confirmed by the fact that an active immunization of mice with myelin peptide gives rise to an experimental animal model called Experimental Autoimmune Encephalomyelitis (EAE), which resembles, in some aspects, human MS.[12]

The pathological hallmark of MS is the presence of focal demyelinating plaques with partial axonal preservation and reactive glial scar formation in the white and gray matter of the CNS. Lesions have a predilection for periventricular and subcortical white matter, optic nerves, cerebellar white matter, pons, medulla, and spinal cord.[13]

In addition to MS plaques, there is also diffuse damage in the normal appearing white and gray matter and global brain atrophy along with disease progression.[14]

Advances in imaging and neuropathology are clarifying that neurodegeneration starts at MS onset and the conversion of RR-MS to SP-MS is due, likely, to a strong neuronal injury that exceeds the capacity of compensatory mechanisms. Many hypotheses underlie the axonal degeneration during MS, and inflammation seems to have a key role. Immune cells secrete neurotoxic products, including reactive oxygen species (ROS), glutamate, cytokines, and chemokines that alter neuronal metabolism and functions. Inflammation products are important for tissue defense, but in the long-term, the inflammatory response is not self-limiting and triggers neuronal stress response. Among the most common cascades triggered by inflammation and involved in neuronal loss we can find oxidative stress (OS), mitochondrial dysfunction, energy deficit, and ion channel dysfunction.[15]

MRI is the most helpful examination in the diagnosis of MS, because of its ability to reveal symptomatic and asymptomatic plaques. Typical MRI findings include white matter hyperintense lesions on T2/FLAIR sequences which are ovoid-shaped and preferentially located in the periventricular zone, corpus callous, juxtacortical areas, and brainstem.[16]

At the initial phase of the disease lesions are typically thin and appear to be linear. Perivascular infiltrations of lymphocytes and macrophages seem to have an active role in the blood brain barrier (BBB) and myelin disruption, but also in the genesis of new lesions. MRI, thanks to its sensitivity, is able to detect the acute lesions disrupting the BBB, leading to gadolinium enhancement, considered the first detectable events in conventional MRI, but is also able to image the small lesions of the gray matter.[17]

In addition to imaging, clinical evaluation and evoked potential studies and colony-stimulating factor (CSF) analysis provides additional information in the diagnosis of MS, such as the level of immunoglobulin index and oligoclonal bands occurrence.

4.1.5 Immunopathogenesis

MS is considered a classical T cell-mediated autoimmune disease, but its immunopathogenesis is still unclear in many aspects. Most of our knowledge about the involvement of the immune system in MS comes from its experimental model EAE. The role of an autoimmune response in this model was demonstrated by adoptive transfer of immune cells from a diseased animal to a healthy one. Transferred T cells were able to transmit the disease. A series of myelin proteins were identified as potential disease-causing antigens and T cells were considered the main disease transmitters.[18] Despite thymic negative selection, our mature T cells repertoire physiologically contains autoreactive T cells, which can recognize antigens like myelin basic protein, proteolipid protein, and myelin oligodendrocyte glycoprotein. Two mechanisms have been hypothesized to explain autoimmunity in MS: molecular mimicry and bystander activation.[19] In the initial phase of the inflammatory process encephalitogenic T cells activate in the periphery and migrate to the CNS. After their entry, T cells start to secrete pro-inflammatory cytokines, like interferon-γ (IFN-γ) and osteopontin, which activate microglia. Activated microglia/macrophages secrete chemokines and contribute to the recruitment of T cells and antigen presenting cells (APCs). APCs expose myelin antigens on MHC II, thus activating infiltrating lymphocytes. The inflammatory environment supported by microglia secretion of ROS, pro-inflammatory cytokines mainly IL-17[20] and proteolytic enzymes amplifies T cells activation.[21] Different subsets of T cells have a role in the immunopathogenesis of MS. Several authors have reported regulatory T cells deficiency in human autoimmune diseases, including MS.[22,23] Despite the fact that EAE-driven data have induced researchers to consider MS a CD4+ T cell-mediated disease, the frequency of CD8+ cell is greater than CD4+ in the active plaques.

4.1.6 Mechanism Underlying MS Progressive Forms

Many efforts have been made in the last century in understanding disease mechanisms of the relapsing—remitting phase of MS. A series of anti-inflammatory and immunomodulatory drugs have been developed to reduce the severity and frequency of relapses. Despite this, once patients enter the progressive phase of MS, therapeutic treatments are only symptomatic and ineffective in stopping disease progression. It is necessary to investigate the progressive nature of MS and other neurodegenerative disorders and thus search for novel causative mechanisms and future therapeutic targets. Unfortunately animal models of MS cannot reproduce the progressive phase of the disease, thus limiting our understanding of the pathogenesis. Several hypothetical mechanisms have been proposed to explain the progressive phase of MS. The first states that brain damage is triggered by an inflammatory process differing from those of the RR-MS. The second hypothesis states that

MS is a "two stage" disease in which the first part is characterized by autoimmunity and consequent inflammation, while the second part is characterized by progressive neurodegeneration. A third hypothesis postulates that MS is a neurodegenerative disorder in which inflammation has a secondary role in the progression of the disease. These three hypothetical mechanisms are not necessarily mutually exclusive, but may be intertwined in a complex manner.

We have earlier described how RR-MS differs from PP-MS and SP-MS in the clinical course, but we do not know how RR-MS patients convert to the progressive forms. It appears that patients have to reach a threshold of irreversible neurological symptoms exceeding the capacity of compensatory mechanisms to repair the brain damage. Many speculate that prolonged chronic inflammation in the CNS triggers this conversion, which generally occurs in a well-defined age window of 35–50 years. Beyond inflammation, neurodegeneration is a key feature of MS, especially for the progressive form. Chronic neurodegenerative changes accumulate over time in focal lesions of MS, but the relationship between MS and brain atrophy has never been found. Among the great number of attempts made to explain progressive MS pathogenesis, four of them seem to be the most credible:

- *Microglia activation*: In all MS forms active tissue injury is associated with microglial activation, which can contribute to neurodegenerative mechanism. Activated microglia can secrete proteases, pro-inflammatory cytokines and nitric oxide (NO), thus leading to oligodendrocytes and myelin damage followed by axonal injury. The OS induced by microglia, through the production of ROS, can also cause reversible conduction block in axons. It is important to notice that microglia also has a beneficial role, providing the first line of defense in our CNS.[24]
- *Iron accumulation*: It is physiologically normal in the aged human brain, but also occurs in MS. Iron can amplify ROS-mediated injury by generating toxic reactants. Further, Fe^{2+} is taken up by microglia after the degeneration of oligodendrocytes, which are the main storage of iron in the CNS. After the uptake of iron, microglia degenerate thus leading to its accumulation in the extracellular space and in neurons.
- *Mitochondrial injury*: The similarities in terms of demyelination and axonal injury between MS and stroke have suggested also that in

MS energy deficiency and hypoxia could have a pathogenetic role. Mitochondrial dysfunction was assessed in MS thanks to the impairment of NADH deydrogenase activity and to the increase of complex IV activity.[24] An excessive ROS production in CNS could lead to mitochondrial DNA mutations, which can compromise oxidative phosphorylation and other important mitochondrial functions. Mitochondria are also an important defense mechanism against the OS.[25]

- *Ion channel dysfunction:* The energy imbalance and demyelination occurring during MS lead to a dysfunction and misdistribution of several ion channels, thus triggering a common result, Ca^{2+} overload. Calcium levels are extremely regulated in physiological conditions, because this ion has strong neurotoxic properties. Aberrant expression of Na^+ channels, glutamate receptors, and voltage-gated Ca^{2+} channels have been observed in demyelinated axons in MS and other demyelinating disorders.[24,25]

4.1.7 Current Therapy of MS

Since the first disease modifying drugs (DMDs) were registered for MS in the early 1990s any medication aimed at modulating MS has been endowed with anti-inflammatory properties. Most of them interfere with the immune system by T cell depletion (Alemtuzumab, Teriflunomide), CNS lymphocytes migration (Natalizumab), or recirculation (FTY) blocking, and leukocyte ablation (total body irradiation). Other drugs reeducate immune cells [glatiramer acetate (GA), stem cells], halt inflammatory pathways [interferon-β (IFN-β), dymethilfumarate, Laquinimod], and deplete specifically B cells (Rituximab, Ocrelizumab) or activated T cells (Daclizumab).

This huge body of data brought drugs to the market, in the 1990s, that were able to slow the progression of disease and reduce clinical and MRI activity. In the last 8−10 years, new drugs have shifted the therapeutic ambition in such a way that instead of slowing the disease we now expect to give MS patients a life with no evidence of disease activity (NEDA).

On the one hand, "old" drugs (IFN-β, GA) are reliable and long lasting/extensive postmarketing studies demonstrate a good safety profile, although none have a perfectly understood mechanism of action. On the other hand, "new" drugs, resulting from specific chemical-biological design, are clear in terms of the main mechanism of action (off target effects are always a possibility) but uncertain in terms of safety. The choice of the right drug to start with or to switch to, as well as the timing and the duration of the treatment can only be the result of the balance between the known risks, side effects, and the potential benefits for that individual patient, and constitutes one of the best examples of personalized medicine.

4.1.8 Current Therapies: Mechanism of Action, Efficacy, and Safety Concerns

4.1.8.1 Interferon-β

IFN-β 1b was the first disease DMD approved for MS (July 1993).[26] There are three subcutaneous and one intramuscular registered preparations. The main focus of IFN-β is the modulation of the immune system. IFN-β decreases expression of matrix-metalloproteases, reverses BBB disruption, decreases pro-inflammatory cytokines production, and modulates B and T cells activity. Clinical trials leading to IFN-β registration have shown a 30% reduction in the annual relapse rate and in MRI disease activity in patients affected by RR-MS.[27] The safety profile of IFN-β is quite fair. Flu-like syndrome, injection site reactions, mild leukocyte and liver abnormalities are the most common side effects. An important drawback of IFN-β treatment is the development of neutralizing antibodies (NAb) in up to 44% of treated patients. Recently, a pegilated form of IFN-β, allowing administration every 15 days and apparently decreasing Nabs formation, has been registered, but postmarketing experience confirming possible advantages is missing.

4.1.8.2 Glatiramer Acetate

GA was registered for MS in 1997. GA is a mixture of synthetic peptides possibly working as an altered peptide ligand for MHC class II molecules, stimulating a regulatory circuit instead of activating autoreactive T cells. Daily subcutaneous injections of GA reduce the annual relapse rate by 30%, and prevent inflammatory lesions on MRI. Erythema and skin induration at injection site are reported. GA can occasionally give rise to a systemic reaction characterized by dyspnea, palpitations, anxiety, and chest pressure.[28]

4.1.8.3 Natalizumab

The watershed line of MS treatment was drawn in 2003 with the registration of Natalizumab. Natalizumab is a humanized monoclonal antibody recognizing alpha 4 integrin on leukocytes. It blocks interaction with cognate ligand on vascular endothelium cells preventing leukocytes migration into the CNS. Natalizumab was shown to reduce the annual relapse rate by 68% and active MRI lesions by 92%, compared to placebo.

The early safety profile of this drug was favorable: anxiety, fatigue, pharyngitis were common side effects. The key safety concern of Natalizumab is the increased risk of developing progressive multifocal leukoencephalopathy (PML), a serious opportunistic infection of oligodendrocytes caused by reactivation of latent John Cunningham polyomavirus, potentially leading to neurological deficits, and often lethal.[29]

4.1.8.4 Fingolimod
Approved in 2009 by the FDA as the first oral treatment for MS, Fingolimod is a sphingosin-1 phosphate receptor modulator. Its main mechanism of action relies on blocking the egression of activated T cells from lymphoid tissues. Fingolimod reduces MRI and clinical activity (reduction of 82% of new active MRI lesions, and annual relapse rate decrease of 54%, respectively). Fingolimod raises safety concerns. Possible side effects encompass "first-dose" bradycardia, Herpes virus dissemination, macular edema, increased blood pressure, and liver abnormalities. Uncommon but recently reported is also PML appearance during Fingolimod treatment.[30]

4.1.8.5 Teriflunomide
Teriflunomide is a specific inhibitor of mitochondrial dihydroorotate dehydrogenase, blocking the replication of rapidly dividing cells. Sparing the salvage pathway of pyrimidine synthesis, it specifically acts on activated T and B cells. It reduces annual relapse rate (37%) and MRI activity (gadolinium positive lesions reduction of 80%).

Hair thinning, hepatic enzyme increase, back pain, and gastrointestinal symptoms are the most common side effects. The main drawback of this drug is its potential teratogenicity and its prolonged half-life.[31]

4.1.8.6 Dimethyl Fumarate
Dimethyl fumarate is the last oral treatment for MS, registered by the FDA 2 years ago with the trade name BG12. BG12 contains only dimethyl ester fumarate in coated microtablets, and is supposed to display reduced gastrointestinal symptoms. BG12 modulates T lymphocyte phenotype, inducing a Th2 profile, and reduces T cell migration through

the BBB by downregulation of adhesion molecules. As well as this anti-inflammatory effect, BG12 induces transcription of nuclear factor-erythroid-2-related factor (Nrf-2). Through the effect on Nrf-2, BG12 fosters antioxidative pathways, first of all increasing glutathione, the most important cellular antioxidant. The treatment effect of BG12 reduced the annual relapse rate by 53%. MRI activity was reduced by 90%. The safety profile is very good: abdominal pain, diarrhea, nausea, and flushing are the most common side effects and only occasionally do they lead to drug drop-out. Nevertheless, one PML case was also reported.[32]

4.1.8.7 Alemtuzumab
Alemtuzumab is a humanized leukocyte-depleting monoclonal antibody approved in 2013 by the FDA only for refractory MS. It binds CD52 leading to the depletion of both lymphocytes and monocytes. Alemtuzumab showed a reduction of 55% in the annual relapse rate. New Gadolinium enhancing lesions and T2 enlarging lesions in MRI were statistically lower in the Alemtuzumab group compared to IFN-β 1a. Moreover, brain atrophy progressed more slowly in the Alemtuzumab group.

Serious infections reactions occurred only in 3% of patients; common but not serious were upper respiratory and urinary infections as well as herpetic infections. Safety concerns have risen regarding the development of severe autoimmune diseases.[33]

4.1.8.8 Cyclophosphamide and Mitoxantrone
Cyclophosphamide and mitoxantrone and other immunosuppressant drugs like azathioprine (AZA), have been commonly used for refractory MS over the last 20 years. Since the introduction of drugs of proven efficacy in severe MS cases, their regular use has been relatively limited, with the exception of induction strategies. Despite their indubitable efficacy, the high-risk profile (malignancies and infections above all) makes the risk-benefit ratio unfavorable.[34]

4.1.9 Treatment Strategies
The continuously growing range of drugs to choose from for MS treatment, the lack of uniformly accepted algorithms to follow, and the absence of reliable and handy biomarkers of treatment efficacy (MRI is a reliable biomarker but cannot be performed weekly), makes the choice of the correct therapeutic strategy extremely difficult. In this uncertain scenario, however, a few concepts have been clearly demonstrated (Fig. 4.1).

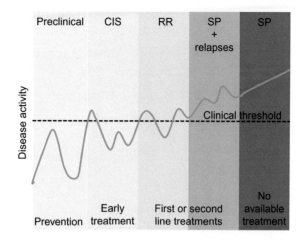

*Figure 4.1 **Treatment opportunities during MS course.** Disease may start several years before becoming clinically evident and being diagnosed. In the preclinical phase prevention (ie, vitamin D administration or nonspecific prevention for autoimmune diseases) is conceivable. After the first clinical episode (CIS) in the presence of negative prognostic markers, early treatment with DMD is highly recommended. Immunomodulatory or, if needed, immunosuppressive treatment is used as long as there is evidence of inflammatory activity, namely during the RR phase, or during the SP phase if it still displays relapses. At the moment, no treatments are available for the purely progressive phases of the disease.*

4.1.9.1 Early Treatment

Histopathological data, and functional and structural MRI imaging, unequivocally show that neurodegeneration is not exclusively related to the later steps of disease or some peculiar disease courses but is already present in the first phases of MS. Axonal degeneration and oligodendrocyte loss have been shown in early lesions. Unblinded extension phases of original randomized placebo-controlled trials, run in order to assess efficacy of first DMDs registration,[35–37] clearly show a slower disease progression in patients treated earlier and continuously compared to those starting active drugs later during the disease course.

4.1.9.2 Escalation Therapy

For a first-diagnosed MS patient, or for CIS patients with evidence of temporal dissemination but without negative prognostic factors, an escalation therapy may be an ideal strategy. First line drugs such as IFN-β or GA may be started early on, shifting to second line treatments whenever a clinical or significant MRI activity is detected (Fig. 4.2). Unfortunately, shifting to second line drugs is not always enough to regain control on disease in overactive patients.

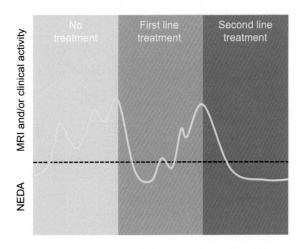

*Figure 4.2 **Ideal escalation therapy**. After a CIS or clinically defined MS diagnosis without negative prognostic markers is made, a first line treatment is started. Usually clinical and MRI evidence of disease activity disappear rapidly (NEDA). Minimal evidence of disease activity might not be sufficient to shift to second line treatments, but if consistent clinical or MRI disease activity is documented under first line treatment, a second line treatment is immediately started. Most MS patients respond to second line treatments, at least initially, going back to NEDA.*

4.1.9.3 Induction Therapy

Some patients display negative prognostic markers (active clinical relapses, MRI lesions in strategic brain areas, age, gender, multisymptomatic onset) that make it mandatory to start with a more aggressive approach. For these patients an early and complete shut off of the immune reaction in the CNS is highly desirable. This outcome is (partially) achievable with immunosuppressants such as mitoxantrone and cyclophosphamide but also with several recent drugs such as Fingolimod, Natalizumab, Rituximab (RX), and Alemtuzumab. After an induction period of variable length, usually a first generation DMD is used for maintenance (Fig. 4.3). This aggressive approach implies important drawbacks, including exposure of patients to the severe side effects of immunesuppressants, and the difficult management of nonresponders.

4.1.9.4 Other Neurodegenerative Diseases

Despite the peculiarities of each neurodegenerative disease, disorders like MS, neuromyelitis optica (NMO), Parkinson's disease (PD), Alzheimer's disease (AD), and amyotrophic lateral sclerosis (ALS) share some common pathogenic features, such as inflammation, genetic predisposition, protein aggregations, OS, and mitochondrial dysfunction. One of the possible common pathways to neurodegeneration involves

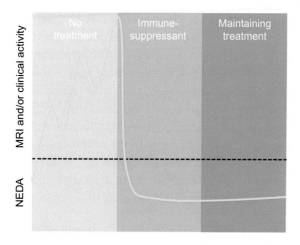

*Figure 4.3 **Ideal induction therapy**. After a CIS or clinically defined MS diagnosis with very negative prognostic markers is made, the patient undergoes immune-suppressive treatment. After a limited time of heavy immune-suppression, usually yielding NEDA, patients are shifted back to a first line treatment able to control residual disease activity for maintenance.*

caspase-1. This caspase has been found to mediate cell death in several neurologic diseases. Any kind of stress, like ROS, Ca^{2+}, or iron accumulation, can lead to an enhancement of mitochondria permeability and a decline in mitochondrial membrane potential. Changes in membrane potentials trigger the release of apoptotic factors, like caspases, and eventually to cellular death. Much experimental evidence suggests that caspase-1 is an early initiator of neuronal death. In neurodegenerative diseases there is no single causative dysfunction, thus characterizing every factor involved in the pathogenesis is not easy.

Until recently, NMO was thought to be a clinical variant of MS. However, clinical features, neuroimaging, immunological, and histopathological characteristics have now been identified which distinguish NMO from MS;[38] for these reasons we have dedicated a "specific space" to NMO in this chapter.

NMO is an autoimmune disorder of the CNS in which the immune system classically attacks the myelin of neurons located at the optic nerves and spinal cord, thus producing a simultaneous or sequential extensive inflammation of the optic nerve and spinal cord.[39]

Clifford and Gault reviewed the relevant features of the disease in 1894, though descriptions of the disease appeared much earlier. The typically long spinal cord segmental involvement, longitudinally extensive transverse myelitis, and neutrophilic pleocytosis in CSF became incorporated into the first Wingerchuk diagnostic criteria for NMO in 1999.[40] Subsequently, the discovery of a serum immunoglobulin (Ig) G autoantibody specific for the AQP4 water channel led to the revised Wingerchuk criteria in 2006[41] unifying a spectrum of NMO-related disorders and distinguished them from MS. The new nomenclature defines the unifying term NMO spectrum disorders (NMOSD), which is stratified further by serologic testing (NMOSD with or without AQP4-IgG). The core clinical characteristics required for patients with NMOSD with AQP4-IgG include clinical syndromes or MRI findings related to optic nerve, spinal cord, area postrema, other brainstem, diencephalic, or cerebral presentations.[42]

Population-based studies from Europe, South East and Southern Asia, the Caribbean, and Cuba suggest that the incidence and prevalence of NMO ranges from 0.05 to 0.4 and 0.52 to 4.4 per 100,000, respectively. Mean age at onset (32.6−45.7) and median time to first relapse (8−12 months) is similar. Most studies reported an excessive disease rate in women and a relapsing course, particularly in anti-AQP4-IgG-positive patients.[43]

4.1.9.5 Pathogenesis of NMO
NMO attacks are not mediated by T cells but rather by B cells. Clinical and laboratory-based studies support a prominent role for B cells in NMO pathogenesis.[44] NMO is recognized as a distinct disease notable for the presence of serum anti-AQP4-IgG.[38] These autoantibodies are predominantly IgG_1, and considerable evidence supports their pathogenicity,[45] presumably by binding to AQP4 on CNS astrocytes, resulting in astrocyte injury and inflammation.

NMO-IgG/anti-AQP4 antibodies (Abs) may compromise the integrity of the BBB and allow NMO-IgG to reach the CNS, bind AQP4, and induce their pathogenic effector functions. Anti-AQP4 Abs induce the internalization of AQP4 and Excitatory Amino Acid Transporter 2astrocyte proteins resulting in excitotoxicity and increasing BBB permeability.[46] Anti-AQP4 Abs can result in astrocyte injury by antibody dependent cellular cytotoxicity and complement dependent cytotoxicity. Chemotactic factors, such as anaphylatoxins C3a and C5a, are released after complement activation and induce the recruitment and activation of inflammatory cells.[47] All these mechanisms further contribute to BBB disruption enhancing Abs and cell entry to the CNS and propagating NMO lesion formation.

In addition to the production of AQP4-IgG in the bone marrow and CNS, plasma cells and plasmablasts may have additional pro-inflammatory and anti-inflammatory functions. Plasmablasts may secrete factors such as IL-17, tumor necrosis factor alpha (TNF-α)/NO, and granulocyte-macrophage CSF, facilitating neutrophil and macrophage CNS infiltration and heightening pro-inflammatory immune cell activity.

Alternatively, anti-inflammatory plasma cells may suppress disease activity in part through the production of IL-10 or IL-35.[48] Memory B cells may further promote disease activity by antigen presentation, secretion of the pro-inflammatory cytokines lymphotoxin and TNFα, or facilitation of Th17 differentiation.[49] IL-10-producing B regulatory cells may limit the immune response through antigen-specific or bystander suppression of pro-inflammatory T cell function. Circulating AQP4-specific anergic B cells may provide a pool of autoreactive disease-relevant B cells that contribute to disease activity. These cells may be enhanced by deficient B cell tolerance; the release of anergic B cells may be enhanced by antigen-complement adducts or decreased levels of IL-6.[44]

Furthermore, the immune release of ROS has been involved in demyelination and axonal damage; while the weak cellular antioxidant defense systems in the CNS and its vulnerability to ROS may increase damage.[50]

We have demonstrated that malondialdehyde, peroxidation potential, advanced oxidation protein products, superoxide dismutase, and catalase (CAT) enzymes were upregulated in NMO patients, suggesting the activation of a detoxification feedback mechanism to abolish the excess of superoxide radicals as a result of the CNS inflammatory process.[51]

4.1.9.6 Therapies
The main treatment goals are: remission and improvement of relapse-associated symptoms; long-term stabilization of disease course by means of relapse prevention; and symptomatic therapy of residual symptoms.[52]

4.1.10 Treatment of Acute Disease Attacks
After standard neurological examination and the exclusion of infection, steroids are applied on five consecutive days.[53] If the patient's condition does not improve sufficiently or the neurological symptoms worsen, therapeutic plasma exchange (TPE) can be performed. Early initiation of TPE might be associated with better clinical outcome.[54]

4.1.11 Long-Term Treatment of NMO

Long-term immunosuppressive treatment should be initiated once the diagnosis of NMO has been confirmed.

Azathioprine: Several studies, including a large retrospective review of 99 patients with NMO/NMOSD, have shown AZA to reduce relapse rate and ameliorate neurological disability in NMO.[55]

Rituximab: B cell depletion with RX has been demonstrated as effective in the treatment of NMO in several clinical case series and retrospective analyses.[56]

Mycophenolate mofetil (MMF): In a retrospective analysis of 24 patients, treatment with MMF was associated with a reduction in relapse frequency and stable or reduced disability in patients with NMOSD.[57]

Immunoglobulins (IVIg): Individual case reports and a 2012 case series have shown that high-dose IVIg are potentially beneficial.[58]

Case reports with *Mitoxantrone, Cyclophosphamide, IFN-β/GA, Methotrexate, Natalizumab, Fingolimod* have been reported.

Other new therapies: Studies have shown a favorable effect of the IL-6 receptor-blocking antibody *tocilizumab* in NMO patients who have failed to respond to other therapies.[59] The monoclonal antibody *eculizumab*, which is directed against the complement component 5, showed considerable efficacy in a small, open-label study of 14 NMO/NMOSD patients with disease activity.[60]

4.1.12 Future Therapies for MS and Neurodegenerative Diseases

At the time of this review, the website www.Clinicaltrials.gov lists more than 1255 studies investigating drugs for MS. Several of these drugs are in the infancy of their development, others, such as Autologous Mesenchimal Stem Cell Transplantation, Rituximab, Laquinimod, Daclizumab, Ocrelizumab, and Ofatumumab, are already in advanced clinical testing. Only 174 of them are tested also for progressive MS courses, reflecting the lack of reliable therapeutic targets for neurodegeneration. If in the early stages of disease, neurodegeneration is unequivocally inflammation driven, later on different mechanisms may be instrumental. Mitochondrial failure, glutamate excitotoxicity, OS, and activation of injurious Na and Ca are major actors.

As for other neurodegenerative diseases, such asPD, AD, ALS, and fronto-temporal lobe degeneration, the desired treatment outcome should be the arrest of the detrimental mechanisms involved or triggering the pathogenic cascade. Among drugs already registered for MS or other diseases and now tested in primary and SP-MS are Laquinimod, BG12, Rituximab, Lithium, Domperidone, Hydroxyurea, Lamotrigine.

For future therapeutic perspectives it will be useful to identify more common mechanisms underlying neurodegenerative disorders, in order to develop new therapeutic agents.[61] Interestingly, therapeutics targeting inflammation or mitochondria dysfunction are beneficial in animal models of different neurodegenerative disorders. Another interesting alternative is to target both inflammation and neurodegeneration by combination therapies.

4.1.13 Conclusions

For several decades any inflammatory response disclosed in neurodegenerative diseases, such as progressive MS, AD, PD, ALS, and adrenoleukodystrophy, has been indiscriminately considered deleterious for the CNS.[62,63] Together with traditional immune cells (T and B cells), microglia releasing inflammatory cytokine and chemokines, neurotoxic and excitotoxic factors (ie, oxygen free radicals, NO, glutamate) have been considered guilty in sustaining a vicious inflammatory circuit. Epidemiological studies show a reduced risk of developing AD or PD later in life for people using an unspecific anti-inflammatory treatment.[64] On the other hand, the failure of anti-inflammatory drugs in arresting neurodegenerative diseases[65] mirrors paradoxical results achieved in MS by using drugs previously showing benefits in EAE or other human autoimmune disease. Lessons coming from TNF blockade (TNF neutralizing antibodies and TNF-receptor−IgG fusion protein) or IL12 and IL23 antagonists (Ustekinumab) or using Atacicept, a fusion protein that inhibits B cell activity, suggest that the role of inflammation in neurodegenerative diseases, such as MS, is still an unsolved conundrum.[66−68] Studies showing the protective role of the immune system in the CNS were pioneered by the group of Michal Schwartz, who reported that boosting CNS-specific autoimmune responses can promote recovery and protect against pathological features ofAD.[69] Thus, considering the induction strategy in very active MS, classical and biological immune-suppressants still might have an important role in future treatments. In classical neurodegenerative diseases, however, such as progressive MS, NMO, AD, PD, and ALS, the use of immune-suppressants does not appear to be justified, at least until the role, protective or detrimental, of inflammation has been elucidated in these diseases. In this uncertain scenario, only a perfectly timed and controlled immunomodulation may help in regaining tissue homeostasis for MS as well as for other neurodegenerative diseases.

REFERENCES

1. Msif. Atlas of MS 2013: Mapping multiple sclerosis around the world; 2013. <www.msif. org/about-us/advocacy/atlas>.

2. Melcon MO, Correale J, Melcon CM. Is it time for a new global classification of multiple sclerosis? *J Neurol Sci* 2014;**344**(1−2):171−81. Available from: http://dx.doi.org/10.1016/j.jns.2014.06.051.

3. Mitchell AJ, Benito-León J, González JM, Rivera-Navarro J. Quality of life and its assessment in multiple sclerosis: integrating physical and psychological components of wellbeing. *Lancet Neurol* 2005;**4**(9):556−66. Available from: http://dx.doi.org/10.1016/S1474-4422(05)70166-6.

4. Miltenburger C, Kobelt G. Quality of life and cost of multiple sclerosis. *Clin Neurol Neurosurg* 2002;**104**(3):272−5. Available from: http://dx.doi.org/10.1016/S0303-8467(02)00051-3.

5. Sawcer S, Franklin RJM, Ban M. Multiple sclerosis genetics. *Lancet Neurol* 2014;**13**(7): 700−9.

6. Compston A, Coles A. Multiple sclerosis. *The Lancet* 2008;**372**(9648):1502−17. Available from: http://dx.doi.org/10.1016/S0140-6736(08)61620-7.

7. Gourraud P-A, Harbo HF, Hauser SL, Baranzini SE. The genetics of multiple sclerosis: an up-to-date review. *Immunol Rev* 2012;**248**(1):87−103. Available from: http://dx.doi.org/10.1111/j.1600-065X.2012.01134.

8. Ramagopalan SV, Dobson R, Meier UC, Giovannoni G. Multiple sclerosis: risk factors, pro-dromes, and potential causal pathways. *Lancet Neurol* 2010;**9**(7):727−39. Available from: http://dx.doi.org/1016/S1474-4422(10)70094-6.

9. Noseworthy JH, Lucchinetti C, Rodriguez M, Weinshenker BG. Multiple sclerosis. *N Engl J Med* 2000;**343**:938−52. Available from: http://dx.doi.org/10.1056/NEJM200009283431307.

10. Lublin FD, Reingold SC, Cohen JA, Cutter GR, Sørensen PS, Thompson AJ, et al. Defining the clinical course of multiple sclerosis. The 2013 revisions. *Neurology* 2014;**83**(3):278−86. Available from: http://dx.doi.org/10.1212/WNL.0000000000000560.

11. Legroux L, Arbour N. Multiple sclerosis and T lymphocytes: an entangled story. *J Neuroimm Pharmacol* 2015. Available from: http://dx.doi.org/10.1007/s11481-015-9614-0.

12. Trapp BD, Nave K-A. Multiple sclerosis: an immune or neurodegenerative disorder? *Ann Rev Neurosci* 2008;**31**:247−69. Available from: http://dx.doi.org/10.1146/annurev.neuro. 30.051606.094313.

13. Kutzelnigg A, Lassmann H. *Pathology of multiple sclerosis and related inflammatory demye-linating diseases.* 1st ed. *Handbook of clinical neurology*, vol. 122. Elsevier B.V; 2014. Available from: http://dx.doi.org/10.1016/B978-0-444-52001-2.00002-9.

14. Frohman EM, Racke MK, Raine CS. Multiple sclerosis. The plaque and its pathogenesis. *N Engl J Med* 2006;**354**(9):942−55. Available from: http://dx.doi.org/10.1056/NEJMra052130.

15. Friese M, Schattling B, Fugger L. Mechanisms of neurodegeneration and axonal dysfunction in multiple sclerosis. *Nat Rev Neurol* 2014;**10**(4):225−38. Available from: http://dx.doi.org/10.1038/nrneurol.2014.37.

16. Deangelis TM, Miller A. *Diagnosis of multiple sclerosis*. 1st ed. *Handbook of clinical neurology*, vol. 122. Elsevier B.V; 2014. Available from: http://dx.doi.org/10.1016/B978-0-444-52001-2.00013-3.

17. Ge Y. Multiple sclerosis: the role of MR imaging. *Am J Neurorad* 2006;**27**:1165–76. <www.ajnr.org/content/27/6/1165.full>.

18. Hemmer B, Archelos JJ, Hartung H-P. New concepts in the immunopathogenesis of multiple sclerosis. *Nat Rev Neurosci* 2002;**3**(4):291–301. Available from: http://dx.doi.org/10.1038/nrn784.

19. Sospedra M, Martin R. Molecular mimicry in multiple sclerosis. *Autoimmunity* 2006;**39**(1):3–8. Available from: http://dx.doi.org/10.1080/08916930500484922.

20. Hofstetter HH, Gold R, Hartung H-P. Th17 cells in MS and experimental autoimmune encephalomyelitis. *Int MS J* 2009;**16**:12–18 PMID:19413921.

21. Sospedra M, Martin R. Immunology of multiple sclerosis. *Ann Rev Immunol* 2005;**23**(1):683–747. Available from: http://dx.doi.org/10.1146/annurev.immunol.23.021704.115707.

22. Haas J, Hug A, Viehöver A, Fritzsching B, Falk CS, Filser A, et al. Reduced suppressive effect of CD4 + CD25 high regulatory T cells on the T cell immune response against myelin oligodendrocyte glycoprotein in patients with multiple sclerosis. *Eur J Immunol* 2005;**35**(11):3343–52. pubmed/16206232.

23. Costantino CM, Baecher-Allan C, Hafler DA. Multiple sclerosis and regulatory T cells. *J Clin Immunol* 2008;**28**(6):697–706. Available from: http://dx.doi.org/10.1007/s10875-008-9236-x.

24. Lassmann H, van Horssen J, Mahad D. Progressive multiple sclerosis: pathology and pathogenesis. *Nat Rev Neurol* 2012;**8**(11):647–56. Available from: http://dx.doi.org/10.1038/nrneurol.2012.168.

25. Friese MA, Schattling B, Fugger L. Mechanisms of neurodegeneration and axonal dysfunction in multiple sclerosis. *Nat Rev Neurol* 2014;**10**:225–38. Available from: http://dx.doi.org/10.1038/nrneurol.2014.37.

26. The IFNB Multiple Sclerosis Study Group. Interferon beta-1b is effective in relapsing-remitting multiple sclerosis. I. Clinical results of a multicenter, randomized, double-blind, placebo-controlled trial. *Neurology* 1993;**43**(4):655–61. pubmed/8469318.

27. Freedman MS. Efficacy and safety of subcutaneous interferon-β-1a in patients with a first demyelinating event and early multiple sclerosis. *Exp Op BiologTher* 2014;**14**(8):1207–14. Available from: http://dx.doi.org/10.1517/14712598.2014.924496.

28. Johnson KP, Brooks BR, Cohen JA, Ford CC, Goldstein J, Lisak RP, et al. Copolymer 1 reduces relapse rate and improves disability in relapsing-remitting multiple sclerosis: results of a phase III multicenter, double-blind placebo-controlled trial. The Copolymer 1 Multiple Sclerosis Study Group. *Neurology* 1995;**45**(7):1268–76. pubmed/7617181.

29. Plavina T, Subramanyam M, Bloomgren G, Richman S, Pace A, Lee S, et al. Anti-JC virus antibody levels in serum or plasma further define risk of natalizumab-associated progressive multifocal leukoencephalopathy. *Ann Neurol* 2014;**76**(6):802–12. Available from: http://dx.doi.org/10.1002/ana.24286.

30. Killestein J., Vennegoor A., van Golde A.E.L., Bourez RLJH, Wijlens M.L.B. et al. PML-IRIS during Fingolimod diagnosed after Natalizumab discontinuation. *Case reports in neurological medicine* 2014; 2014. Available from: http://dx.doi.org/10.1155/2014/307872.

31. Confavreux C, O'Connor P, Comi G, Freedman MS, Miller AE, Olsson TP, et al. Oral teriflunomide for patients with relapsing multiple sclerosis (TOWER): a randomised, double-blind, placebo-controlled, phase 3 trial. *Lancet Neurol* 2014;**13**(3):247–56. Available from: http://dx.doi.org/10.1016/S1474-4422(13)70308-9.

32. Van Kester MS, Bouwes Bavinck JN, Quint KD. PML in patients treated with dimethyl fumarate. *N Engl J Med* 2015;**373**(6):583–4. Available from: http://dx.doi.org/10.1056/NEJMc1506151#SA2.

33. Coles AJ, Compston DAS, Selmaj KW, Lake SL, Moran S, Margolin DH, et al. Alemtuzumab vs. interferon beta-1a in early multiple sclerosis. *N Engl J Med* 2008;**359** (17):1786–801. Available from: http://dx.doi.org/10.1056/NEJMoa0802670.

34. Cocco E, Marrosu MG. The current role of mitoxantrone in the treatment of multiple sclerosis. *Exp Rev Neurotherap* 2014;**14**(6):607–16. Available from: http://dx.doi.org/10.1586/14737175.2014.915742.

35. Beck RW, Chandler DL, Cole SR, Simon JH, Jacobs LD, Kinkel RP, et al. Interferon beta-1a for early multiple sclerosis: CHAMPS trial subgroup analyses. *Ann Neurol* 2002;**51** (4):481–90. pubmed/11921054.

36. Kappos L, Freedman MS, Polman CH, Edan G, Hartung H-P, Miller DH, et al. Effect of early versus delayed interferon beta-1b treatment on disability after a first clinical event suggestive of multiple sclerosis: a 3-year follow-up analysis of the BENEFIT study. *Lancet* 2007;**370**(9585):389–97. Available from: http://dx.doi.org/10.1016/S0140-6736(07)61194-5.

37. Stüve O, Cutter GR. Multiple sclerosis drugs: how much bang for the buck? *Lancet Neurol* 2015;**14**(5):460–1. Available from: http://dx.doi.org/10.1016/S1474-4422(15)00016-2.

38. Lennon VA, Wingerchuk DM, Kryzer TJ, Pittock SJ, Lucchinetti CF, Fujihara K, et al. A serum autoantibody marker of neuromyelitis optica: distinction from multiple sclerosis. *Lancet* 2004;**364**:2106–12. pubmed/15589308.

39. Habek M, Adamec I, Pavliša G, Brinar VV. Diagnostic approach of patients with longitudinally extensive transverse myelitis. *Acta Neurol Belg* 2012;**12**:39–43. Available from: http://dx.doi.org/10.1007/s13760-012-0006-4.

40. Wingerchuk DM, Hogancamp WF, O'Brien PC, Weinshenker BG. The clinical course of neuromyelitis optica (Devic'ssyndrome). *Neurology* 1999;**53**:1107–14. pubmed/10496275.

41. Wingerchuk DM, Lennon VA, Pittock SJ, Lucchinetti CF, Weinshenker BG. Revised diagnostic criteria for neuromyelitis optica. *Neurology* 2006;**66**:1485–9. pubmed/16717206.

42. Wingerchuk DM, Banwell B, Bennett JL, Cabre P, Carroll W, Chitnis T, et al. International consensus diagnostic criteria for neuromyelitis optica spectrum disorders. *Neurology* 2015;**85**:177–89. Available from: http://dx.doi.org/10.1212/WNL.0000000000001729.

43. Pandit L, Asgari N, Apiwattanakul M, Palace J, Paul F, Leite, et al. Demographic and clinical features of neuromyelitis optica: a review. *Mult Scler J* 2015;**21**(7):845–53. Available from: http://dx.doi.org/10.1177/1352458515572406.

44. Bennett JL, O'Connor KC, Bar-Or A, Zamvil SS, Hemmer B, Tedder TF, et al. B lymphocytes in neuromyelitis optica. *Neurol Neuroimmunol Neuroinflamm* 2015;**2**:e104. Available from: http://dx.doi.org/10.1212/NXI.0000000000000104.

45. Saikali P, Cayrol R, Vincent T. Anti-aquaporin-4 auto-antibodies orchestrate the pathogenesis in neuromyelitis optica. *Autoimmun Rev* 2009;**9**132–5. Available from: http://dx.doi.org/10.1016/j.autrev.2009.04.004.

46. Hinson SR, Roemer SF, Lucchinetti CF, Fryer JP, Kryzer TJ, Chamberlain JL, et al. Aquaporin-4-binding autoantibodies in patients with neuromyelitis optica impair glutamate transport by down-regulating EAAT2. *J Exp Med* 2008;**205**(11):2473–81. Available from: http://dx.doi.org/10.1084/jem.20081241.

47. Alberdi E, Sanchez-Gomez MV, Torre I, Domercq M, Pérez-Samartín A, Pérez-Cerdá F, et al. Activation of kainate receptors sensitizes oligodendrocytes to complement attack. *J Neurosci* 2006;**26**(12):3220–8. Available from: http://dx.doi.org/10.1523/JNEUROSCI.3780-05.2006.

48. Shen P, Roch T, Lampropoulou V, O'Connor RA, Stervbo U, Hilgenberg E, et al. IL-35-producing B cells are critical regulators of immunity during autoimmune and infectious diseases. *Nature.* 2014;**507**(7492):366–70. Available from: http://dx.doi.org/10.1038/nature12979.

49. Wang HH, Dai YQ, Qiu W, Lu ZQ, Peng FH, Wang YG, et al. Interleukin-17- secreting T cells in neuromyelitis optica and multiple sclerosis during relapse. *J Clin Neurosci* 2011;**18**:1313–17. Available from: http://dx.doi.org/10.1016/j.jocn.2011.01.031.

50. Gilgun-Sherki Y, Melamed E, Offen D. The role of oxidative stress in the pathogenesis of multiple sclerosis: the need for effective antioxidant therapy. *J Neurol* 2004;**251**(3):261–8. pubmed/15015004.

51. Penton-Rol G, Cervantes-Llanos M, Martínez-Sánchez G, Cabrera-Gómez JA, Valenzuela-Silva CM, Ramírez-Nuñez O, et al. TNF-α and IL-10 downregulation and marked oxidative stress in Neuromyelitis Optica. *J Inflamm* 2009;**6**:18 <http://www.journal-inflammation.com/content/6/1/18>.

52. Trebst C, Jarius S, Berthele A, Friedemann P, Schippling S, Wildemann B, et al. Update on the diagnosis and treatment of neuromyelitis optica: recommendations of the Neuromyelitis Optica Study Group (NEMOS). *J Neurol* 2014;**261**:1–16. Available from: http://dx.doi.org/10.1007/s00415-013-7169-7.

53. Wingerchuk DM, Weinshenker BG. Neuromyelitis optica. *Curr Treat Options Neurol* 2008;**10**:55–66 <http://rd.springer.com/article/10.1007%2Fs11940-008-0007-z>.

54. Bonnan M, Cabre P. Plasma exchange in severe attacks of neuromyelitis optica. *Mult Scler Int* 2012;787630. Available from: http://dx.doi.org/10.1155/2012/787630.

55. Costanzi C, Matiello M, Lucchinetti CF, Weinshenker BG, Pittock SJ, Mandrekar J, et al. Azathioprine: tolerability, efficacy, and predictors of benefit in neuromielitis optica. *Neurology* 2011;**77**:659–66. Available from: http://dx.doi.org/10.1212/WNL.0b013e31822a2780.

56. Jacob A, Weinshenker BG, Violich I, et al. Treatment of neuromyelitis optica with rituximab: retrospective analysis of 25 patients. *Arch Neurol* 2008;**65**:1443–8. Available from: http://dx.doi.org/10.1001/archneur.65.11.noc80069.

57. Jacob A, Matiello M, Weinshenker BG, Wingerchuk DM, Lucchinetti C, Shuster E, et al. Treatment of neuromyelitis optica with mycophenolate mofetil: retrospective analysis of 24 patients. *Arch Neurol* 2009;**66**:1128–33. Available from: http://dx.doi.org/10.1001/archneurol.2009.175.

58. Bakker J, Metz L. Devic's neuromyelitis optica treated with intravenous gamma globulin (IVIG). *Can J Neurol Sci* 2004;**31**:265–7. pubmed/15198456.

59. Araki M, Aranami T, Matsuoka T, Nakamura M, Miyake S, Yamamura T. Clinical improvement in a patient with neuromyelitis optica following therapy with the anti-IL-6 receptor monoclonal antibody tocilizumab. *Mod Rheumatol* 2013;**23**:827–31. Available from: http://dx.doi.org/10.1007/s10165-012-0715-9.

60. Pittock SJ, Lennon VA, McKeon A, Mandrekar J, Weinshenker BG, Lucchinetti CF, et al. Eculizumab in AQP4-IgG-positive relapsing neuromyelitis óptica spectrum disorders: an open-label pilot study. *Lancet Neurol* 2013;**12**:554–62. Available from: http://dx.doi.org/10.1016/S1474-4422(13)70076-0.

61. Dhib-Jalbut S, Arnold DL, Cleveland DW, Fisher M, Friedlander RM, Mouradian MM, et al. Neurodegeneration and neuroprotection in multiple sclerosis and other neurodegenerative diseases. *J Neuroimmunol* 2006;**176**(1–2):198–215. Available from: http://dx.doi.org/10.1016/j.jneuroim.2006.03.027.

62. Gao HM, Hong JS. Why neurodegenerative diseases are progressive: uncontrolled inflammation drives disease progression. *Trends Immunol* 2008;**29**(8):357–65. Available from: http://dx.doi.org/10.1016/j.it.2008.05.002.

63. Moser HW, Raymond GV, Dubey P. Adrenoleukodystrophy: new approaches to a neurodegenerative disease. *JAMA* 2005;**294**(24):3131–4. Available from: http://dx.doi.org/10.1001/jama.294.24.3131.

64. Marchetti B, Abbracchio MP. To be or not to be (inflamed)—is that the question in anti-inflammatory drug therapy of neurodegenerative disorders? *Trends Pharmacol Sci* 2005;**26** (10):517–25. Available from: http://dx.doi.org/10.1016/j.tips.2005.08.007.

65. No authors listed. Anti-inflammatory drugs fall short in Alzheimer's disease. *Nat Med* 2008; **14**(9): 916. Available from: http://dx.doi.org/10.1038/nm0908-916.

66. Van Oosten BW, Barkhof F, Truyen L, Boringa JB, Bertelsmann FW, von Blomberg BM, et al. Increased MRI activity and immune activation in two multiple sclerosis patients treated with the monoclonal anti-tumor necrosis factor antibody cA2. *Neurology* 1996;**47**(6):1531–4 <www.ncbi.nlm.nih.gov/pubmed/8960740>.

67. Segal BM, et al. Repeated subcutaneous injections of IL12/23 p40 neutralising antibody, ustekinumab, in patients with relapsing–remitting multiple sclerosis: a phase II, double-blind, placebo-controlled, randomised, dose-ranging study. *Lancet Neurol* 2008;**7**:796–804.

68. Lulu S, Waubant E. Humoral-targeted immunotherapies in multiple sclerosis. Neurotherapeutics. *J Am Soc Exp NeuroTherap* 2013;**10**(1):34–43. Available from: http://dx.doi.org/10.1007/s13311-012-0164-3.

69. Schwartz M, Shechter R. Systemic inflammatory cells fight off neurodegenerative disease. *Nat Rev Neurol* 2010;**6**(7):405–10. Available from: http://dx.doi.org/10.1038/nrneurol.2010.71.

CHAPTER 5

Therapeutic Approaches in Allergic Diseases

Ilaria Puxeddu[1], Francesca Levi-Schaffer[2] and Paola Migliorini[1]

[1]Immuno-Allergology Unit, Department of Clinical and Experimental Medicine, Pisa University, Pisa, Italy [2]Pharmacology Unit, Faculty of Medicine, School of Pharmacy, Institute for Drug Research, Hebrew University of Jerusalem, Jerusalem, Israel

5.1 GENERAL ASPECTS OF ALLERGIC DISEASES

Allergic diseases are common pathological conditions caused by an IgE-dependent immunological reaction to an innocuous environmental antigen (allergen), that can occur in different anatomical locations (nose, lung, eye, gastrointestinal tract, and skin).[1]

During the first contact with the allergen, specific IgE are produced (sensitization phase); upon subsequent exposure to the same allergen, the sensitized subject develops an IgE-mediated hypersensitivity reaction.

Individuals with a predisposition to allergic diseases (atopy) may or may not have clinical symptoms. In developed countries 30–40% of individuals are atopic, whereas only a proportion has allergic diseases, including asthma (5–10%), rhinitis (10–20%), food allergy (1–3%),[1] and atopic dermatitis (10–20%).[2]

In population studies allergic diseases peak at different ages: food allergy and atopic dermatitis are predominant in early childhood, whereas asthma shows a biphasic peak, and rhinitis peaks in the second or third decade.

Allergic reactions are typically characterized by the emergence of T helper (Th) 2-type cytokines, including interleukin (IL)-4, IL-5, IL-9, IL-13, IL-25, and IL-31, which favor antibody isotype class switching to IgE.[3,4] Once IgE is produced by B cells during the sensitization phase, it binds to the high-affinity FcεRI receptors expressed on the surface of mast cells and basophils, creating a multivalent binding site for the allergen. Following subsequent allergen exposure, the allergen

Immune Rebalancing. DOI: http://dx.doi.org/10.1016/B978-0-12-803302-9.00005-1

cross-links the bound IgE, stimulates the release of preformed mediators (eg, histamine and tryptase), and induces within a few minutes
vasodilation, bronchial and smooth muscle contraction, glandular
secretion, and pruritus. Following activation, mast cells synthesize
newly generated mediators (eg, leukotrienes, prostaglandins, kinins,
cytokines, and chemokines) responsible for the perpetuation of the
allergic inflammation (AI). Thus, the IgE-dependent hypersensitivity
reaction takes place in two temporal patterns: an immediate reaction
or "early phase reaction," which develops within seconds or minutes
after allergen exposure of a sensitized individual, and a "late phase
reaction," which develops a few hours later.

The preformed mediators induce a response within minutes,
whereas inflammation due to newly generated mediators develops after
several hours, the time lag required for protein synthesis and recruitment of immune cells into the tissue.

Many cell types contribute to the development and perpetuation of
AI. Current data suggest that the imbalance between the T helper lymphocytes (Th) 1 and Th2 phenotypes with a predominance of Th2
results in AI. Th2 lymphocytes via IL-5 production coordinate the
recruitment and activation of eosinophils to the site of inflammation,
and via IL-4 promote the switching of B-cell to the synthesis of
IgE and activation of mast cells (Fig. 5.1).

Mast cells are found particularly around blood vessels and peripheral
nerves, located strategically beneath epithelial surfaces exposed to the
external environment, such as those of the respiratory and gastrointestinal tracts and skin. These cells have a clear and pivotal role in IgE-
mediated hypersensitivity reactions: following release of performed and
newly synthesized mediators into the extracellular milieu, they interact
with a variety of cell types to elicit and perpetuate proinflammatory
responses.[4]

The main cells involved in the late phase of AI are eosinophils, blood
granulocytes produced in the bone marrow under the influence of IL-3,
IL-5, and GM-CSF, that infiltrate the tissue in various pathological
situations, such as allergic diseases, parasitic infections, and neoplastic
diseases.[5] Mature eosinophils have small, primary and secondary or
"specific" granules. The secondary granules attract the greatest interest
since they store different inflammatory mediators such as the granule

Allergic inflammation

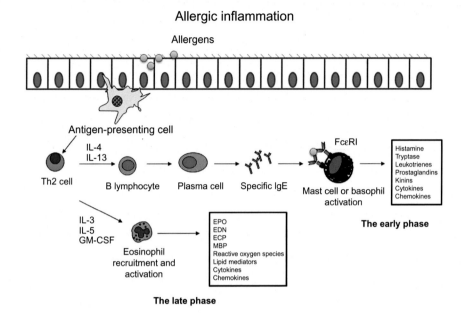

Figure 5.1 *Development and Perpetuation of Allergic Inflammation (AI).*

basic proteins (major basic protein, eosinophil peroxidase, eosinophil cationic protein, and eosinophil-derived neurotoxin), reactive oxygen species, lipid mediators, and a wide array of cytokines and chemokines. Through their preformed and newly synthesized mediators, eosinophils can contribute to AI, damaging airway epithelium and associated nerves, recruiting and activating other inflammatory cells, and promoting tissue remodeling. Increasing evidence indicates that tissue eosinophilia during allergic diseases may be intimately related to Th2-derived cytokines, including IL-5 and GM-CSF and eosinophil chemoattractant chemokines, such as Eotaxin, RANTES, and MCP-1, which prolong the viability and enhance the effector responses of mature eosinophils.[6]

A cross-talk among mast cells, basophils, eosinophils, T lymphocytes, dendritic cells (DC), neutrophils, monocytes, and structural cells (eg, fibroblasts, endothelial cells, and epithelial cells) occurs at sites of AI, leading to the amplification and perpetuation of the allergic process. Thus, the past 10 years have witnessed the development and evaluation of a number of biologics that target the Th2 cytokines involved in AI during allergic diseases, particularly IL-5 and IL-4/IL-13.[7]

5.2 MODULATION OF ALLERGEN-SPECIFIC RESPONSES

The first attempt to downmodulate allergic responses was published 1 century ago, when Noon and Cantoor conducted a trial using grass pollen extracts for desensitization of patients with hay fever.[8] At the time, little was known of the immune mechanisms underlying allergic diseases and the efficacy of such a treatment was unexplained. The first hint of the possible mechanisms of action of desensitization was published in 1935 by Cooke, who described a protective allergen-specific serum factor induced by allergen-specific immunotherapy (SIT).[9]

SIT is characterized by the repeated administration of the causative allergen at progressively increasing doses, subcutaneously or sublingually; oral administration is used for food allergy, while intranodal or cutaneous routes are presently under investigation. SIT reduces mediator release in the immediate phase of allergic reaction and inhibits cellular recruitment, thus resolving AI.

It is now well established that SIT represents an allergen-specific and disease-modifying treatment of allergic diseases. SIT works by different mechanisms not all completely clear but mostly centered on the modulation of T cell responses to allergens, leading to a reduction in Th2 responses and induction of IL-10-producing T and B regulatory cells. In parallel, allergen-specific IgE are either unchanged or reduced and IgG, mainly of the IgG4 subclass, are induced.

Thus, the result of SIT is a rebalancing of the immune response, obtained with the administration of allergens in adjuvant: the route of entry of allergens and the presence of adjuvant distinguish the physiological exposure from the immunotherapeutic one. Safety has been a major concern in SIT, for the high risk of serious adverse events, up to anaphylactic reactions, mostly due to IgE-mediated responses. Thus, the main goal of research in this field has been to improve the efficacy of SIT while limiting its side effects.

The chemical modification of allergens by formaldehyde or glutaraldehyde was the first approach, used in the 1970s. These agents, acting as cross-linkers, lead to the formation of high molecular weight polymers (allergoids) where the epitopes recognized by IgE antibodies have been destroyed. This approach is effective, but limited by the difficult characterization and standardization of allergoids, because the amount of allergens contained is difficult to measure after the chemical modification. In this respect, the availability of recombinant allergens has been a major improvement and has allowed the production of hypoallergens, that is allergens modified in the critical residues for IgE binding, retaining or not retaining T cell reactivity.

An example of a hypoallergen coupled to a carrier protein is the modified Der p 23, a major dust mite allergen, proposed for a new immunotherapy of allergy to house dust mites. Inside the C terminal region of Der p 23, that bears the epitopes recognized by IgE from allergic patients, short sequences have been identified that do not bind IgE but induce IgG in rabbits when coupled to hepatitis B pre-S protein. IgG induced by immunization with these recombinant antigens block Der p 23-induced basophil degranulation. Moreover, the recombinant antigens elicit from peripheral blood mononuclear cells of atopic patients the release of lower amounts of IL-13 and higher amounts of IL-10 and IFNγ when compared with the native allergen.[10]

In the design of hypoallergens for grass pollen vaccine, hybrid molecules have been constructed with fragments of allergens that are not recognized by IgE in atopic patients and induce the production of IgG when administered subcutaneously.[11] Interestingly, depending on the arrangement of allergen fragments, hybrid molecules displayed a variable IgE binding activity. A few recombinant proteins induced proliferation of T cells from atopic patients, elicited in mice IgG antibodies that blocked IgE binding to native allergens and reduced airway hyperresponsiveness in a murine model of grass pollen allergy, thus displaying all the features of a potential vaccine.

Most allergens so far known bear both T and B epitopes, but some of them may also elicit primarily a T cell response. An alternative approach for immunotherapy is the use of synthetic peptides corresponding to allergen sequences that represent pure T epitopes. Targeting T cells specific for one epitope, the immune response to other epitopes of the same molecule can be downregulated by a mechanism of linked epitope suppression, associated with the induction of IL-10-producing T cells.[12] This approach is used for cat allergy SIT: a mix of peptides of 13−17 aminoacids, administered intradermally, proved to be safe and effective in phase II clinical trials.[13]

Similarly, the subcutaneous administration of peptides representing major T cell epitopes of bee venom allergen phospholipase induced peripheral T cell anergy and the production of IgG4 similarly to conventional immunotherapy.[14] The results were confirmed using long synthetic peptides, in a double-blind placebo-controlled phase I clinical trial in patients hypersensitive to bee venom, indicating that long peptides may represent a novel and safe SIT.[15]

In the case of Timothy grass pollen allergens, an extensive bioinformatic and proteomic approach has allowed the identification of T epitopes on newly discovered proteins that are not recognized by IgE or IgG from allergic patients. These molecules, and in particular the promiscuous HLA binding sequences, may represent new candidates for immunotherapy.[16]

Toll like receptors (TLRs) targeting has also been exploited in the development of new forms of immunotherapy.

The role of TLRs in allergic disorders is complex. Allergens can interact with TLRs expressed on epithelia, inducing the production of cytokines, such as thymic stromal lymphopoietin (TLSP), that triggers a Th2-mediated AI.

This mechanism has been demonstrated for Der p 2 from mite dust, Fel d 1, a cat dander protein, and Can f 6, a dog dander protein, that enhance TLR4 and TLR2 signaling either acting on the coreceptor MD2 or complexing with bacterial lipids.[17]

The activation of TLR4 on airway epithelial cells causes the production of several pro-allergic cytokines, such as TLSP, GM-CSF, IL-25, and IL-33, driving allergic airway inflammation. The intrapulmonary administration of a functional TLR4 antagonist, together with allergen, reduced airway lymphocytosis, eosinophilia, local production of Th2 cytokines, and reversed airway hyperresponsiveness.[18]

Activation of TLR4 and 8, expressed on myeloid DC (mDC), has been reported to break allergen-specific T cell tolerance in human peripheral and tonsil T cells via MyD88 signaling.[19]

On the other hand, it has been reported that DC from allergic subjects produce higher amounts of proinflammatory cytokines such as

IL-6 and lower amounts of IFNα, following TLR7 and 9 stimulation.[20,21] IL-6 secretion by mDC is responsible for the skewing to Th2 response, while IFNα acts on mDC increasing the production of IL-10 that downregulates FcεRI-dependent inflammatory responses.

SLIT and oral immuno-therapy (OIT) may partially correct these abnormalities, modulating either mDC or plasmacytoid DC function and restoring the cytokine milieu that characterizes the condition of tolerance to allergens.[22] It is also well accepted that TLR stimulation by infectious agents in early childhood may shape adaptive immunity allowing the development of Th1 and regulatory T cells (Treg). On the basis of these observations, agonists of either cell surface or intracellular TLRs have been used both in animal models and in clinical trials in humans, mainly subcutaneously or sublingually.

Some TLR2/6 agonists, like Pam3CSK4, a synthetic triacylated lipoprotein, the macrophage-activating liprotein-2, or lipoprotein 1, reduced Th2 response and airway eosinophilia in murine asthma models.[23–25] In murine models, the administration of these molecules reduced CD4+ T cell proliferation and Th2 cytokine production, while increasing IL-10 and Th1 cytokines and in some cases expanding Treg.

At variance with TLR2/6 agonists, TLR4 ligands have been used in humans and the results of a number of clinical trials are already available. Monophosphoryl lipid A has been widely tested in immunotherapy with pollens, demonstrating efficacy and lack of side effects; on the contrary, only a few data are available for mite antigens. Other TLR4 ligands have only been tested in experimental models of allergy.[26]

As far as intracellular TLRs are concerned, TLR7/8 and TLR9 agonists showed promising results in animal models. For example, it has been shown that TLR7 stimulation by R848 prevents AI in mice activating iNKT that produce high levels of IFNγ.[27] Interestingly, TLR9 ligands can be administered either subcutaneously or via the mucosal route and are effective on both new-onset and established asthma. A few clinical trials, mainly phases I and II, have so far been conducted.

A novel strategy in immunotherapy is the conjugation of allergens with TLR ligands, resulting in targeted codelivery of both antigen and adjuvant to the same Antigen Presenting Cells (APC).

A fusion protein of flagellin, a TLR5 ligand, and Ova has been used for intranasal and intraperitoneal immunization in a mouse model of food allergy. Administration of the fusion protein prevented allergic sensitization and decreased IgE production. The immune modulating properties of the fusion protein, which is taken up by DC, are mediated by a TLR5-dependent stimulation of IL-10 production.[28]

5.3 TARGETING TH2 CYTOKINES: IL-5, IL-4, AND IL-13

Given the importance of IL-5 in maturation, mobilization, activation, recruitment, proliferation, survival, and suppression of apoptosis in eosinophils, IL-5 has been chosen as a pharmacological target for blocking the eosinophil influx into the tissue. Since the year 2000 several clinical trials have evaluated the therapeutic relevance of anti-IL-5 biologics in asthma treatment and symptoms management. Several monoclonal antibodies (mAb) were engineered to neutralize free circulating IL-5 and/or target receptor α (IL-5Rα) and are now in different phases of development.[29,30]

The first results obtained with anti-IL-5 Ab were contradictory. A single infusion of anti-IL-5 Ab in asthmatics resulted in a significant reduction in both blood and induced-sputum eosinophils, without changes in either the late asthmatic reaction or airway hyperreactivity.[31] A later study employing 3 infusions of Mepolizumab, a humanized mAb (IgG$_1$) with a high affinity for binding free IL-5, indicated that such a treatment is unable to deplete eosinophils from the bronchial mucosa.[32] Recently, two proof-of-concept studies in asthmatic patients with persistent blood and sputum eosinophilia treated with Mepolizumab suggested that this drug is effective as a steroid-sparing agent, reduces the frequency of severe exacerbations, and improves quality of life in patients with severe refractory eosinophilic asthma.[33,34] These data have been confirmed in a multicenter, double-blind, placebo-controlled trial in patients with severe eosinophilic asthma. Mepolizumab was shown to be an effective and well tolerated treatment, able to reduce the risk of asthma exacerbations[35] along with depletion of blood eosinophils. Another anti-IL-5 mAb (IgG$_{4/k}$), Reslizumab, showed a similar reduction in sputum eosinophils, a significant improvement in lung function and a trend towards improved asthma score in patients with severe refractory eosinophilic asthma.[36,37]

IL-5Rα, expressed by both mature eosinophils and eosinophil-lineage progenitor cells, is targeted by Benralizumab, a humanized afucosylated mAb. This drug induces apoptosis in its target cells via enhanced antibody-mediated cellular toxicity and is considered to have an increased efficacy of eosinophil depletion in comparison with the other anti-IL-5 biologics.[38]

The variable outcomes from anti-IL-5 clinical trials highlight the need for careful endotyping of patients, since the therapy is deemed effective on those patients whose asthma is dependent on the eosinophilic inflammatory pathway.[39] The reduction of eosinophils in bone marrow and peripheral blood, but not in airway mucosa/submucosa observed in the clinical trials with Benralizumab suggests an alternative mechanism of eosinophil recruitment, activation, and survival in the tissue, independent of the IL-5 and the classical Th2 pathway activation triggers.

The control of airway eosinophilia may require targeting multiple factors that stimulate eosinophils recruitment, differentiation, or prolonged tissue survival.

Clinical trials conducted with a mAb targeting IL-4, IL-13, and their shared receptors, similarly to anti-IL-5, met with a mixed response in improving clinical symptoms in refractory asthma.[29] However, a combination therapy with drugs like Dupilumab, a fully human mAb to the IL-4 receptor α subunit, that inhibits both IL-4 and IL-13 signaling,[40] and an anti-IL-5 mAb, could synergistically affect the mechanisms of in situ eosinophilia in severe asthmatics, responsible for the maintenance of clinical symptoms.

Beyond asthma, small pilot studies have documented the potential efficacy of targeting IL-5 in other eosinophil-depending diseases such as hypereosinophilic syndrome (HES) and eosinophilic granulomatosis and polyangitis (EGPA).[30] As suggested from clinical trials conducted in severe eosinophilic asthmatic patients, targeting IL-5 and other Th2 cytokines such as IL-4 and IL-13 in HES and EGPA might be useful to reduce eosinophils in infiltrated tissues and successfully control eosinophil-derived clinical symptoms.

Epigenetic regulation represents one important mechanism by which environmental factors might interact with genes involved in allergy and asthma development.[41] Recently, the concept of

Table 5.1 Emerging Biological Drugs in the Treatment of Allergic Diseases

Drug Name	Molecular Format	Target	Clinical Indications
Mepolizumab	Humanized IgG1	IL-5	Severe eosinophilic asthma; COPD; HES; EGPA; EE; Nasal polyps (phase 3)
Reslizumab	Humanized IgG4	IL-5	Severe eosinophilic asthma (phase 2/3)
Benralizumab	Humanized IgG1	IL-5Rα	Severe eosinophilic asthma COPD (phase 3)
Dupilumab	Human IgG4	IL-4Rα	Severe asthma; atopic dermatitis
Omalizumab	Humanized IgG1	IgE	Severe asthma; allergic rhinitis; bronchopolmonary allergic aspergillosis; chronic urticaria; Kimura's disease (phase 3)
Ligelizumab	Humanized IgG1	IgE	Severe asthma; atopic dermatitis, food allergy
XmAb7195	Humanized IgG1 (FcγRIIb-interacting)	IgE	Severe asthma; atopic dermatitis (phase 1/2)

Note: COPD, chronic obstructive pulmonary disease; HES, hypereosinophilic syndrome; EGPA, eosinophilic granulomatosis and polyangitis; EE, eosinophilic esophagitis.

epigenetic regulation in asthma development has gained increasing attention.[42] In mice and human subjects, a number of studies have provided evidence for the pivotal role of INFγ in allergy protection and T cells from subjects at risk of allergic diseases generally produce lower INFγ levels.[43] Brand et al. showed that induction of allergic airway inflammation in mice was associated with methylation of the promoter of the gene encoding INFγ in CD4+ T cells, which consequently led to a decrease of INFγ expression. Reversal of INFγ promoter methylation in CD4+ T cells inhibited Th2 polarization, reducing production of IL-4, IL-5, and IL-13 and consequently allergic airway inflammation.[44] These observations may open new perspectives for the modulation of cytokine production in allergic diseases (Table 5.1).

5.4 TARGETING IgE AND FcεRI

IgE are well known therapeutic targets for allergic diseases, but the main difficulty has been to select agents that do not trigger cross-linkage of IgE when bound to its high affinity receptor (FcεRI) on mast cells and basophils.[45]

A major breakthrough occurred when the interaction between IgE and FcεRI was fully elucidated at the molecular level.[46] In fact, it was shown that the Cε3 region of the Fc fragment of IgE binds very selectively to one side of the D2 domain at the top of the D1−D2 interface of the α-chain of the tetrameric FcεRI, and is not exposed on receptor-bound IgE.[47] Thus, targeting specifically the Cε3 region poses no risk of cross-linking the IgE bound to the high affinity receptor. A chimeric IgG mAb specific for the human Cε3 region was developed and shown to be effective in reducing circulating IgE without causing an anaphylactic response.[48]

Omalizumab is the first humanized IgG1 antihuman IgE mAb containing mouse sequences only in the antigen binding site, able to neutralize free IgE and the IgE-hypersensitivity reaction without activating mast cells and basophils.[49] Following Phase II studies, Omalizumab successfully entered the clinic for the treatment of severe allergic asthma in both adults and children over the age of 12 years. With a good safety profile, clinical studies confirmed efficacy in severe asthma which have now extended to "real world" studies.[50]

High levels of circulating IgE result in an increase of FcεRI on effector cells, whereas removal of IgE with Omalizumab causes downregulation of FcεRI on these cells, contributing to the efficacy of the treatment.[51] The infusion of this drug leads to the formation of IgG/IgE trimeric and hexameric immune complexes that do not activate complement, thus explaining efficacy in the absence of side effects.

The reduction in IgE affects allergen sensing and processing by airway DC, thus reducing the AI cascade, including the recruitment of eosinophils and basophils.[52] Omalizumab has been shown to be effective not only in downregulating the early and the late phase of allergic airway inflammation, but also in reducing reticular basement membrane thickening, suggesting an effect also on airway remodeling.[53]

A systemic anti-IgE therapy has been shown to exert powerful effects on other allergic manifestations in addition to asthma. Some randomized and observational studies have demonstrated that Omalizumab is efficacious in patients with allergic rhinitis, broncho-pulmonary allergic aspergillosis, urticaria, Kimura's disease, food allergy and idiopathic and exercise-induced anaphylaxis, atopic dermatitis, protection from anaphylaxis during allergen immunotherapy, latex allergy, cutaneous mastocytosis, eosinophilic gastroenteritis, nasal polyposis, and even some cases of intrinsic asthma. The beneficial effect of anti-IgE therapy in chronic urticaria and angioedema is especially valuable since the therapeutic options for such patients are limited to antihistamines, oral corticosteroids, and immunosuppressants. While urticaria can occur with asthma when it is associated with atopy, especially food allergy, it most frequently occurs as an independent entity.

Even when allergens or auto-Ab against IgE or FcεRI play no role in causing chronic urticaria, anti-IgE therapy can still be highly effective. The clinical efficacy of anti-IgE therapy in chronic spontaneous urticaria[54] suggests that quietening mast cells activation with loss of the cell surface FcεRI during Omalizumab treatment raises the threshold for mast cell activation independent of the stimulus.

New more potent anti-IgE mAb are presently in the development phase. The QGE031 (Ligelizumab) has been demonstrated to be at least 12 times more potent than Omalizumab for the treatment of IgE-driven diseases where a unmet need exists such as severe uncontrolled asthma, atopic dermatitis, and food allergies.[55] Chu et al. compared Omalizumab with a novel anti-IgE Ab called XmAb7195 that not only binds free IgE effectively, but also inhibits plasma cell differentiation and human IgE production as a result of its ability to coengage transmembrane IgE on the B-cell along with FcγRIIb[56] (Table 5.1).

5.5 TARGETING MAST CELLS AND EOSINOPHILS

Given the importance of mast cells and eosinophils respectively in the early and late phases of AI, targeting of their soluble mediators, adhesion molecules, surface-activating (AR), or inhibiting (IR) receptors and intracellular enzymes show promising approaches for the treatment of allergic diseases.

Mast cells activation and consequent degranulation can be prevented by mast cell stabilizers such as cromolyn sodium and nedocromil sodium. Recently, it has been demonstrated that some H1 antihistamines (anti-H1R) have dual-action of both anti-histaminic and mast cell stabilizing activities.[57] Anti-H1R together with anti-H4R exert therapeutic effects on both the allergic symptoms, eosinophil chemotaxis, and proliferation of fibroblasts in a mouse model of chronic dermatitis. Clinical trials are underway for asthma and other allergic diseases.[58]

Besides histamine, other mast cell-preformed mediators, such as tryptase and chymase, released following mast cell activation, were identified as targets for downregulating AI.

The JNJ-27390467, a β-tryptase inhibitor, has been shown to reduce AI in experimental models of asthma, while several potent chymase inhibitors display anti-inflammatory and antifibrotic effects in a variety of animal and ex vivo models.[59]

As discussed above, a well-established approach to prevent mast cell degranulation during IgE-hypersensitivity reactions is to interfere with the IgE-FcεRI binding, either blocking the FcεRI or the Fc portion of the IgE. Since the viability of mast cells in the tissue is tightly regulated by stem cell factor (SCF), the inhibition of the SCF/c-kit pathway by using anti-SCF or anti-c-kit Ab was proposed and found to be useful in the treatment of mastocytosis and in severe nonglucocorticoid responsive allergy.[60]

Since eosinophils are the main player in the late/chronic stages of allergy, strategies to control their tissue recruitment and activation have been proposed as an alternative approach for treating allergic diseases. One possible strategy is to inhibit differentiation, maturation, and survival of eosinophils by targeting IL-5 as previously discussed. However, eosinophil trafficking into the tissue is regulated not only by IL-5, but also by various adhesion molecules, such as VLA-4, VCAM-1, ICAM-1, ICAM-2, ICAM-3, and integrins, such as a4b7 (a4b1), cytokines (GM-CSF, IL-3, and IL-5), prostaglandins (PGD2), chemokines (Eotaxin, RANTES, MCP-1), and chemoattractant receptors (CRTH2, CCR3, CCR5). Therefore, selective antagonists mainly for chemoattractant receptors have been recently proposed. The OC000459, a selective CRTH2 antagonist, was found to inhibit PGD2 mediated eosinophil chemotaxis in addition to preventing the activation of Th2 lymphocytes.[61] This antagonist was able to improve lung function and asthma control in allergic asthmatics,[62] to induce beneficial clinical effects in adult patients with active, corticosteroid-dependent or corticosteroid-refractory eosinophilic esophagitis,[63] and to ameliorate the clinical symptoms in allergic rhinoconjunctivitis patients.[61]

The effect of the compound GW766994, a small molecule antagonist of the CCR3 receptor, was recently evaluated on sputum eosinophil counts in patients with eosinophilic asthma. However, the CCR3 antagonist did not significantly reduce eosinophils or eosinophil progenitor cells (CD34+ CD45+ IL-5Rα+) in sputum or in blood, suggesting that other cellular mechanisms mediated by the CCR3 receptor may contribute to airway hyperresponsiveness.[64] Other CCR3 compounds are currently under evaluation. In parallel to antagonists of chemokine receptors, Ab against adhesion molecules, such as VLA-4 and integrins, have been reported to reduce eosinophil recruitment and airway eosinophilic inflammation in animal models of airway AI but not in human asthma.[65]

Recently the stimulation of IR expressed on the surface of mast cells and eosinophils, such as CD300a, FcγRIIB, or Siglec-8, using mAb or specific ligands, has been proposed as innovative strategy for inhibiting the activation of these cells.[60] In a mouse model of cutaneous anaphylaxis, cross-linking of CD300a with c-kit on mast cells by a bispecific Ab fragment was shown to abrogate mast cells degranulation.[66] Linking of CD300a with FcϵRI inhibited AI in the two animal models: IgE-dependent PCA and OVA-induced acute experimental asthma.[67] Since mast cells and eosinophils in addition to IR also express on their membrane AR (eg, CD48 and 2B4) used in their physical cross-talk ("the Allergic Effector Unit"), the specific blocking of one or both receptors can prevent their proinflammatory cross-talk. In a mouse model of allergen-induced asthma, CD48 was found to be critically involved in allergic eosinophilic airway inflammation: neutralization of this receptor in allergen-challenged mice abrogated airway eosinophilic inflammation.[68] Based on the results obtained in preclinical studies, drugs targeting membrane AR and IR of mast cells and eosinophils hold promising therapeutic possibilities for allergic diseases.[69]

5.6 CONCLUSIONS

- A safe and cost-effective therapy of allergic diseases such as asthma, atopic dermatitis, allergic rhinitis, and food allergy is currently an unmet need.
- Emerging therapeutic options for allergic diseases are intended to target the different steps of IgE hypersensitivity reactions.
- A deeper understanding of cellular and humoral circuits involved in IgE responses has allowed new approaches to allergen immunotherapy, which remains the only disease-modifying therapy.
- Several biological drugs have been developed against mediators and cellular components that are involved in the development and perpetuation of AI; their usefulness could be further increased when used in combination.
- Randomized clinical trials will establish their place in therapeutic guidelines and possibly open the way to a personalized therapy for allergic diseases.

REFERENCES

1. Holgate ST, Church MK, Lichtenstein LM. *Allergy.* 2nd ed. London: Mosby International; 2001.

2. Totri CR, Diaz L, Eichenfield LF. 2014 update on atopic dermatitis in children. *Curr Opin Pediatr* 2014;**26**:466−71.

3. Holgate ST. Innate and adaptive immune responses in asthma. *Nat Med* 2012;**18**:673−83.

4. Akdis CA. Therapies for allergic inflammation: refining strategies to induce tolerance. *Nat Med* 2012;**18**:736−49.

5. Akuthota P, Weller PF. Eosinophils and disease pathogenesis. *Semin Hematol* 2012;**49**:113−19.

6. Davoine F, Lacy P. Eosinophil cytokines, chemokines, and growth factors: emerging roles in immunity. *Front Immunol* 2014;**5**:570.

7. Wynn TA. Type 2 cytokines: mechanisms and therapeutic strategies. *Nat Rev Immunol* 2015;**15**:271−82.

8. Noon L, Cantar BO. Prophylactic inoculation against hay fever. *Lancet* 1911;1572−3.

9. Cooke RA, Barnard JH, Hebald S, Stull A. Serolological evidence of immunity with coexisting sensitization in a type of human allergy (hay fever). *J Exp Med* 1935;**62**:733−50.

10. Banerjee S, Weber M, Blatt K, Swoboda I, Focke-Tejkl M, Valent P, et al. Conversion of Der p 23, a new major house dust mite allergen, into a hypoallergenic vaccine. *J Immunol* 2014;**192**:4867−75.

11. Linhart B, Focke-Tejkl M, Weber M, Narayanan M, Neubauer A, Mayrhofer H, et al. Molecular evolution of hypoallergenic hybrid proteins for vaccination against grass pollen allergy. *J Immunol* 2015;**194**:4008−18.

12. Campbell JD, Buckland KF, McMillan SJ, Kearley J, Oldfield WL, Stern LJ, et al. Peptide immunotherapy in allergic asthma generates IL-10-dependent immunological tolerance associated with linked epitope suppression. *J Exp Med* 2009;**206**:1535–47.

13. Creticos PS. Advances in synthetic peptide immuno-regulatory epitopes. *World Allergy Organ J* 2014;**7**:30.

14. Müller U, Akdis CA, Fricker M, Akdis M, Blesken T, Bettens F, et al. Successful immunotherapy with T-cell epitope peptides of bee venom phospholipase A2 induces specific T-cell anergy in patients allergic to bee venom. *J Allergy Clin Immunol* 1998;**101**:747–54.

15. Fellrath JM, Kettner A, Dufour N, Frigerio C, Schneeberger D, Leimgruber A, et al. Allergen-specific T-cell tolerance induction with allergen-derived long synthetic peptides: results of a phase I trial. *J Allergy Clin Immunol* 2003;**111**:854–61.

16. Schulten V, Peters B, Sette A. New strategies for allergen T cell epitope identification: going beyond IgE. *Int Arch Allergy Immunol* 2014;**165**:75–82.

17. Herre J, Grönlund H, Brooks H, Hopkins L, Waggoner L, Murton B, et al. Allergens as immunomodulatory proteins: the cat dander protein Fel d 1 enhances TLR activation by lipid ligands. *J Immunol* 2013;**191**:1529–35.

18. Hammad H, Chieppa M, Perros F, Willart MA, Germain RN, Lambrecht BN. House dust mite allergen induces asthma via Toll-like receptor 4 triggering of airway structural cells. *Nat Med* 2009;**15**:410–16.

19. Kucuksezer UC, Palomares O, Ruckert B, Jartti T, Puhakka T, Nandy A. Triggering of specific Toll-like receptors and proinflammatory cytokines breaks allergen-specific T-cell tolerance in human tonsils and peripheral blood. *J Allergy Clin Immunol* 2013;**131**:875–85.

20. Frischmeyer-Guerrerio PA, Guerrerio AL, Chichester KL, Bieneman AP, Hamilton RA, Wood RA, et al. Dendritic cell and T cell responses in children with food allergy. *Clin Exp Allergy* 2011;**41**:61–71.

21. Tulic MK, Hodder M, Forsberg A, McCarthy S, Richman T, D'Vaz N, et al. Differences in innate immune function between allergic and nonallergic children: new insights into immune ontogeny. *J Allergy Clin Immunol* 2011;**127**:470–8.

22. Frischmeyer-Guerrerio PA, Keet CA, Guerrerio AL, Chichester KL, Bieneman AP, Hamilton RG, et al. Modulation of dendritic cell innate and adaptive immune functions by oral and sublingual immunotherapy. *Clin Immunol* 2014;**155**:47–59.

23. Patel M, Xu D, Kewin P, Choo-Kang B, McSharry C, Thomson NC, et al. TLR2 agonist ameliorates established allergic airway inflammation by promoting Th1 response and not via regulatory T cells. *J Immunol* 2005;**174**:7558–63.

24. Weigt H, Nassenstein C, Tschernig T, Muhlradt PF, Krug N, Braun A. Efficacy of macrophage-activating lipopeptide-2 combined with interferon-gamma in a murine asthma model. *Am J Respir Crit Care Med* 2005;**172**:566–72.

25. Aumeunier A, Grela F, Ramadan A, Pham Van L, Bardel E, Gomez Alcala A, et al. Systemic toll-like receptor stimulation suppresses experimental allergic asthma and autoimmune diabetes in NOD mice. *PLoS One* 2010;**5**:e11484.

26. Aryan Z, Holgate ST, Radzioch D, Rezaei N. A new era of targeting the ancient gatekeepers of the immune system: toll-like agonists in the treatment of allergic rhinitis and asthma. *Int Arch Allergy Immunol* 2014;**164**:46–63.

27. Grela F, Aumeunier A, Bardel E, Van LP, Bourgeois E, Vanoirbeek J, et al. The TLR7 agonist R848 alleviates allergic inflammation by targeting invariant NKT cells to produce IFN-gamma. *J Immunol* 2011;**186**:284–90.

28. Schülke S, Wolfheimer S, Gadermaier G, Wangorsch A, Siebeneicher S, Briza P, et al. Prevention of intestinal allergy in mice by rflaA:Ova is associated with enforced antigen processing and TLR5-dependent IL-10 secretion by mDC. *PLoS One* 2014;**9**:e87822.

29. Hambly N, Nair P. Monoclonal antibodies for the treatment of refractory asthma. *Curr Opin Pulm Med* 2014;**20**:87–94.

30. Mukherjee M, Sehmi R, Nair P. Anti-IL5 therapy for asthma and beyond. *World Allergy Organ J* 2014;**7**:32.

31. Leckie MJ, ten Brinke A, Khan J, Diamant Z, O'Connor BJ, Walls CM, et al. Effects of an interleukin-5 blocking monoclonal antibody on eosinophils, airway hyper-responsiveness, and the late asthmatic response. *Lancet* 2000;**356**:2144–8.

32. Flood-Page PT, Menzies-Gow AN, Kay AB, Robinson DS. Eosinophil's role remains uncertain as anti-interleukin-5 only partially depletes numbers in asthmatic airway. *Am J Respir Crit Care Med* 2003;**167**:199–204.

33. Nair P, Pizzichini MM, Kjarsgaard M, Inman MD, Efthimiadis A, Pizzichini E, et al. Mepolizumab for prednisone-dependent asthma with sputum eosinophilia. *N Engl J Med* 2009;**360**:985–93.

34. Haldar P, Brightling CE, Hargadon B, Gupta S, Monteiro W, Sousa A, et al. Mepolizumab and exacerbations of refractory eosinophilic asthma. *N Engl J Med* 2009;**360**:973–84.

35. Pavord ID, Korn S, Howarth P, Bleecker ER, Buhl R, Keene ON, et al. Mepolizumab for severe eosinophilic asthma (DREAM): a multicentre, double-blind, placebo-controlled trial. *Lancet* 2012;**380**:651–9.

36. Castro M, Mathur S, Hargreave F, Boulet LP, Xie F, Young J, et al. Reslizumab for poorly controlled, eosinophilic asthma: a randomized, placebo-controlled study. *Am J Respir Crit Care Med* 2011;**184**:1125–32.

37. Castro M, Zangrilli J, Wechsler ME, Bateman ED, Brusselle GG, Bardin P, et al. Reslizumab for inadequately controlled asthma with elevated blood eosinophil counts: results from two multicentre, parallel, double-blind, randomised, placebo-controlled, phase 3 trials. *Lancet Respir Med* 2015;**3**:355–66.

38. Ghazi A, Trikha A, Calhoun WJ. Benralizumab—a humanized mAb to IL-5Rα with enhanced antibody-dependent cell-mediated cytotoxicity—a novel approach for the treatment of asthma. *Expert Opin Biol Ther* 2012;**12**:113–18.

39. Nair P. What is an "eosinophilic phenotype" of asthma? *J Allergy Clin Immunol* 2013;**132**:81–3.

40. Wenzel S, Ford L, Pearlman D, Spector S, Sher L, Skobieranda F, et al. Dupilumab in persistent asthma with elevated eosinophil levels. *N Engl J Med* 2013;**368**:2455–66.

41. Martino DJ, Prescott SL. Silent mysteries: epigenetic paradigms could hold the key to conquering the epidemic of allergy and immune disease. *Allergy* 2010;**65**:7–15.

42. White GP, Hollams EM, Yerkovich ST, Bosco A, Holt BJ, Bassami MR, et al. CpG methylation patterns in the IFNgamma promoter in naive T cells: variations during Th1 and Th2 differentiation and between atopics and non-atopics. *Pediatr Allergy Immunol* 2006;**17**:557–64.

43. Rowe J, Heaton T, Kusel M, Suriyaarachchi D, Serralha M, Holt BJ, et al. High IFN-gamma production by CD8 + T cells and early sensitization among infants at high risk of atopy. *J Allergy Clin Immunol* 2004;**113**:710–16.

44. Brand S, Kesper DA, Teich R, Kilic-Niebergall E, Pinkenburg O, Bothur E, et al. DNA methylation of TH1/TH2 cytokine genes affects sensitization and progress of experimental asthma. *J Allergy Clin Immunol* 2012;**129**:1602–10.

45. Holgate ST. New strategies with anti-IgE in allergic diseases. *World Allergy Organ J* 2014;**7**:17.

46. Field KA, Holowka D, Baird B. Compartmentalized activation of the high affinity immunoglobulin E receptor within membrane domains. *J Biol Chem* 1997;**272**:4276–80.

47. Garman SC, Wurzburg BA, Tarchevskaya SS, Kinet JP, Jardetzky TS. Structure of the Fc fragment of human IgE bound to its high-affinity receptor Fc epsilonRI alpha. *Nature* 2000;**406**:259–66.

48. Corne J, Djukanovic R, Thomas L, Warner J, Botta L, Grandordy B, et al. The effect of intravenous administration of a chimeric anti-IgE antibody on serum IgE levels in atopic subjects: efficacy, safety, and pharmacokinetics. *J Clin Invest* 1997;**99**:879−87.

49. Easthope S, Jarvis B. Omalizumab. *Drugs* 2001;**61**:253−60.

50. Campbell JD, McQueen RB, Briggs A. The "e" in cost-effectiveness analyses. A case study of omalizumab efficacy and effectiveness for cost-effectiveness analysis evidence. *Ann Am Thorac Soc* 2014;**11**:S105−11.

51. MacGlashan D. Loss of receptors and IgE in vivo during treatment with anti-IgE antibody. *J Allergy Clin Immunol* 2004;**114**:1472−4.

52. Schroeder JT, Bieneman AP, Chichester KL, Hamilton RG, Xiao H, Saini SS, et al. Decreases in human dendritic cell-dependent T(H)2-like responses after acute in vivo IgE neutralization. *J Allergy Clin Immunol* 2010;**125**:896−901.

53. Riccio AM, Dal Negro RW, Micheletto C, De Ferrari L, Folli C, Chiappori A, et al. Omalizumab modulates bronchial reticular basement membrane thickness and eosinophil infiltration in severe persistent allergic asthma patients. *Int J Immunopathol Pharmacol* 2012;**25**:475−84.

54. Maurer M, Rosén K, Hsieh HJ, Saini S, Grattan C, Gimenéz-Arnau A, et al. Omalizumab for the treatment of chronic idiopathic or spontaneous urticaria. *N Engl J Med* 2013;**368**:924−35.

55. Arm JP, Bottoli I, Skerjanec A, Floch D, Groenewegen A, Maahs S, et al. Pharmacokinetics, pharmacodynamics and safety of QGE031 (ligelizumab), a novel high-affinity anti-IgE antibody, in atopic subjects. *Clin Exp Allergy* 2014;**44**:1371−85.

56. Chu SY, Horton HM, Pong E, Leung IW, Chen H, Nguyen DH, et al. Reduction of total IgE by targeted coengagement of IgE B-cell receptor and FcγRIIb with Fc-engineered antibody. *J Allergy Clin Immunol* 2012;**129**:1102−15.

57. Levi-Schaffer F, Eliashar R. Mast cell stabilizing properties of antihistamines. *J Invest Dermatol* 2009;**129**:2549−51.

58. Landolina N, Gangwar RS, Levi-Schaffer F. Mast cells' integrated actions with eosinophils and fibroblasts in allergic inflammation: implications for therapy. *Adv Immunol* 2015;**125**:41−85.

59. Caughey GH. Mast cell tryptases and chymases in inflammation and host defense. *Immunol Rev* 2007;**217**:141−54.

60. Harvima IT, Levi-Schaffer F, Draber P, Friedman S, Polakovicova I, Gibbs BF, et al. Molecular targets on mast cells and basophils for novel therapies. *J Allergy Clin Immunol* 2014;**134**:530−44.

61. Horak F, Zieglmayer P, Zieglmayer R, Lemell P, Collins LP, Hunter MG, et al. The CRTH2 antagonist OC000459 reduces nasal and ocular symptoms in allergic subjects exposed to grass pollen, a randomised, placebo-controlled, double-blind trial. *Allergy* 2012;**67**:1572−9.

62. Pettipher R, Hunter MG, Perkins CM, Collins LP, Lewis T, Baillet M, et al. Heightened response of eosinophilic asthmatic patients to the CRTH2 antagonist OC000459. *Allergy* 2014;**69**:1223−32.

63. Straumann A, Hoesli S, Bussmann Ch, Stuck M, Perkins M, Collins LP, et al. Anti-eosinophil activity and clinical efficacy of the CRTH2 antagonist OC000459 in eosino-philicesophagitis. *Allergy* 2013;**68**:375−85.

64. Neighbour H, Boulet LP, Lemiere C, Sehmi R, Leigh R, Sousa AR, et al. Safety and efficacy of an oral CCR3 antagonist in patients with asthma and eosinophilic bronchitis: a randomized, placebo-controlled clinical trial. *Clin Exp Allergy* 2014;**44**:508−16.

65. Barthel SR, Johansson MW, McNamee DM, Mosher DF. Roles of integrin activation in eosinophil function and the eosinophilic inflammation of asthma. *J Leukoc Biol* 2008;**83**:1–12.

66. Bachelet I, Munitz A, Berent-Maoz B, Mankuta D, Levi-Schaffer F. Suppression of normal and malignant kit signaling by a bispecific antibody linking kit with CD300a. *J Immunol* 2008;**180**:6064–9.

67. Bachelet I, Munitz A, Levi-Schaffer F. Abrogation of allergic reactions by a bispecific antibody fragment linking IgE to CD300a. *J Allergy Clin Immunol* 2006;**117**:1314–20.

68. Munitz A, Bachelet I, Eliashar R, Khodoun M, Finkelman FD, Rothenberg ME, et al. CD48 is an allergen and IL-3-induced activation molecule on eosinophils. *J Immunol* 2006;**177**:77–83.

69. Puxeddu I, Piliponsky AM, Bachelet I, Levi-Schaffer F. Mast cells in allergy and beyond. *Int J Biochem Cell Biol* 2003;**35**:1601–7.

Immunotherapy for Transforming Advanced Cancer into a Chronic Disease: How Far Are We?

Tania Crombet and Agustin Lage
Center of Molecular Immunology, Havana, Cuba

6.1 INTRODUCTION: THE BASIC BIOLOGY OF CHRONIC DISEASES

Common wisdom in medical sciences distinguishes acute diseases (ie, infections, injuries, poisoning) from chronic diseases (ie, cardiovascular diseases, atherosclerosis, diabetes, kidney failure). In acute diseases initiation is sudden, causes are few, mainly external and identifiable, the clinical course is fast, the disease is vulnerable to medical intervention with rather simple technologies, and effective treatments can fully restore previous health. For chronic diseases the initiation is insidious, the causes are often internal and multiple, the clinical course is slow, treatment is complex, full restoration of previous health seldom occurs, and the disease will be there for the lifetime. Health interventions have been successful mainly in acute diseases, for example, environmental hygiene, better nutrition, and vaccinations have brought a drastic decrease of primary incidence in many countries, and antibiotics, surgery, and advances in intensive care have increased cure rates. These advancements have translated into a steep increase in human life expectancy over the past 200 years. In aging populations chronic diseases replaced infections as the first cause of mortality, a shift captured by the term "epidemiological transition."[1] For chronic diseases medical success does not mean cure, but long-term control, improved quality of life (QoL), and better management of complications. Acute and chronic diseases can be seen as the extremes of a continuous spectrum of time course and medical efficacy, with middle ground situations such as chronic infections. Beneath this operational categorization lies a more fundamental biological difference. Acute diseases occur mainly in the prereproductive ages, for which the species' evolution has fixed negative feedback control loops (such as the immune system, DNA-repairing,

Immune Rebalancing. DOI: http://dx.doi.org/10.1016/B978-0-12-803302-9.00006-3

blood clotting, and wound healing) to fight the external aggressions and to guarantee reproductive performance and species survival. Chronic diseases occur mainly in the postreproductive age, when there has been an entropy-driven accumulation of molecular damages and relaxation of homeostatic control loops, protective mutations have not been fixed (because there is no reproductive advantage at advanced ages), and positive feedback loops reinforcing the disease itself are often created by the very same homeostatic mechanisms. For decades cancer research has ignored this dichotomy, and medical intervention has tried to reproduce, in cancer treatment, its past success in achieving cures for infections with antibiotics. Is it time for a review of our undeclared assumptions, and for a shift in our scientific paradigms? Can immunotherapy be instrumental in the transformation of cancer into a chronic disease? This chapter will try to address these questions by reviewing the current approaches to cancer therapy, with a focus on the more innovative therapies. We will also describe some examples, based on our direct experience in Cuba.

6.2 THE EVIDENCE OF A TRANSITION TO CHRONICITY

Leaving aside primary prevention and curative treatments for early stage tumors, we will focus in this article on advanced cancer, a stage reached by approximately half of diagnosed tumors. Three lines of evidence show that a slow but continuous transformation of advanced cancer into a chronic disease is occurring: the trend to increasing survival, the shape of survival curves, and the appearance of second tumors in patients with the primary disease under control.

6.2.1 Increasing Survival in the Advanced Disease

Survival of advanced cancer has increased gradually for most tumor types in the last 20 years.[2] This could be attributed to the improvement in the conventional therapeutic tools like surgery, irradiation and chemotherapy together with the identification of many molecular targets relevant for tumor growth and the consequent emergence of targeted therapies. Immunotherapy has recently started to contribute to this survival increase, after the FDA approval of the first therapeutic vaccine (sipuleucel T)[3] and the first monoclonal antibodies that inhibit "the inhibition" of the effector T cells (ipilimumab, nivolumab, pembrolizumab).[4] The following examples can illustrate this survival shift: advanced colorectal cancer survival had increased from 12 to 26—30 months after the combination of fluoropyrimidines, oxaliplatin, irinotecan, and biologic therapies (bevacizumab, panitumumab, and cetuximab)[5]; the survival of Her-2-positive metastatic breast cancer women had reached 40 months after the combined use of chemotherapy and the sequential introduction of trastuzumab, pertuzumab, lapatinib, and T-DM1 drug conjugate.[6] Before trastuzumab approval, life expectancy was 20 months for these Her-2-positive, metastatic patients.[6] Castration resistant prostate cancer patients can live more than 24 months after sequential use of sipuleucel T followed by docetaxel, cabazitaxel, abiraterone, enzalutamide, and radium 223.[7]

In Cuba, several innovative drugs improving the survival of head and neck cancer, high grade gliomas, esophageal and lung cancers have been approved. Remarkably, the combination of chemo/radiochemotherapy and nimotuzumab, a humanized anti-Epidermal Growth Factor Receptor (EGFR) antibody, has produced a significant improvement in the overall survival of newly diagnosed squamous cell carcinoma of the head and neck (SCCHN)[8] and high grade glioma patients.[9] The approval of Vaxira and Cimavax, two novel therapeutic cancer vaccines, has provided survival improvement for advanced lung cancer patients.[10,11]

6.2.2 The Shape of Survival Curves: Delayed Tails, Probability Functions, and Bimodality

Beyond the mean figures of survival, a closer look at the kinetics of mortality provides additional insight on the transition to chronicity. For several cancers, the relative survival curve will reach a plateau some years after diagnosis, indicating that the mortality among survivors is approaching the expected mortality in the general population. Two populations often compose survival curves: a group of patients with short-term survival (population 1) and a subset of long-term survivors (population 2), from whom the hazard risk after some time is much lower.[12,13] Long-term survivorship even in advanced cancer has been described in patients bearing different tumor types including breast, colorectal, lymphoma, melanoma, and renal cell carcinoma.[5,6,14–16] Our group recently reviewed the survival data of 4944 patients with stages IIIb/IV NSCLC, registered in the National Cancer Registry of Cuba between January 1998 and December 2006. Patients' survival was fitted assuming Gaussian, Log-normal, Weibull, and Gamma models, according to a one-component and a

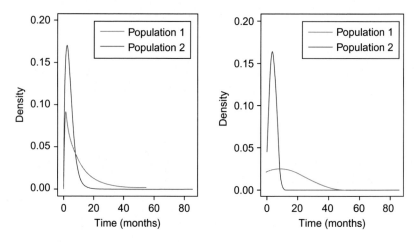

Figure 6.1 Density survival curves for short-term (1) and long-term survival (2) populations assuming Gaussian (a) and Gamma (b) distributions for the survival of nonsmall cell lung cancer patients from the Cuban National Cancer Registry.

two-component model (Fig. 6.1). Best fit was obtained for the two-component pattern. Once more, even for advanced lung cancer, the model comparison demonstrated that there is a subgroup with chronic evolution.[17]

6.2.3 Second Tumors in Long-Term Survivors

The number of patients who survive cancer diagnosis is growing by 2% each year.[18] Second primary neoplasms, particularly solid tumors, are a major cause of mortality and serious morbidity among cancer survivors successfully cured of their first cancer. This could be attributed to several causes: the deregulation of oncogenes and tumor suppressor genes that condition cancer development, a "chronic inflammatory state," and the long-term effect of radiotherapy and chemotherapy. According to US data, 18% of incident malignancies are a second cancer. Multiple etiologies may lead to a second primary neoplasm, including radiotherapy for the first cancer, unhealthy lifestyle behaviors, genetic factors, aging, or an interaction between any of these factors.[18]

The emergence of a second primary neoplasm is well established among patients with prolonged survival after treatment from a primary tumor, describing a chronic trend, which cannot be reversed by the treatment of each particular tumor. Shared risk factors, genetic susceptibility, and the late effects of previous cancer treatments contribute to that condition in diverse proportions according to tumor types.[19–22]

6.3 THE PHARMACOLOGIC CONSEQUENCE: ANTICANCER DRUGS FOR LONG-TERM USE

Chronic diseases require long-term treatments. Anticancer drugs are progressively being used for a prolonged time. Although modern targeted therapies are now an example of this trend, there are precedents in hormone therapy. Increasing evidence supports the use of extended endocrine therapy with either tamoxifen or an aromatase inhibitor after 5 years of initial adjuvant tamoxifen to reduce breast cancer recurrence and mortality.[23] In a recently published meta-analysis involving more than 29,000 breast cancer women, extended endocrine therapy beyond 5 years of tamoxifen significantly improved overall survival compared with 5 years only. Locoregional and distant relapses were reduced by 36% and 13%, respectively. The benefits of long-term androgen deprivation therapy (ADT) in patients with advanced prostate cancer are well established and recent studies have shown that long-term ADT with radiotherapy improves survival in patients with earlier stages of disease.[24,25] Novel compounds like targeted therapies are more efficacious when used long-term in hematological malignancies. Imatinib, one of the first approved targeted therapies for chronic myeloid leukemia, should be used for a prolonged time.[26] The uninterrupted blockade of Her-2 (using trastuzumab, lapatinib, pertuzumab, or T-DM1) is the standard practice for the treatment of advanced Her-2 positive breast cancer patients. In the absence of lapatinib, pertuzumab, or T-DM1, prolonged exposure to trastuzumab, even after the progression of the disease, is recommended for metastatic breast cancer patients.[6] Continuous hampering of the Vascular Endothelial Growth Factor (VEGF)/Vascular Endothelial Growth Factor Receptor (VEGFR) signaling pathway using bevacizumab, regorafenib, or aflibercept is recommended for metastatic colorectal cancer patients.

Data from the Center of Molecular Immunology (CIM) in Cuba also support that prolonged treatment with nimotuzumab, a humanized anti-EGFR antibody, grants better outcomes.[27] We hypothesize that prolonged use of nimotuzumab, even beyond progressive disease, might be needed to exert its maximal clinical effect, since maintaining a prolonged blockade on the Her1 signaling pathways would be crucial for Her1-positive cancer cells throughout all the natural history of disease. Prolonged use of nimotuzumab is safe and there is preliminary evidence on the benefit of maintenance therapy versus short-term in the scenario of advanced SCCHN. In the systematic review of five different trials enrolling unresectable SCCHN patients receiving the same therapy, there was a significant survival advantage for those patients in whom treatment prescription was larger than six doses, as compared to patients receiving less.[27] Cancer vaccines had a larger survival impact after prolonged vaccination. Most cancer antigens are self-proteins or carbohydrates, for which breaking tolerance and keeping immune response, demands frequent antigen challenges. For maintaining antibody titers against self epidermal growth factor (EGF), repeated immunizations with the EGF-Vaccine was required.[28] Another therapeutic vaccine, racotumomab that mimics NGcGM3, has also been used for very a prolonged time in advanced nonsmall cell lung carcinoma patients that were alive after the first year of treatment.[11] In general, for targeted therapies and immunotherapy, prolonged use even after progressive disease or retreatment after a treatment break at the moment of tumor progression is the recommended practice. Chronic treatment with safe drugs is instrumental in transforming cancer into a chronic disease.[29]

6.4 THE EXPANDING ROLE OF IMMUNOTHERAPY

The idea of mobilizing the immune system to control tumor growth is very old. Evidence in laboratory animals indicating that the immune system can be active against tumor cells began to accumulate more than 60 years ago. However, the implementation of this idea in the clinical setting has been characterized by successive waves of enthusiasm and disappointment. Bacillus Calmette -Guérin (BCG) and levamisole nonspecific immunostimulation, interferon, and interleukin-2 (IL-2) provided clinical evidence of antitumor activity but their role in the oncology practice remained limited.[30] Several clinical trials testing active specific immunostimulation (therapeutic vaccines) also failed.[31,32] Nevertheless in the 21st century, with the advent of monoclonal antibodies and the discovery of immune "checkpoints," cancer immunotherapy seems to have matured to become a systematic tool in cancer treatment. Immunotherapy marks an entirely different way of treating cancer by targeting the immune system, not the tumor itself.[33] Based on the very promising results in the clinical setting of the checkpoints inhibitors and adoptive therapy with chimeric receptor-transfected T cells, immunotherapy was appointed as the breakthrough result of the year in 2013 by Science magazine.[34] Blocking the blockers like the CTLA-4 and PD1 molecules would set the immune system free to fight cancer. Antibodies against CTLA-4,

PD1, and PD1-ligands represent a major step forward and are the first examples of efficacious immunotherapies in advanced cancer.[31] Such immune-based therapies would offer two advantages over other cancer drugs: these therapies could be applied to a diverse range of tumor types, and patients would not be expected to develop resistance.[34] In another strategy, researchers are genetically engineering T cells, introducing a chimeric receptor to target tumor cells. Although many clinical trials are still ongoing, the first results are very promising: some patients with end-stage metastatic disease are surviving for much longer than anticipated. At the Memorial Sloan-Kettering Cancer Center in New York, it was reported that the T cell therapy achieved 45 complete remissions in 75 adults and children with leukemia.[35]

At CIM, the cancer therapy pipeline includes several cancer vaccines and monoclonal antibodies against tumor specific antigens, as well as novel drugs to circumvent tumor-induced immunosuppression. A human IL-2 mutant (Fig. 6.2) has been developed with higher antitumor efficacy and lower toxicity than wild type IL-2 (wtIL-2). The mutant induces *in vitro* proliferation of $CD8^+CD44^{hi}$ memory T cells and NK1.1 cells as efficiently as wtIL-2, but it shows a reduced capacity to activate the regulatory T cells. The IL-2 mutant shows a higher antimetastatic effect than wtIL-2 in several transplantable tumor models. In silico simulations, predict that the properties of the IL-2 mutein

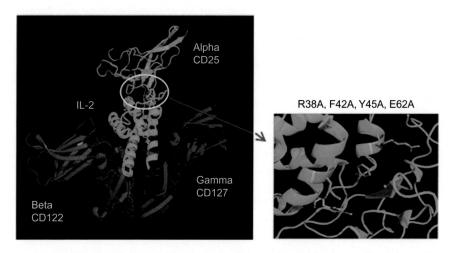

Figure 6.2 *Bioinformatic design of the human IL-2 mutant with decreased affinity for CD25. This IL-2 mutein will acts as an IL-2 agonist. The IL-2 mutant will activate the NK and memory CD8 T cells, but not the regulatory T cells.*

are a consequence of the reduction of two orders of magnitude in its affinity for CD25.[36]

The appeal of cancer immunotherapy has been based in the promises of diversity, specificity, low toxicity, and possible long-term use. The huge size of the immune repertoire (roughly a billion different antibody molecules circulate in a human being) allows a very specific targeting of relevant molecules in a tumor cell with limited damaging of normal cells. The possibility of long-term use due to low toxicity has also been validated in the clinical setting. But there is more than that. Immunotherapy is not just another targeted therapy prone to be used long-term. It has the unique possibility of target spreading and evolution. Although the clonal heterogeneity, genetic instability, and clonal evolution of tumors have always been suspected on experimental and clinical grounds, recent advances in DNA sequencing technology have allowed measuring these phenomena and the emerging numbers are far bigger than anticipated.[37,38] Such a permanent and adaptive generation of cellular heterogeneity is a feature that distinguishes cancer from other chronic diseases. It has therapeutic implications. The regular and fast appearance of resistance to the treatment of melanoma with B-Raf proto-oncogene, serine/threonine kinase (B-RAF) specific inhibitors illustrates the ironic fact that the more specific the treatment is, the more rapidly resistance appears. A naïve strategy would be to do repeated cycles of biopsies, identification of new mutations driving resistance, and change of the specific drug. The recent development of liquid biopsy technology (through circulating DNA) would facilitate the process, but still this man-made evolution of individual treatment will have huge practical limitations. The mobilization of the immune system could be the alternative, providing the simultaneous attack of diverse molecular targets and the evolution of the response coping with the clonal evolution of the tumor itself, as happens in the centuries-old coevolution of the immune system and the microbial environment. This theoretical possibility seems to be verified by the recent description of "antigen-spreading" in the antitumor immune response.[39,40]

At CIM, it has been described that a monoclonal antibody targeting EGFR induces immunogenic apoptosis of cancer cells, as shown by the extracellular exposure of calreticulin, whereas a small molecule tyrosine kinase inhibitor, although also slowing cell proliferation, does not induce immunogenic cell death (Fig. 6.3).[41]

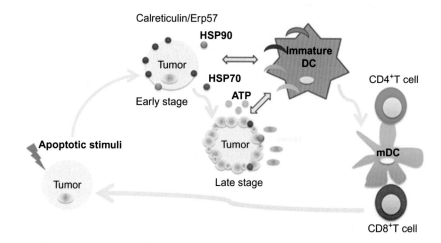

Figure 6.3 How apoptotic cells alert the immune system about danger. Antibodies targeting EGFR induce immunogenic cell death confirmed by the expression of calreticulin, endoplasmic reticulum protein 57 (ERp57), and the secretion of heat shock proteins 70 and 90. Immunogenic death of tumor cells transforms immature dendritic cells into mature dendritic cells that trigger CD4 and CD8 T cells activation.

6.5 A METHODOLOGICAL CONSEQUENCE: THE NEED OF NOVEL APPROACHES TO CLINICAL TRIAL DESIGN AND EVALUATION

The use of targeted therapies, which slow tumor progression and increase survival, but do not dramatically reduce the tumor size, has created a problem for the evaluation of the new drugs. The conventional paradigm of clinical development encompassing Phase I, Phase II, and Phase III trials is not applicable to these kinds of drugs. For conventional chemotherapy drugs, the maximum tolerated dose should be established in Phase I. Drugs might be effective in open populations and only patients with good performance status can be treated with chemotherapy. Additionally, since cytotoxic drugs induce rapid tumor shrinkage, the response rate is the preferred endpoint for Phase II trials for which evaluation tools (such as RECIST or WHO criteria) have been developed. Treatment should be stopped at progressive disease. On the contrary, for targeted therapy and immunotherapy, the optimal biologic dose (which is not the maximal tolerated dose) should be established in Phase I, and trials should be conducted in well-defined populations, including the evaluation of target/antigen expression and immune-competence. Patients with poor performance status can still tolerate and benefit from targeted therapy or immunotherapy. Contrary to chemotherapy, immunotherapy may not cause tumor reduction. As a result, response rate, time to progression, and progression-free survival might not accurately reflect vaccine or antibody activity; overall survival together with QoL are the best endpoints. Finally, a delayed response, which may follow initial progression, might occur, since the immune system needs time to elicit a protective response. Consequently, treatment should be continued beyond clinically irrelevant progression, to allow a late response to occur.[42,43]

Over recent years, several initiatives across the cancer immunotherapy community have been promoted by the Cancer Immunotherapy Consortium. Firstly, as results from T cell immune response assays are highly variable, harmonization of assays can minimize variability and support the investigation of the cellular immune response as a biomarker of clinical efficacy.[44] Secondly, as immunotherapy induces novel patterns of the antitumor response not captured by WHO or RECIST methodologies, new immune-related response criteria were defined.[45] Thirdly, as survival curves in randomized immunotherapy trials often show a delayed separation, there is a need of different statistic tools to assess significance.[46]

Moreover, testing the hypothesis of a transition to chronicity would also require measurements of QoL in the clinical trials. For cancer patients, not only survival is important but also the QoL of the gained months or years. With the gradual survival improvement achieved with immunotherapy and targeted therapy, QoL has an increasing relevance when evaluating a new drug.[47] Contrary to conventional chemotherapy, these types of drugs are very specific and would not generally hamper normal organs. Therefore, all trials evaluating this new class of compounds should incorporate validated questionnaires of QoL.[48,49]

6.6 IMMUNE REBALANCING: THE RESEARCH AGENDA FOR THE AGE OF CHRONICITY

For the first time cancer seems to have transited from an often incurable, rapidly fatal disease, to a "clinically manageable" chronic disease.[50] Research strategies must take note of this transition. New therapies should be amenable for long-term use, should preserve the QoL, and should be useful for elderly patients with comorbidities.

Immunotherapy could be the main tool for accelerating this transition, but this time our theoretical framework must go beyond the reductionists' views of immunity stimulation (as for infectious diseases) or suppression (as for autoimmune diseases or transplants), and foresee a fine "rebalancing" of the immune response, as it can play a dual role in tumors, sometimes inhibiting tumor progression and sometimes promoting it. Research priorities can be formulated at three levels. The first level is the optimization of the use of already available therapeutic weapons. That means producing knowledge for optimal treatment dosage and schedule, duration, and intervals together with the evaluation of treatment beyond progression either as continuous maintenance or rechallenge. The classic dogma in oncology dictates that therapy should be changed at disease progression, because the cancer is assumed to have become drug-resistant. There are circumstances where patients respond to the reintroduction of the same therapy after a drug holiday following disease relapse or progression. Additional evidence suggests that, in certain conditions, continuing a therapy beyond disease progression can also have antitumor activity.[29]

Research priorities should also include the adequate selection of patients for each therapeutic drug. This is extremely important for targeted therapy and immunotherapy, which might not work if the target is not relevant for tumor growth in a given patient. In that sense, clinical trials to prospectively or retrospectively validate predictive biomarkers of drugs efficacy should be designed to personalize therapy. Another relevant research avenue is the development of algorithms to predict optimal combinations. There are a large number of approved drugs for cancer therapy, together with more than 300 antibodies and 300 vaccines under clinical development. Accordingly, it will be impossible to try many combinations in the preclinical and clinical setting without the assistance of computational programs and well-designed algorithms. As immunotherapy must work in many cases with senescent immune system, the study of markers of immune-senescence and their relationships with treatment outcomes will be mandatory.

Cancer programs should include "complex packages" encompassing primary and secondary prevention, early diagnosis, better therapeutic as well as palliative drugs more than isolated interventions, which are less likely to modify cancer survival. Beyond biology and clinical research, a scientific approach will be needed for the study of the performance of health systems in handling chronic diseases. It will demand operational research, including social sciences. In summary, the reality of an increasing population of patients living (and socially active) with advanced cancer is already here, demanding adjustment of both cancer control strategies and research agendas. In a second level comes the continuous discovery of new therapeutic targets, which will provide novel drugs and novel predictive biomarkers. Living species have evolved adding successive layers of complexity in molecular regulatory networks. This means that there are numerous redundant regulatory loops both in cell proliferation control, and in the immune response control. Novel fast and cheap DNA sequencing techniques will provide many more actionable molecular targets and emerging evidence suggests that we cannot expect the discovery of widespread molecular lesions, but instead many possible targets, each one relevant for a smaller proportion of tumors. This cumulative process of new molecular markers and new drugs for small patient niches will soon overwhelm the capacity of the industry to manufacture and the capacity of the health system to absorb and deliver. Then a third and more basic research level should address the intrinsic complexity of the immune system and the evolutionary mechanisms that have created it for protecting life until the reproductive age, and not beyond. We guess that these mechanisms are related to chronic inflammation. Chronic inflammation is a complex process that underlies most chronic diseases, including atherosclerosis, autoimmune diseases, cognitive disorders, and surely cancer. Moreover, it is a hallmark of senescence even in the absence of any "disease" as we classify them. As frequently happens in complex systems, there is a "dual role" for inflammation. It is required for the immune reaction to be effective, as has recently been ratified by the relationship between tumor infiltration by inflammatory cells and sensitivity to treatment with checkpoints inhibiting antibodies. But on the other side, inflammation brings cells and molecules inhibiting the immune system and facilitating tumor escape. This is not a contradiction. The immune system has been selected for short-term responses and rapid in-built contraction,[51] which makes evolutionary sense by protecting individuals successfully in handling acute infections and discarding the others. As humans (not other primates) enjoy a long postreproductive life in the pathogen-free and nutrition abundant environment built by themselves, chronic inflammation becomes deleterious in advanced ages, so creating a genome—environment mismatch. Perhaps cancer incidence in the elderly is a downside of evolution itself.[52]

Using the immune system for chronic control of tumor growth will demand action on the fine-tuning between its tumor fighting and its tumor facilitating capabilities. Good news is that tools for such a rebalancing are starting to appear through the discovery of molecules regulating the size and duration of the immune response. The recent success of monoclonal antibodies targeting molecules that regulate the immune response, such as CTLA-4 on helper T lymphocytes and PD1 on effector T lymphocytes,[53] illustrate the potential of that strategy. The development of muteins of IL-2 and Transforming Growth Factor beta (TGFβ) at CIM is also in line with that goal. We will see in the near future the emergence of treatments aiming to handle simultaneously the concentration of several molecular mediators of the immune response, and the size of several cell subpopulations. But regulatory loops in the immune system can be expected to be too many and also redundant. Redundancy is a property of multicomponent complex systems and a requirement for robustness facing external perturbations. The role of each molecular component of regulatory loops will be dependent on the context given by the status of other components, and cannot be captured by dose-effect curves of conventional pharmacology. Mathematical modeling should step into cancer immunotherapy research. Imagine for example the possibility to use five biotechnology drugs able to modulate five cytokines, and another five antibodies tackling regulatory molecules in immune cells, and modulating cell population sizes. This scenario will place us walking in a 10-dimension space, with regions driving either to tumor growth or to tumor inhibition. Empiric design of therapeutic regimes will be simply impossible.

Progress in the practical goal of rebalancing the immune system to control cancer chronically will be connected to the emergence of a new fundamental biology with improved capacity to handle floods of molecular information coming from high throughputs measurement technologies and to understand the emergence of order and structure in complex and apparently chaotic systems. Such a convergence of sciences to fight cancer is starting to occur.

REFERENCES

1. Santosa A, Wall S, Fottrell E, Högberg U, Byass P. The development and experience of epidemiological transition theory over four decades: a systematic review. *Glob Health Action* 2014;7:235–74.

2. Coleman MP. Cancer survival: global surveillance will stimulate health policy and improve equity. *Lancet* 2014;**383**(9916):564–73.

3. Gomella LG, Gelpi-Hammerschmidt F, Kundavram C. Practical guide to immunotherapy in castration resistant prostate cancer: the use of sipuleucel-T immunotherapy. *Can J Urol* 2014;**21**(2 Suppl. 1):48–56.

4. Sanlorenzo M, Vujic I, Posch C, Dajee A, Yen A, Kim S, et al. Melanoma immunotherapy. *Cancer Biol Ther* 2014;**15**(6):665–74.

5. Tonini G, Imperatori M, Vincenzi B, Frezza AM, Santini D. Rechallenge therapy and treatment holiday: different strategies in management of metastatic colorectal cancer. *J Exp Clin Cancer Res* 2013;**32**(1):92.

6. Verma S, Joy AA, Rayson D, McLeod D, Brezden-Masley C, Boileau JF, et al. HER story: the next chapter in HER-2-directed therapy for advanced breast cancer. *Oncologist* 2013; **18**(11):1153–66.

7. Gomella LG, Petrylak DP, Shayegan B. Current management of advanced and castration resistant prostate cancer. *Can J Urol* 2014;(2 Suppl. 1):1–6.

8. Reddy BK, Lokesh V, Vidyasagar MS, Shenoy K, Babu KG, Shenoy A, et al. Nimotuzumab provides survival benefit to patients with inoperable advanced squamous cell carcinoma of the head and neck: a randomized, open-label, phase IIb, 5-year study in Indian patients. *Oral Oncol* 2014;**50**(5):498–505.

9. Solomón MT, Selva JC, Figueredo J, Vaquer J, Toledo C, Quintanal N, et al. Radiotherapy plus nimotuzumab or placebo in the treatment of high grade glioma patients: results from a randomized, double blind trial. *BMC Cancer* 2013;**13**:299.

10. Crombet T, Neninger E, Acosta S, Amador R, Mendoza S, Santiesteban E, et al. EGF-based cancer vaccine for advanced NSCLC: results from a phase III trial. *J Clin Oncol.* 2012;**30**:114 (Suppl.; abstr 2527).

11. Alfonso S, Valdes-Zayas A, Santiesteban ER, Flores YI, Areces F, Hernandez M, et al. A randomized, multicenter, placebo-controlled clinical trial of racotumomab-alum vaccine as switch maintenance therapy in advanced non-small-cell-lung cancer patients. *Clin Cancer Res* 2014;**20**(14):3660–71.

12. Andersson TM, Dickman PW, Eloranta S, Lambert PC. Estimating and modelling cure in population-based cancer studies within the framework of flexible parametric survival models. *BMC Med Res Methodol* 2011;**11**:96.

13. Lambert PC, Thompson JR, Weston CL, Dickman PW. Estimating and modeling the cure fraction in population-based cancer survival analysis. *Biostatistics* 2007;**8**:576–94.

14. Hiddemann W, Cheson BD. How we manage follicular lymphoma. *Leukemia* 2014; **28**(7):1388–95.

15. Eggermont A, Robert C, Soria JC, Zitvogel L. Harnessing the immune system to provide long-term survival in patients with melanoma and other solid tumors. *Oncoimmunology* 2014;**3**(1):e27560.

16. Pracht M, Berthold D. Successes and limitations of targeted therapies in renal cell carcinoma. *Prog Tumor Res* 2014;**41**:98–112.

17. Sanchez L, Lorenzo-Luaces P, Viada C, Galan Y, Ballesteros J, Crombet T, et al. Is there a subgroup of long-term evolution among patients with advanced lung cancer?: hints from the analysis of survival curves from cancer registry data. *BMC Cancer* 2014;**14**:933.

18. Oeffinger KC. Introduction: the science of survivorship: moving from risk to risk reduction. *Semin Oncol* 2013;**40**(6):662–5.

19. Caini S, Boniol M, Botteri E, Tosti G, Bazolli B, Russell-Edu W, et al. The risk of developing a second primary cancer in melanoma patients: a comprehensive review of the literature and meta-analysis. *J Dermatol Sci* 2014;**75**(1):3–9.

20. Sun LC, Tai YY, Liao SM, Lin TY, Shih YL, Chang SF, et al. Clinical characteristics of second primary cancer in colorectal cancer patients: the impact of colorectal cancer or other second cancer occurring first. *World J Surg Oncol* 2014;**12**:73.

21. Martin A, Schneiderman J, Helenowski IB, Morgan E, Dilley K, Danner-Koptik K, et al. Secondary malignant neoplasms after high-dose chemotherapy and autologous stem cell rescue for high-risk neuroblastoma. *Pediatr Blood Cancer* 2014;**61**(8):1350–6.

22. Petrucci MS, Brunori V, Masanotti GM, Bianconi F, La Rosa F, Stracci F. Incidence of multiple primary cancers following respiratory tract cancer in Umbria, Italy. *Ig Sanita Pubbl* 2013;**69**(5):629–38.

23. Jankowitz RC, McGuire KP, Davidson NE. Optimal systemic therapy for premenopausal women with hormone receptor-positive breast cancer. *Breast* 2013;**22**(Suppl. 2):S165–70.

24. Schulman C, Irani J, Aapro M. Improving the management of patients with prostate cancer receiving long-term androgen deprivation therapy. *BJU Int* 2012;**109**(Suppl. 6):13–21.

25. Daskivich TJ, Oh WK. Recent progress in hormonal therapy for advanced prostate cancer. *Curr Opin Urol* 2006;**16**(3):173–8.

26. Avilés-Vázquez S, Chávez-González A, Mayani H. Tyrosine kinase inhibitors (TKI): a new revolution in the treatment of chronic myeloid leukemia (CML). *Gac Med Mex* 2013;**149**(6):646–54.

27. Morejón O, Piedra P. Report of the fifth nimotuzumab global meeting. *Biotecnol Aplicada* 2009;**26**(4):1–6.

28. Gonzalez G, Crombet T, Torres F, Catala M, Alfonso L, Osorio M, et al. Epidermal growth factor-based cancer vaccine for non-small-cell lung cancer therapy. *Ann Oncol* 2003;**14**(3):461–6.

29. Kuczynski E, Sargent D, Grothey A, Kerbel R. Drug rechallenge and treatment beyond progression—implications for drug resistance. *Nat Rev Clin Oncol* 2013;**10**:571–87.

30. Dillman RO. Cancer immunotherapy. *Cancer Biother Radiopharm* 2011;**26**(1):1–64.

31. Ruiz R, Hunis B, Raez LE. Immunotherapeutic agents in non-small-cell lung cancer finally coming to the front lines. *Curr Oncol Rep* 2014;**16**(9):400.

32. Cuppens K, Vansteenkiste J. Vaccination therapy for non-small-cell lung cancer. *Curr Opin Oncol* 2014;**26**(2):165–70.

33. Couzin-Frankel J. Breakthrough of the year 2013. Cancer immunotherapy. *Science* 2013;**342**(6165):1432–3.

34. McNutt M. Cancer immunotherapy. *Science*; 2013;20;**342**(6165):1417.

35. Kalos M, June CH. Adoptive T cell transfer for cancer immunotherapy in the era of synthetic biology. *Immunity* 2013;**39**(1):49–60.

36. Carmenate T, Pacios A, Enamorado M, Moreno E, Garcia-Martínez K, Fuente D, et al. Human IL-2 mutein with higher antitumor efficacy than wild type IL-2. *J Immunol* 2013;**190**(12):6230–8.

37. Thompson BA, Spurdle AB. Microsatellite instability use in mismatch repair gene sequence variant classification. *Genes* 2015;**6**(2):150.

38. Bosman F, Yan P. Molecular pathology of colorectal cancer. *Pol J Pathol* 2014;**65**(4):257–66.

39. Singh BH, Gulley JL. Therapeutic vaccines as a promising treatment modality against prostate cancer: rationale and recent advances. *Ther Adv Vaccines* 2014;**2**(5):137–48.

40. Hu Y, Petroni GR, Olson WC, Czarkowski A, Smolkin ME, Grosh WW, et al. Immunologic hierarchy, class II MHC promiscuity, and epitope spreading of a melanoma helper peptide vaccine. *Cancer Immunol Immunother* 2014;**63**(8):779–86.

41. Garrido G, Rabasa A, Sánchez B. Linking oncogenesis and immune system evasion in acquired resistance to EGFR-targeting antibodies: lessons from a preclinical model. *Oncoimmunology* 2013;**2**(12):e26904.

42. Hoos A, Britten CM, Huber C, O'Donnell-Tormey J. A methodological framework to enhance the clinical success of cancer immunotherapy. *Nat Biotechnol* 2011;**29**(10):867−70.

43. Hoos A, Eggermont AM, Janetzki S, Hodi FS, Ibrahim R, Anderson A, et al. Improved endpoints for cancer immunotherapy trials. *J Natl Cancer Inst* 2010;**102**(18):1388−97.

44. Hoos A, Janetzki S, Britten CM. Advancing the field of cancer immunotherapy: MIATA consensus guidelines become available to improve data reporting and interpretation for T-cell immune monitoring. *Oncoimmunology* 2012;**1**(9):1457−9.

45. Wolchok JD, Hoos A, O'Day S, Weber JS, Hamid O, Lebbé C, et al. Guidelines for the evaluation of immune therapy activity in solid tumors: immune-related response criteria. *Clin Cancer Res* 2009;**15**(23):7412−20.

46. Hoos A. Evolution of end points for cancer immunotherapy trials. *Ann Oncol* 2012;**23** (Suppl. 8):viii47−52.

47. Efficace F, Jacobs M, Pusic A, Greimel E, Piciocchi A, Kieffer JM, et al. Patient-reported outcomes in randomised controlled trials of gynaecological cancers: investigating methodological quality and impact on clinical decision-making. *Eur J Cancer.* 2014;**50**(11):1925−41.

48. Leppert W, Majkowicz M, Forycka M, Mess E, Zdun-Ryzewska A. Quality of life assessment in advanced cancer patients treated at home, an inpatient unit, and a day care center. *Onco Targets Ther* 2014;**7**:687−95.

49. Bergman J, Laviana A. Quality-of-life assessment tools for men with prostate cancer. *Nat Rev Urol* 2014;**11**(6):352−9.

50. Dömling A, Holak TA. Programmed death-1: therapeutic success after more than 100 years of cancer immunotherapy. *Angew Chem Int Ed Engl* 2014;**53**(9):2286−8.

51. Garrod KR, Moreau HD, Garcia Z, Lemaître F, Bouvier I, Albert ML, et al. Dissecting T cell contraction *in vivo* using a genetically encoded reporter of apoptosis. *Cell Rep* 2012; **2**(5):1438−47.

52. Vasto S, Carruba G, Lio D, Colonna-Romano G, DiBona D, Candore G, et al. Inflammation, ageing and cancer. *Mech Ageing Dev* 2009;**130**:40−5.

53. Harshman LC, Drake CG, Wargo JA, et al. Cancer immunotherapy highlights from the 2014 ASCO meeting. *Cancer Immunol Res* 2014;**2**(8):714−19.

Biologics as Immunosuppressive Agents

CHAPTER 7

Modulation of Macrophage Activation

Paola Italiani, Elfi Töpfer and Diana Boraschi
Institute of Protein Biochemistry, National Research Council, Napoli, Italy

7.1 INTRODUCTION

Macrophages (from Greek "macro" and "phage," meaning "large" and "to eat," respectively) were traditionally seen as the cells that provide the first line of defense to infections by removing pathogens via phagocytosis, and accordingly were tagged as "the garbage men" of the immune system, or "trash disposal units" serving at the bequest of T and B cells. Over the past two decades, macrophages have been recognized as having a central defensive and homeostatic role, as main effector cells of inflammatory reactions, in maintaining tissue homeostasis, in supporting tissue development, and in repairing tissue damage. To fulfill this plethora of functions, macrophages exhibit a spectrum of transient polarization statuses that are influenced by varying microenvironmental cues. Current evidence has uncovered a series of immune and ontogenic features of macrophages, such as their embryonic origin, tissue heterogeneity, proliferative potential, polarization or plasticity, and memory (reviewed in Refs[1−5]).

Macrophages reside in all tissues of the body, and originate from circulating monocytes (until recently considered the only source of tissue-resident macrophages) and from precursors that seed the tissue during embryonic development (as recently described).[6−8]

The pool of tissue-resident macrophages is sustained by self-renewal and by their ability to proliferate during injury events.[9] Tissue macrophages acquire distinct morphological and physiological characteristics according to the organs and microenvironment in which they are present.[10] On the other hand, monocytes are generated in the bone marrow (BM) and released into the bloodstream, where they circulate for a few days. Monocytes can differentiate into macrophages after extravasation through the endothelium and infiltration into a tissue,

Immune Rebalancing. DOI: http://dx.doi.org/10.1016/B978-0-12-803302-9.00007-5

an event that occurs for steady state turnover (ie, tissue homeostasis) or for taking part into an inflammatory reaction in response to an infection or a trauma. These macrophages are called monocyte-derived macrophages.[11] Thus, tissue-resident macrophages and recruited monocyte-derived macrophages react to inflammatory stimuli in the inflamed tissue, and exhibit a spectrum of functional activities related to their functional diversity[12] and to the microenvironmental conditions.[13,14] This ability is called macrophage polarization (synonymous with macrophage activation).

In this review we refer to both tissue-resident macrophages and monocyte-derived macrophages using simply the word "macrophages." In fact, the mechanisms and implications of macrophage activation/polarization are valid for both cell types.

Among macrophage features, plasticity (ie, the capacity to polarize in different functional phenotypes) confers to macrophages the role of key players within the different phases of innate inflammatory responses (from the initiation to resolution). Thereby, macrophages are able to steer the adaptive immune cells according to circumstances, driving a Th1-type or Th2-type response, depending on the microenvironmental conditions and surrounding signals that are generated by different antigens.[15,16]

The aim of this review is to focus on macrophage polarization and its mechanisms during the course of an immune response, leaving the issues of the heterogeneity and plasticity due to tissue-specific signals during homeostasis to some recent excellent reviews.[2,9-14,17] We will describe how macrophage phenotypes can be integrated into the design of a new generation of immunomodulatory molecules/compounds and therapeutic strategies (eg, therapy of solid tumors), rebalancing the immune responses that have been altered by a pathological condition.

7.2 AN OVERVIEW ON MACROPHAGE POLARIZATION/ACTIVATION

As briefly mentioned in the introduction, macrophages are able to respond with appropriate functions in distinct contexts, and functional diversity becomes the key feature of these cells. Two main types of macrophage functions have been identified in vivo, the killing/inhibitory activity and the heal/growth-promoting function.[18,19] Accordingly, macrophages programmed to fulfill these functions are broadly classified as classical or M1-type macrophages, and alternative or M2-type macrophages. The main functions of M1 and M2 macrophages are the production of microbicidal and harmful reactive species such as nitric oxide (NO), in the case of M1 cells, and the production of the healing molecule ornithine, in the case of M2 macrophages. The M1/M2 macrophage subsets are most commonly distinguished based on the catabolism of Arginine (Arg). While classically activated macrophages express increased levels of inducible NO synthase (iNOS), which converts Arg to citrulline and NO, alternatively activated macrophages express Arginase I, which catabolizes Arg to ornithine, a precursor of polyamines and proline.[20,21]

The M1 functional phenotype emerges as a result of macrophage stimulation by inflammatory signals such as pathogen-associated molecular patterns [PAMPs; eg, the lipopolysaccharide (LPS) of Gram-negative bacteria], or damage-associated molecular patterns (DAMPs; such as HMGB1), or T cell cytokines, such as IFNγ. M1 macrophages are efficient producers of toxic effector molecules, such as reactive oxygen/nitrogen species, as well as inflammatory cytokines such as IL-1β, IL-6, IL-12, IL-23, and TNFα. M1 macrophages promote T lymphocyte activation/polarization in the Th1 direction and Th1 inflammatory cytokine production (eg, IFNγ and IL-2); and they mediate resistance against tumors.[15,22]

In the case of M2 macrophages, the large majority of studies has been conducted in vitro by exposing macrophages to the Th2-related cytokines IL-4 or IL-13, by the concomitant triggering of Fcγ receptors (eg, with immune complexes) and Toll-like receptors (TLRs), by exposure to anti-inflammatory molecules, such as IL-10, TGF-β, and glucocorticoids. These in vitro polarized M2 macrophages are characterized by high expression levels of scavenger receptors (eg, CD163), mannose receptors (eg, CD206), and galactose-type receptors. M2 macrophages take part in polarized Th2 responses, allergy, parasite clearance, dampening of inflammation, tissue remodeling, angiogenesis, immunoregulation, and tumor promotion.[4,20] In vivo, the M2 functional phenotype (healing/growth promotion) is the "default" program adopted by resident macrophages.[23] Fig. 7.1 summarizes the main features of M1 and M2 macrophages and their interplay with lymphocytes.

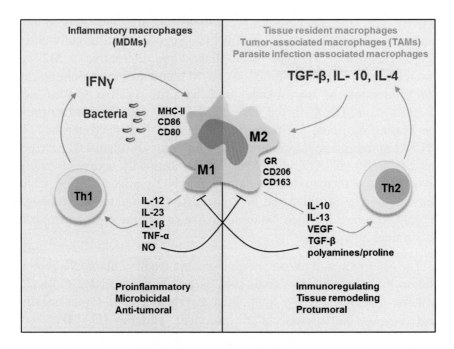

Figure 7.1 M1 and M2 macrophage activation and interplay with Th1 and Th2 lymphocytes. In the presence of bacterial infections and/or the Th1 cytokine IFNγ, macrophages polarize into an M1 phenotype, characterized by microbicidal and antitumor activity and by the production of inflammatory cytokines (eg, IL-12, IL-23, TNFα, IL-1β) and reactive species, such as NO generated upon transformation of Arg by iNOS. In the presence of the Th2-derived cytokines IL-4 and IL-13, or TGF-β and IL-10, macrophages polarize into an M2 phenotype, characterized by immune-regulating, tissue remodeling, and protumoral activities and by the production of anti-inflammatory cytokines (eg, IL-10, TGF-β), growth factors (eg, VEGF), and polyamines/proline generated upon transformation of Arg by Arg1. M1 and M2 macrophages activate Th1 and Th2 lymphocytes thereby triggering an adaptive immune response against microbial infections and tumors, or against parasite infections and allergies, respectively. In turn, Th1 and Th2 lymphocytes keep macrophages in active M1 and M2 functional states. Moreover, NO and TGF-β inhibit M2-like and M1-like phenotype development, respectively. M1 are inflammatory macrophages, mostly originating from circulating monocytes recruited into damaged tissues upon infection or trauma. On the other hand, M2 macrophages are tissue-resident macrophages, TAMs, and monocyte-derived macrophages recruited during parasite infection or homeostatic turnover. GR, galactose-type receptor; MDMs, monocyte-derived macrophages.

For a thorough understanding of macrophage polarization, one should bear in mind the following considerations. TLR agonists and other stimuli can induce M1- or M2-type polarization in vitro, but the original description of M1/inhibit and M2/heal-type macrophage responses was in vivo, specifically in sterile wounds and in supporting or rejecting tumors (reviewed in Ref.[24]). Neither one of these responses requires the contribution of T cells or adaptive immunity. Indeed, while Th1 and Th2 cytokines promote M1 and M2 macrophage activation in vitro, the M1 and M2 phenotypes can be observed in T cell-deficient mice, suggesting that T helper cells are not required to drive macrophage polarization in vivo.[19,25] Thus, M1 and M2 macrophages do not need to be activated by T cell cytokines, like IFNγ or IL-4.[25] Actually, PAMPs and DAMPs are the major polarizing signals in vivo. The in vitro work shows a variety of M1 and M2 polarization phenotypes in response to a variety of different stimuli and their combinations. This has led to the concept, possibly misleading, that M1 and M2 polarization are the extremes of a functional continuum, that is, a spectrum of diverse functional states.[26] David Mosser with his "color wheel"[26] and more recently Joachim Schultze's group[27] with his "spectrum" model of macrophages, have proposed vast or even seamless heterogeneity in macrophages "types." In fact, in order to organize this broad spectrum of phenotypes, Murray and coworkers attempted a reclassification of polarized macrophages in response to a range of stimuli,[28] while Martinez and Gordon[29] suggest it is time for reassessing the concept of macrophage activation.

George Mackaness[30] discovered macrophage "activation" in vivo in the 1960s, though macrophages were believed at that time to be dependent on T cells for their activation. Siamon Gordon[31] observed in the 1990s that macrophages incubated with IL-4 displayed an increase in different activities and markers, such as scavenger receptors. Now, these activities are typically referred to as M2-type, although, as mentioned above, there is evidence that the contribution of T cell cytokines is not necessary. Indeed, in all tissues examined resident macrophages are M2-type (as defined by their ability to produce ornithine, but not NO). Also, there is no IL-4 in either sterile wounds or most tumors, both of which are strongly M2-type inflammatory events. Thus, M2 is the default functional program in macrophages, and it can be amplified in T cell-independent inflammation. From this viewpoint, the continuum mentioned above is not really a continuum of diverse functional states but a series of variations in functional phenotypes. We personally support a recently proposed attempt at explaining this alleged heterogeneity,[24] which is summarized below. If one takes resident macrophages that express M2/heal-type activity and expose them to M1 activating stimuli, like IFNγ or LPS, massive changes occur in macrophage physiology in order to adopt a different function. During the transition from M2-dominance to M1-dominance over several hours, one will necessarily find macrophages of "intermediate" type. Thus, examining macrophages at different times during this transition, one will of course detect different functional profiles in terms of gene upregulation and secretion of factors and cytokines.

The M1/M2 polarization/activation that occurs during infection or inflammation also occurs under homeostatic conditions or during stress in the tissue. This polarization involves both resident macrophages and monocyte-derived macrophages. The macrophages residing in tissues constantly exposed to stress (eg, mucosae, skin, heart) all come from circulating monocytes (continuous recruitment due to a sort of low grade inflammation?), while in other tissues (eg, brain, liver) they are mostly yolk sac-derived and self-maintaining cells with an M2-like phenotype.

The tissue provides endless combinations of different signals, which change with changes in the tissue functions, age, diseases, and stress. Macrophages are prepared to react to such combinations of tissue signals by taking either a killing/inhibitory phenotype (M1) for defense, or a healing phenotype (M2) for tissue repair.

It is worth reminding that the M2/heal-type activity (ornithine, TGF-β production, etc.) evolved long before the M1/inhibit-type activity (NO production).[32] Indeed, the ability to repair is a primordial function, exhibited by even simple multicellular animals. Most people think of immunity as "killing stuff." But one should bear in mind that the normal day-by-day function of macrophages is to repair and replace cells and matrices lost to senescence or injury. The body does not routinely produce toxic molecules (like NO), because these molecules are nonspecifically toxic and will damage the body's cells and tissues (unlike adaptive effectors such as CTL or antibodies that can kill specifically, with limited collateral damage). Thus, a tight control of their activation mechanisms is necessary in order to keep macrophages/innate immunity in a "constructive" mode.

7.3 M1/M2 SKEWING: DETRIMENTAL AND BENEFICIAL CONSEQUENCES

Important questions in macrophage polarization are whether polarized macrophage populations can switch from one to the other in response to different conditions; whether these activation states involve recruitment of circulating monocyte precursors or the re-education of cells in situ or both; and whether M1 and M2 polarization is reversible.

The answers for all these issues seem to be positive. Indeed, according to a model of functional adaptation proposed by Stout and Suttles,[33] macrophages are capable not only of adapting to microenvironmental signals by adopting different functional programs, but also of changing their functional phenotype in response to progressive variations of these signals or their temporal presentation.[34] Data from in vitro studies demonstrate that human monocytes can acquire the phenotype of polarized M1 macrophages and then mature into M2 repair macrophages upon exposure to sequential changes in the microenvironmental conditions.[35] Furthermore, the induction of TNFα and IL-12 production by the inflammatory (M1 polarizing) cytokines or LPS can be significantly dampened in the presence of the M2 polarizing cytokines IL-4 or TGF-β.[25]

The best proof of functional M1/M2 phenotype switching comes from observations in tissues such as brain, liver, and adipose tissue, where the number of M1 and M2 macrophages changes during homeostatic and inflammatory conditions, and from observations in severe pathological disorders such as cancer and obesity. Tissue-resident macrophages as well as monocyte-derived macrophages appear to have the capability of adopting both M1 and M2 phenotypes. However, the relative contribution of these macrophage subsets to the progression and resolution of chronic inflammation remains unclear. An attempt to clarify the role of these two macrophage populations in the tissue, and their similarities and differences during homeostasis and inflammatory conditions, is reported elsewhere.[11,12]

Here we want to underline how the shift or the imbalance between M1 and M2 phenotypes can induce beneficial effects, but also have detrimental consequences if not appropriately regulated (Fig. 7.2). The involvement of an altered M1/M2 ratio with the development or progression of diseases has been widely observed. Following are some examples.

An increase in both M1 and M2 phenotypes is observed in experimental models of chronic diseases of the central nervous system, for example, Alzheimer's disease and experimental autoimmune encephalitis (an experimental model of multiple sclerosis).[36] In these diseases, M1 cells outnumber the M2 cells in the early stages of chronic inflammation, disrupting normal neuronal/glial cross-talk, and promoting a proinflammatory milieu implicated in the progression of disease.[37,38]

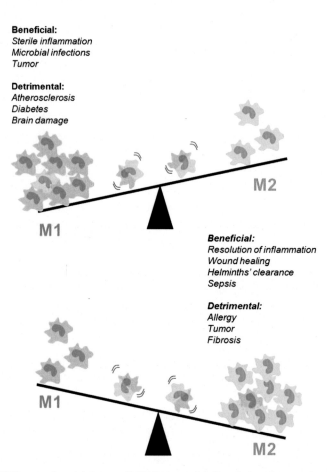

Figure 7.2 *M1/M2 macrophage imbalance or "M1/M2 skewing." Polarized macrophage populations can switch from one to the other in response to different environmental conditions. Thus, M1 inflammatory macrophages can mature into M2 repair macrophages and vice versa in response to molecular changes in the surrounding microenvironment. An imbalance towards a predominance of M2 or M1 phenotypes can be beneficial or detrimental depending on the pathological circumstances. For example, M1 macrophages are required in the protective inflammatory response against microbial infections, tissue injury, or tumors. However, M1 macrophages cause destructive inflammation in atherosclerosis, diabetes, or brain damage. Likewise, the M2 macrophage response is beneficial as it contributes to resolution of inflammation, wound healing, and protection against parasite infections. On the other hand, M2 activity is detrimental in exacerbated allergic responses and in pathological fibrosis, and it can contribute to the progression of neoplasias by promoting tumor survival.*

Moreover, the classically activated M1 phenotype is predominant in acute pathological conditions such as traumatic brain injury, spinal cord injury, stroke, and ischemic reperfusion injury, as well as in experimental LPS-induced systemic inflammation.[38,39]

Increasingly evident is also the involvement of inflammation and macrophage polarization in the development of the metabolic syndrome. For example, the progression of obesity implies a shift in the phenotype of adipose tissue macrophages from M2/heal (as in healthy nonobese humans) to classically activated M1 macrophages.[40] The same shift has been observed in type-2 diabetes, where M1 macrophages contribute to glucose intolerance and insulin resistance through mechanisms that are still unclear.[41] Another syndrome linked to obesity or metabolism is atherosclerosis, where it is now well established that atherosclerotic plaques contain both M1 and M2 macrophages. However, this M1/M2 balance seems to be dynamic, with M1 predominating in plaque progression and M2 in regression.[42]

In the liver, M1 macrophages are involved in hepatic steatosis or nonalcoholic fatty liver disease, while M2 macrophages promote the development of fibrosis.[12,43]

Macrophage polarization is responsible for the host response to bacteria, with M1-type macrophages being protective (killing bacteria), whereas M2-type macrophages are exploited by pathogens for intracellular survival, and are therefore associated with bacterial persistence.[44,45] When a systemic inflammatory response occurs following an infection, for instance in sepsis, both M1 and M2 macrophages are involved, but in different phases: M1 during the early phase and M2 at a later stage. However, enrichment of M2 macrophages has no impact on sepsis prognosis,[46] and sepsis does not exhibit a characteristic profile of macrophage polarization. In order to understand the contribution of macrophages to the human infectious disease development, it has been recently proposed that the type of myeloid cells (monocytes vs macrophages) and the kinetics of the immune response (early vs late responses) are critical variables.[47] Finally, in cancer, tumor-infiltrating classically activated macrophages have the potential to counteract the early stages of neoplasia, and then, as the tumor progresses, they progressively differentiate to a regulatory phenotype and eventually become cells that share the characteristics of both regulatory and wound healing macrophages.[48]

Macrophage polarization also occurs in the course of pathologies such as chronic inflammation in rheumatoid arthritis or lupus nephritis, where there is an imbalance of the M1/M2 ratio in favor of M1.[49,50]

In all the above cases, signals present in the surrounding microenvironment at a given time drive the changes in the functional phenotype of macrophages and at a given stage of the disease. This suggests that the presence of macrophages in different states of polarization in the same microenvironment can be harnessed to induce appropriate functions thereby minimizing the harmful effect of the M1/M2 disequilibrium.

As mentioned above, it is now generally recognized that the M1/M2 polarization of macrophages plays a central role in the progression of chronic inflammation in a wide range of diseases. This leads researchers to exploring the regulation of macrophage polarization as a possible therapeutic approach to chronic inflammatory diseases. To this end, the knowledge of the mechanisms underlying macrophage polarization becomes a central issue.

7.4 MECHANISMS OF MACROPHAGE ACTIVATION

Extensive research has provided important clues in identifying the molecular mechanisms underlying the M1 and M2 activation of macrophages. As shown in Fig. 7.3, these mechanisms encompass: (1) Local activation by exogenous and endogenous molecules, such as cytokines, myelopoietic growth factors, DAMPs (eg, HMGB1, adenosine, uric acid), PAMPs (eg, LPS, peptidoglycans, β-glucans, nucleic acids), interferons, and complement components; (2) triggering of different signaling pathways upon pathogen recognition receptors activation; (3) subsequent activation of different transcription factors; (4) a wide microRNA (miRNA) network; (5) gene expression reprogramming by epigenetic mechanisms; and (6) reprogramming of metabolism. Recent excellent reviews have been published on each of these mechanisms, and we invite the reader to refer to them for more detailed information.[51,52] Herein we will only provide a brief summary of them. All these mechanisms strictly cooperate in a network of interactions that culminates in specific patterns of gene expression that determine the macrophage functional phenotype.

7.4.1 Signaling

As mentioned before, TLR signaling (as for instance TLR4 stimulated by LPS and other microbial molecules) or type-I interferons drive macrophages towards an M1 phenotype, while cytokines like IL-4, IL-13, and IL-10 promote M2 polarization.[31,53] Canonical IRF/STAT/SOCS signaling is a major regulatory pathway in modulating M1 and M2

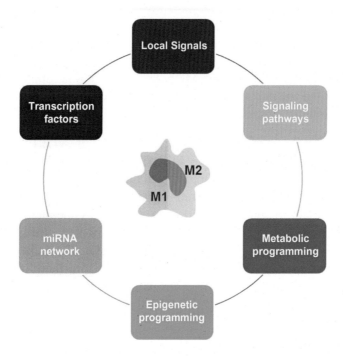

Figure 7.3 Mechanisms of macrophage polarization. Initiation and modulation of macrophage polarization towards M1 or M2 encompass tissue-generated signals/molecules arising from microbial infections, tissue injury (upon trauma or disease), and during tissue homeostatic processes (local signals); different signaling pathways triggered by DAMPs and PAMPs or cytokines such as IFNγ, IL-4, IL-13 (signaling pathways); a metabolic shift from oxidative phosphorylation towards glycolysis or vice versa (metabolic reprogramming); post-translational modifications at the gene promoting and enhancing regions (epigenetic reprogramming); regulation of gene expression by miRNAs (miRNA network); and activation of different transcription factors (transcription factors).

polarization. Indeed, activation of IRF/STAT signaling by LPS or IFNγ via STAT1 skews macrophage functions toward the M1 phenotype, while activation via STAT6 and STAT3 by IL-4/IL-13 and IL-10, respectively, skews macrophage functions toward M2 phenotype.[22,51,54] Upon TLR4 activation by LPS, the two adapters MyD88 and TRIF mediate the downstream signaling by triggering a cascade of kinases, including IRAK4, TRAF6, and IKKβ, which finally leads to the activation of the transcription factor NF-κB. Transcription factors IRF3 and IRF5 are also critically involved in directing macrophages toward M1 polarization by upregulating proinflammatory genes and dampening expression of M2 markers.[55,56] These transcription factors in turn regulate the expression of a large number of inflammatory genes, such as IL-1β, TNFα, IL-6, IL-12p40, IL-8, and cycloxygenase 2 (COX2). In contrast, alternative stimulation of macrophages with IL-4 and IL-13 leads to activation of JAK1 and JAK3,[57] and then to STAT6 activation and translocation.[58] M2 polarization is promoted by several other transcription factors including PPARγ, KLF-4, and IRF4. All these transcription factors coordinate the M2 polarization of macrophages thereby protecting the host from parasite infection and inhibiting the development of insulin resistance.[59,60]

SOCS family members are key regulators of STAT activity in macrophages.[61] IL-4 and IFNγ/TLR ligands upregulate SOCS1 and SOCS3, which, in turn, inhibit the action of STAT1 and STAT3, respectively.[62,63] Recently, Notch signaling has been implicated in regulating macrophage polarization in a SOCS3-dependent manner,[64] by increasing translation of the transcription factor IRF8.[24,65] Furthermore, it was shown that SOCS2 and SOCS3 are key opposite regulators of M1 and M2 macrophage polarization, therefore controllers of the inflammatory response.[66] The role of transcription factors in M1 and M2 polarization has been recently reviewed.[67,68]

7.4.2 Endogenous Factors

In vivo and in vitro studies have demonstrated a role for the myeloid colony-stimulating factors M-CSF and GM-CSF in macrophage functional polarization. GM-CSF amplifies the response to M1 polarizing stimuli, while M-CSF potentiates responses to M2 stimuli. The role of these growth factors in macrophage polarization has been detailed in a recent review.[69]

Complement has an important role in driving the macrophage polarization (reviewed in Ref.[70]). Indeed complement components, such as anaphylatoxins, C3a and C5a, and opsonins C3b, C1q, and mannan binding lectin, significantly influence macrophage responses. The anaphylatoxins trigger inflammasome activation, while opsonins downregulate inflammation by inhibiting proinflammatory and promoting anti-inflammatory cytokine production, and upregulating engulfment of apoptotic cells (consistent with a resolving or M2 macrophage phenotype).[70]

7.4.3 microRNA

The macrophage polarization may be modulated also at the post-transcriptional level by miRNAs.[51,71,72] miRNAs pair with partially complementary sequences in target mRNAs increasing their stability and/or inhibiting their translation.[73] Different miRNAs have been identified that are associated with polarized macrophages, for example, miR-155, miR-125b, miR-146, and miR-9. All of them are induced by LPS and in turn inhibit TLR4/IL-1R signaling thereby contributing to the switching of inflammatory macrophages to an immunosuppressive phenotype, needed for resolution.[51] Among these noncoding RNAs, miR-155 is apparently a key molecule in M1 polarization, since its overexpression or depletion drives macrophages to M1 or M2 phenotypes, respectively.[74,75] Conversely, the recently identified miRNA let-7c seems to be expressed at a higher level in M2 macrophages as opposed to M1 cells.[76] LPS stimulation reduced let-7c expression in M2 macrophages, suggesting that this miRNA might play an inhibitory role in modulating the macrophage inflammatory response. Growing evidence of new miRNAs involved in innate immunity response in general, and in macrophage polarization in particular, support the hypothesis that these can strongly regulate macrophage functional phenotypes.[51,72]

7.4.4 Metabolic Reprogramming

One of major differences between M1 and M2 macrophages is their metabolism (reviewed in Ref.[77]). For iron metabolism, it is known that M1 macrophages have high levels of iron retention, while M2 cells show high levels of iron export. Regarding glutathione and redox metabolism, M1 cells have high glutathione levels, which on the other hand are low in M2 macrophages. For amino acid metabolism, as already mentioned, iNOS metabolizes Arg to NO and citrulline in M1, while in M2 Arg1 metabolizes Arg to ornithine and urea. NO is an important effector of macrophage microbicidal activity, while ornithine initiates the polyamine production necessary for collagen synthesis, cell proliferation, and tissue remodeling. Regarding lipid metabolism, fatty acid oxidation is enhanced in M2 macrophages. For glucose metabolism, M1 macrophages show increased glycolysis.

The metabolic reprogramming of macrophages has experienced an increasing interest in the last years with studies that have highlighted the tight link between metabolism and function/cellular phenotype. Authors like Luke O'Neill have published extensively in the area.[78,79] M1 macrophages show the same glucose metabolic profile as tumor cells in normoxic conditions, a situation known as the "Warburg effect" or aerobic glycolysis. This occurs when glycolysis predominates, even though enough oxygen is available for oxidative metabolism to proceed. In this situation, glucose is metabolized to pyruvate, and pyruvate is converted to lactate for rapid ATP production, to fuel activation in acute inflammation or in defense against pathogens. In contrast, M2 macrophages draw upon oxidative phosphorylation to produce ATP in the more long-term process of resolution and repair, or in defense against parasites. Metabolic intermediates of the Krebs cycle, such as citrate and succinate, can also act as signaling molecules in macrophage activation.[78,80,81] Succinate, produced during glutamine metabolism upon TLR4 stimulation, stabilizes hypoxia-inducible factor (HIF)-1α, which in turn increases the expression of inflammatory genes such as IL-1β.[82] Moreover, succinate produced during ischemia induces the production of reactive oxygen species (ROS) after reperfusion, promoting inflammation and damage in the infarcted tissue.[83] On the other hand, the accumulation of citrate out of mitochondria upon LPS stimulation increases ROS, which in turn stabilizes HIF-1α.[78]

7.4.5 Epigenetic Reprogramming

Similarly to metabolic reprogramming, epigenetic reprogramming is raising great interest in the field of macrophage polarization/activation. Emerging evidence on a key role for epigenetic mechanisms in modulating macrophage polarization is reviewed in Refs.[84,85] Epigenetic mechanisms are mediated by post-translational modifications such as methylation and acetylation of histones, by methylation and hydroxymethylation of CpG DNA motifs, and by noncoding RNAs. The epigenetic arrangement, known as "epigenetic landscape," is a snapshot of chromatin modifications, DNA methylation, and proteins prebound to promoters and enhancers, which determine basal transcription rates of the genes *"hic et nunc"* by reducing or allowing chromatin accessibility of genes. The epigenetic landscape can be remodeled in response to microenvironmental polarizing signals, and consequently the gene expression can be altered.

In the case of histone modification, trimethylation of H3K4 is associated with active gene transcription (positive histone marker), whereas trimethylation of H3K9, H3K27, and H4K20 is linked to silencing of gene expression,[86] so they are considered negative histone markers. Epigenetic reprogramming is also one of the mechanisms that possibly underlie the memory of monocytes during their differentiation into macrophages, in LPS tolerance and in trained immunity.[87,88] Some epigenetic markers have been identified that are associated with the acquisition of a trained or a tolerant phenotype, such as H3K4me3 and acetylation of the H3 lysine at position 27 (H3K27ac).[89]

All the mechanisms mentioned above can be important factors determining the degree and duration of macrophage activation and of its modulation. Therefore, all of them are potential targets for therapeutic manipulation in specific human disease settings.

7.5 LOCAL CONDITIONS AND CELL–CELL INTERACTIONS: OTHER CUES IN MACROPHAGE POLARIZATION

We have discussed how macrophages receive a diverse range of signals from their surrounding environment, and the fact that the integral effect of these signals on macrophages is to direct their future behavior. In this section we introduce two other important components in macrophage polarization, that is, the special local conditions arising during the inflammatory reaction, which encompass changes in the microenvironment (such as hypoxia), and interaction with other cells, in particular mesenchymal stem cells or multipotent stromal cells (MSCs).

7.5.1 Hypoxia

Among the several microenvironmental changes that occur during a local inflammatory reaction, hypoxia acts as a link between environmental conditions in infected, inflamed, or damaged tissues and metabolism via HIFs, which are activated by mTOR and Akt signaling.[90]

Microenvironmental conditions in inflamed or tumor tissue are generally characterized by decreased availability of oxygen and nutrients. Macrophages recruited into hypoxic environments release prohealing, proangiogenic, and metastasis-promoting factors such as VEGF, PDGF, FGF2, and metalloproteinases (eg, MMP7 and MMP9).[91] Most likely, hypoxia does not directly influence the behavior of macrophages and affect their polarization, but it seems to direct the preferential homing of M2-like macrophages [in particular the tumor-associated macrophages (TAMs)], from the perivascular area to hypoxic areas, where the growth-promoting protumoral activities of these cells are boosted.[92,93] While the role of M2 macrophages in a hypoxic wound environment is beneficial, as they promote vascularization and cell proliferation during repair, hypoxia-induced recruitment of TAMs in a tumor would promote tumor progression. In addition, hypoxia can induce inflammatory factors like TNFα, IL-1β, MIF, CCL3, and

COX2, as well as M2-related factors like IL-10 and Arg1.[94] The response of macrophages in hypoxic conditions is mediated HIF-1α and HIF-2α.[95,96] HIF-1α promotes the switch to glycolysis when oxygen is limited both in cancer[97] and during inflammation.[98] A recent study[99] suggested that HIF-1α and HIF-2α might also drive macrophage polarization, with HIF-1α upregulating iNOS and M1-related NO production, and HIF-2α upregulating Arg1 and correlating with tumor microvessel density.

A key mechanism for HIF-1α activation by LPS involves the serine-threonine kinase mTOR, a key regulator of cellular metabolism, highly active in proliferating cells and in metabolically demanding situations, such as during inflammation or cancer.[100] The mTOR network reconfigures cellular metabolism and regulates translation, cytokine responses, antigen presentation, macrophage polarization, and cell migration.[101] In mammals, mTOR exists in two complexes, mTORC1 and mTORC2. mTORC1 and Akt regulate glycolysis in tumor cells and proliferating cells,[102,103] and apparently also in M1 macrophages, by increasing HIF-1α expression, which in turn increases the expression of glycolytic and inflammatory genes. The integration of Akt and mTORC1 signaling into the canonical signaling JAK-STAT pathway activated by IL-4 and LPS controls cellular metabolism and function during both M1 and M2 activation.

However, many questions remain outstanding about how mTORC1 and Akt support the metabolism of M1 and M2 macrophages, and accordingly their activation. All the knowledge and open issues on this topic have been tackled in an excellent recent review.[90]

7.5.2 Interaction with MSCs in the Microenvironment

The main cell types known to play an important role in macrophage activation are lymphocytes and mesenchymal stem cells. As already mentioned, the bidirectional interaction between lymphocytes and macrophages is well established[104] (Fig. 7.1). Indeed, both M1 and M2 polarization could be favored in vivo and activated in vitro by interaction with lymphocytes. Th1 lymphocytes release IFNγ, which can help macrophage polarization toward an M1 phenotype. Then, M1 macrophages enhance the inflammatory response by recruiting more Th1 lymphocytes.[48] Likewise, Th2 lymphocyte-derived signals, such as IL-4 and IL-13, promote M2 polarization of macrophages, which in turn enhance the recruitment of Th2 lymphocytes.[48]

In addition to the well-known interaction between lymphocytes and macrophages, more recent evidence has highlighted the important involvement, in the modulation of macrophage polarization, of the cross-talk between macrophages and MSCs.

MSCs are adult stem cells that are found in tissues such as the BM and in the connective tissues of most organs, and that can differentiate toward a multitude of lineages including fat, bone, cartilage, muscle, and skin.[105] Due to their ability to home to sites of injury and secrete anti-inflammatory cytokines, such as IL-10 and VEGF, MSCs are additionally endowed with broad immunoregulatory properties.[106,107]

MSCs from BM release chemokines CCL2 and CCL3, which recruit more monocytes in the tissues.[108] It has also been shown that MSCs are early regulators of inflammation.[109]

Currently, one of the main proposed mechanisms for the MSC reparative/regenerative effects after tissue damage is their ability to polarize macrophages from the classic inflammatory M1 phenotype toward the anti-inflammatory M2 phenotype. Moreover, many studies have demonstrated that MSCs interfere with the acquisition of an M1 phenotype, while promoting M2 polarization.[110,111] Macrophages cocultured with MSCs consistently show high expression of M2 markers, and high production of anti-inflammatory cytokines,[110] although they differ from monocyte-derived M2 macrophages for their increased production of IL-6.[112] MSCs produce paracrine factors such as PGE$_2$, IDO, and TGF-β1, when stimulated with inflammatory molecules such as LPS and TNFα. These paracrine factors promote M2 polarization, which leads to increased Th2 response, upregulation of regulatory T cells, immunosuppression, and tissue remodeling.

The beneficial effects of the elevated MSC-induced M2 macrophages in wound healing, brain/spinal cord injuries, and diseases of heart, lung, and kidney, have been recently reviewed in Ref.[113] Despite these promising experimental results, however, more investigation is still required for understanding the in vivo functionality of the M2 phenotype, and for shedding light on macrophage–MSC interactions, before a clinical application might be foreseen.

7.6 THERAPEUTIC APPLICATIONS BASED ON MODULATION OF MACROPHAGE POLARIZATION/ACTIVATION IN THE TUMOR

Modulation of innate immune responses is a promising avenue that is currently explored in the therapeutic approaches to many diseases, as well as in the design of new effective preventive strategies. The most striking example of how the plasticity of macrophages can be exploited for clinical applications comes from TAMs, which provide a paradigm for macrophage plasticity and an example of how immunotherapy can affect their function.[48]

M1 macrophages recruited during the early phase of tumor development are able to kill tumor cells and provoke destruction of the surrounding tissue. At advanced stages of tumor development and progression, distinct tissue-specific signals found in tumor microenvironment (eg, M-CSF, CCL2, IL-10, and TGF-β) and changes such as hypoxia, drive macrophage polarization to a "trophic" M2-like phenotype. M2-like TAMs have poor antigen-presenting ability and inhibit T cell proliferation and activity.[48] They secrete the chemokine CCL22, responsible for recruitment of Treg cells,[114] which in turn promote M2 polarization through IL-10 release, thus creating a self-amplifying loop for suppressed adaptive immunity and protumor activities. M2-polarized TAMs are able to stimulate angiogenesis (by producing VEGF and other angiogenic factors) and further tumor cell invasion (by producing metalloproteinases), and their number in a solid tumor is associated with a poor clinical prognosis.[115] Therefore, a new strategy for antitumor therapy is based on counteracting macrophage tumor-promoting activities and re-educating them to express tumoricidal activity. This strategy involves different therapeutic approaches: (1) blockage of macrophages recruitment; (2) suppression of TAM survival; (3) re-education TAMs towards a M1-like cytocidal phenotype; and (iv) use of antibodies to enhance TAM antitumoral activity. All these strategies have been recently reviewed in Refs.[116,117] The efficiency of these strategies has been demonstrated either concomitantly with chemotherapy and/or radiotherapy in clinical trials,[118,119] or alone in preclinical models. Promising data for therapy of prostate and breast cancer come with the use of antibodies against CCL2 and its receptor CCR2, or against M-CSF and its receptor CSF-1R, factors known to recruit macrophages to the site of inflammation.[120] Furthermore, recent work has shown that shifting macrophage polarization towards M1 by inhibiting CSF-1R signaling is therapeutically efficient in a mouse model of glioblastoma.[121] Strategies adopted for TAM depletion within the tumor include induction of macrophage apoptosis, using for example immunotoxin-conjugated mAbs targeting TAM-specific surface proteins such as the folate receptor,[122] or activation of TAM-specific cytotoxic T lymphocytes with a DNA vaccine against TAM membrane molecules, such as legumain.[123] Repolarization of TAMs towards an M1-like phenotype has been obtained with anti-IL-10R mAbs, or with agents capable of activating NF-κB, such as TLR agonists (eg, PolyI:C, monophosphoryl lipid A, CpG-oligodeoxynucleotide), or anti-CD40 mAbs. CD40 is a costimulatory molecule expressed on the macrophage membrane that, upon stimulation with agonist anti-CD40 mAbs, induces NF-κB activation[124,125] and increases serum levels of inflammatory cytokines in pancreatic carcinoma, correlating with tumor regression.[124] Another approach for repolarizing TAMs towards M1 involves the expression of miRNA such as miR-125b and miR-155. The former is higher in macrophages with improved ability to induce T cell activation,[126] while the latter is upregulated in macrophages in response to inflammatory stimuli.[127] Yet another strategy is based on the use of tumor antigen-specific mAbs. Macrophages can engage the antibodies through their different types of Fc receptors and come in contact with tumor cells. Possible mechanisms of action employed by mAbs include the antibody-dependent cell-mediated cytotoxicity, in which antibodies link macrophages to tumor cells thereby promoting tumor cell killing by macrophages; antibody-dependent cell-mediated phagocytosis, where tumor cells are opsonized by antibodies and readily taken up by phagocytes; and complement-dependent cytotoxicity by mAbs of IgG1 subclass, capable of activating the complement cascade.[128] To give some examples, it has been demonstrated that TAMs can efficiently kill tumor cells in the presence of mAbs against Tissue Factor (CD142)[129] in a mouse model of breast cancer. Furthermore, macrophage depletion abrogates the therapeutic efficiency of tumor-targeting anti-CD20 and anti-CD30 antibodies in murine models of lymphoma and severe combined immunodeficiency.[130,131]

7.7 CONCLUSIONS

It is well established that microenvironmental cues represented by tissue-specific, microbial, or danger signals play a crucial role in

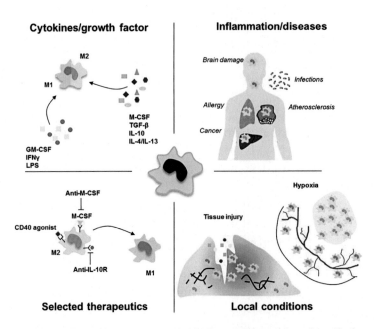

Figure 7.4 Modulation of macrophage activation. M1 and M2 macrophages can be modulated by four groups of agents/events. (1) Inflammatory molecules and growth factors. Inflammatory molecules, such as IFNγ and LPS, or growth factors, such as GM-CSF, polarize macrophages towards an M1 phenotype, while anti-inflammatory cytokines IL-4 or IL-10 and growth factor M-CSF polarize macrophages towards an M2 phenotype. (2) Pathology-related events can facilitate the polarization towards the M1 or M2 phenotypes. For example, M1 macrophages are predominant upon brain damage, bacterial or viral infections, or during atherosclerosis, and contribute to exacerbate the pathological conditions. On the other hand, in allergy or cancer development there is a predominance of M2 macrophages that correlates with poor prognosis. (3) Macrophage targeting with immunomodulating compounds that can repolarize (re-educate) M2 cells into an M1-like phenotype (eg, mAbs to M-CSF or IL-10R, or CD40 agonists). (4) Local conditions. Danger signals released during tissue injury can polarize macrophages towards an M1 phenotype. Later, during the phases of resolution of inflammation and tissue repair, changes in the microenvironment re-educate macrophages towards an M2 phenotype. As a consequence of the recruitment from perivascular to hypoxic areas (eg, within a wound or tumor), macrophages polarize towards an M2 phenotype.

modulating the response of macrophages and driving their functional polarization in M1 and M2 directions. Macrophage plasticity is also the outcome of a complex interplay/interaction between macrophages and other cells (stromal and immune cells) through soluble signals released in the local microenvironment (summarized in Fig. 7.4). Our deeper understanding of macrophage polarization in health and in diseases such as cancer is leading to the development of strategies for harnessing macrophage polarization for therapeutic goals. Thus, current and future research should aim at obtaining a precise knowledge and control of factors and mechanisms involved in macrophage polarization, with the ultimate goal of exploiting macrophage plasticity for rebalancing anomalous responses and re-establishing fully protective immunological functions in a series of different disease conditions.

ACKNOWLEDGMENTS

We are particularly grateful to Charles D. Mills for his precious advice and inspiring discussion.

This work was supported by EU grants HUMUNITY (FP7-PEOPLE-INT-2012 GA n. 316383) and BioCog (FP7-HEALTH-2013-INNOVATION-1 GA n. 602461), and by the Cluster project Medintech of the Italian Ministry of Education, University and Research.

CONFLICT OF INTEREST

The authors declare no commercial or financial conflict of interest.

REFERENCES

1. Italiani P, Boraschi D. New insights into tissue macrophages: from their origin to the development of memory. *Immune Netw* 2015;**15**:167–76.

2. Epelman S, Lavine KJ, Randolph GJ. Origin and function of tissue macrophages. *Immunity* 2014;**41**:21–35.

3. Haldar M, Murphy KM. Origin, development, and homeostasis of tissue-resident macrophages. *Immunol Rev* 2014;**262**:25–35.

4. Mantovani A, Sozzani S, Locati M, Allavena P, Sica A. Macrophage polarization: tumor-associated macrophages as a paradigm for polarized M2 mononuclear phagocytes. *Trends Immunol* 2002;**23**:549–55.

5. Netea MG, Latz E, Mills KHG, O'Neill LAJ. Innate immune memory: a paradigm shift in understanding host defense. *Nat Immunol* 2015;**16**:675–9.

6. Yona S, Kim KW, Wolf Y, Mildner A, Varol D, Breker M, et al. Fate mapping reveals origins and dynamics of monocytes and tissue macrophages under homeostasis. *Immunity* 2013;**38**:79–91.

7. Gomez Perdiguero E, Klapproth K, Schulz C, Busch K, Azzoni E, Crozet L, et al. Tissue-resident macrophages originate from yolk-sac-derived erythromyeloid progenitors. *Nature* 2015;**518**:547–51.

8. Schulz C, Gomez Perdiguero E, Chorro L, Szabo-Rogers H, Cagnard N, Kierdorf K, et al. A lineage of myeloid cells independent of Myb and hematopoietic stem cells. *Science* 2012;**336**:86–90.

9. Gentek R, Molawi K, Sieweke MH. Tissue macrophage identity and self-renewal. *Immunol Rev* 2014;**262**:56–73.

10. Varol C, Mildner A, Jung S. Macrophages: development and tissue specialization. *Annu Rev Immunol* 2015;**33**:643–75.

11. Italiani P, Boraschi D. From monocytes to M1/M2 macrophages: phenotypical vs. functional differentiation. *Front Immunol* 2014;**5**:514.

12. Dey A, Allen J, Hankey-Giblin PA. Ontogeny and polarization of macrophages in inflammation: blood monocytes versus tissue macrophages. *Front Immunol* 2014;**5**:683.

13. Gosselin D, Link VM, Romanoski CE, Fonseca GJ, Eichenfield DZ, Spann NJ, et al. Environment drives selection and function of enhancers controlling tissue-specific macrophage identities. *Cell* 2014;**159**:1327–40.

14. Lavin Y, Winter D, Blecher-Gonen R, David E, Keren-Shaul H, Merad M, et al. Tissue-resident macrophage enhancer landscapes are shaped by the local microenvironment. *Cell* 2014;**159**:1312–26.

15. Gordon S, Taylor PR. Monocyte and macrophage heterogeneity. *Nat Rev Immunol* 2005;**5**:953–64.

16. Taylor PR, Gordon S. Monocyte heterogeneity and innate immunity. *Immunity* 2003;**9**:2–4.

17. Okabe Y, Medzhitov R. Tissue-specific signals control reversible program of localization and functional polarization of macrophages. *Cell* 2014;**157**:832–44.

18. Mills CD. M1 and M2 macrophages: oracles of health and disease. *Crit Rev Immunol* 2012;**32**:463–88.

19. Mills CD, Ley K. M1 and M2 macrophages: the chicken and the egg of immunity. *J Innate Immun* 2014;**6**:716–26.

20. Mills CD. Macrophage arginine metabolism to ornithine/urea or nitric oxide/citrulline: a life or death issue. *Crit Rev Immunol* 2001;**21**:399–425.

21. Rath M, Müller I, Kropf P, Closs EI, Munder M. Metabolism via arginase or nitric oxide synthase: two competing arginine pathways in macrophages. *Front Immunol* 2014;**5**:532.

22. Sica A, Mantovani A. Macrophage plasticity and polarization: in vivo veritas. *J Clin Invest* 2012;**122**:787–95.

23. Murray PJ, Wynn TA. Protective and pathogenic functions of macrophage subsets. *Nat Rev Immunol* 2011;**11**:723–37.

24. Mills CD, Thomas A, Lenz LL, Munder M. Macrophage: SHIP of immunity. *Front Immunol* 2014;**5**:620.

25. Mills CD, Kincaid K, Alt JM, Heilman MJ, Hill AM. M-1/M-2 macrophages and the Th1/Th2 paradigm. *J Immunol* 2000;**164**:6166–73.

26. Mosser DM, Edwards JP. Exploring the full spectrum of macrophage activation. *Nat Rev Immunol* 2008;**8**:958–69.

27. Xue J, Schmidt SV, Sander J, Draffehn A, Krebs W, Quester I, et al. Transcriptome-based network analysis reveals a spectrum model of human macrophage activation. *Immunity* 2014;**40**:274–88.

28. Murray PJ, Allen JE, Biswas SK, Fisher EA, Gilroy DW, Goerdt S, et al. Macrophage activation and polarization: nomenclature and experimental guidelines. *Immunity* 2014;**41**:14–20.

29. Martinez FO, Gordon S. The M1 and M2 paradigm of macrophage activation: time for reassessment. *F1000Prime Rep* 2014;**6**:13.

30. Mackaness GB. The phagocytosis and inactivation of Staphylococci by macrophages of normal rabbit. *J Exp Med* 1960;**112**:35–53.

31. Gordon S. Alternative activation of macrophages. *Nat Rev Immunol* 2003;**3**:23–35.

32. Dzik JM. Evolutionary roots of arginase expression and regulation. *Front Immunol* 2014;**5**:544.

33. Stout RD, Suttles J. Functional plasticity of macrophages: reversible adaptation to changing microenvironments. *J Leukoc Biol* 2004;**76**:509–13.

34. Stout RD, Jiang C, Matta B, Tietzel I, Watkins SK, Suttles J. Macrophages sequentially change their functional phenotype in response to changes in microenvironmental influences. *J Immunol* 2005;**175**:342–9.

35. Italiani P, Mazza EM, Lucchesi D, Cifola I, Gemelli C, Grande A, et al. Trascriptomic profiling of the development of the inflammatory response in human monocytes in vitro. *PLoS One* 2014;**9**:e87680.

36. Egger BJL, Raj D, Hanisch U-K, Boddeke HWGM. Microglia phenotype and adaptation. *J Neuroimmune Pharmacol* 2013;**8**:807−23.

37. Olah M, Biber K, Vinet J, Boddeke HWGM. Microglia phenotype diversity. *CNS Neurol Disord Drug Targets* 2011;**10**:108−18.

38. Cherry JD, Olschowka JA, O'Banion MK. Neuroinflammation and M2 microglia: the good, the bad, and the inflamed. *J Neuroinflammation* 2014;**11**:98.

39. Boche D, Perry VH, Nicoll JAR. Review: activation patterns of microglia and their identification in the human brain. *Neuropathal Appl Neurobiol* 2013;**39**:3−18.

40. De Heredia FP, Gómez-Martínez S, Marcos A. Obesity, inflammation and the immune system. *Proc Nutr Soc* 2012;**71**:332−8.

41. Kraakman MJ, Murphy AJ, Jandeleit-Dahm K, Kammoun HL. Macrophage polarization in obesity and type 2 diabetes: weighing down our understanding of macrophage function? *Front Immunol* 2014;**5**:470.

42. Peled M, Fisher EA. Dynamic aspects of macrophage polarization during atherosclerosis progression and regression. *Frontiers Immunol* 2014;**5**:579.

43. Sica A, Invernizzi P, Mantovani A. Macrophage plasticity and polarization in liver homeostasis and pathology. *Hepatology* 2014;**59**:2035−43.

44. Motwani PM, Gilroy DW. Macrophage development and polarization in chronic inflammation. *Semin Immunol* 2015. Available from: http://dx.doi.org/10.1016/j.smim.2015.07.002.

45. Muraille E, Leo O, Moser M. Th1/Th2 paradigm extended: macrophage polarization as an unappreciated pathogen-driven escape mechanism? *Front Immunol* 2014;**5**:603.

46. Brunialti MK, Santos MC, Rigato O, Machado FR, Silva E, Salomao R. Increased percentages of T helper cells producing IL-17 and monocytes expressing markers of alternative activation in patients with sepsis. *PLoS One* 2012;**7**:e37393.

47. Ka MB, Daumas A, Textoris J, Mege JL. Phenotypic diversity and emerging new tools to study macrophage activation in bacterial infectious diseases. *Front Immunol* 2014;**5**:500.

48. Biswas SK, Mantovani A. Macrophage plasticity and interaction with lymphocyte subsets: cancer as a paradigm. *Nat Immunol* 2010;**11**:889−96.

49. Li J, Hsu H-C, Mountz JD. Managing macrophages in rheumatoid arthritis by reform or removal. *Curr Rheumatol Rep* 2012;**14**:445−54.

50. Hamilton JA, Tak PP. The dynamics of macrophage lineage populations in inflammatory and autoimmune diseases. *Arthritis Rheum* 2009;**60**:1210−21.

51. NanWang N, Liang H, Zen K. Molecular mechanisms that influence the macrophage M1−M2 polarization balance. *Front Immunol* 2014;**5**:614.

52. Van Overmeire E, Laoui D, Keirsse J, Van Ginderachter JA, Sarukhan A. Mechanisms driving macrophage diversity and specialization in distinct tumor microenvironments and parallelisms with other tissues. *Front Immunol* 2014;**5**:127.

53. Lang R, Patel D, Morris JJ, Rutschman RL, Murray PJ. Shaping gene expression in activated and resting primary macrophages by IL-10. *J Immunol* 2002;**169**:2253−63.

54. Molawi K, Sieweke MH. Transcriptional control of macrophage identity, self-renewal, and function. *Adv Immunol* 2013;**120**:269−300.

55. Krausgruber T, Blazek K, Smallie T, Alzabin S, Lockstone H, Sahgal N, et al. IRF5 promotes inflammatory macrophage polarization and TH1-TH17 responses. *Nat Immunol* 2011;**12**:231−8.

56. Fleetwood AJ, Dinh H, Cook AD, Hertzog PJ, Hamilton JA. GM-CSF- and M-CSF-dependent macrophage phenotypes display differential dependence on type I interferon signaling. *J Leukoc Biol* 2009;**86**:411−21.

57. Kelly-Welch AE, Hanson EM, Boothby MR, Keegan AD. Interleukin-4 and interleukin-13 signaling connections maps. *Science* 2003;**300**:1527−8.

58. Goenka S, Kaplan MH. Transcriptional regulation by STAT6. *Immunol Res* 2011;**50**:87−96.

59. Liao X, Sharma N, Kapadia F, Zhou G, Lu Y, Hong H, et al. Kruppel-like factor 4 regulates macrophage polarization. *J Clin Invest* 2011;**121**:2736−49.

60. Odegaard JI, Ricardo-Gonzalez RR, Goforth MH, Morel CR, Subramanian V, Mukundan L, et al. Macrophage-specific PPARgamma controls alternative activation and improves insulin resistance. *Nature* 2007;**447**:1116−20.

61. Wilson HM. SOCS proteins in macrophage polarization and function. *Front Immunol* 2014;**5**:357.

62. Whyte CS, Bishop ET, Ruckerl D, Gaspar-Pereira S, Barker RN, Allen JE, et al. Suppressor of cytokine signaling (SOCS)1 is a key determinant of differential macrophage activation and function. *J Leukoc Biol* 2011;**90**:845−54.

63. Liu Y, Stewart KN, Bishop E, Marek CJ, Kluth DC, Rees AJ, et al. Unique expression of suppressor of cytokine signaling 3 is essential for classical macrophage activation in rodents in vitro and in vivo. *J Immunol* 2008;**180**:6270−8.

64. Wang YC, He F, Feng F, Liu XW, Dong GY, Qin HY, et al. Notch signaling determines the M1 versus M2 polarization of macrophages in antitumor immune responses. *Cancer Res* 2010;**70**:4840−9.

65. Xu H, Zhu J, Smith S, Foldi J, Zhao B, Chung AY, et al. Notch-RBP-J signaling regulates the transcription factor IRF8 to promote inflammatory macrophage polarization. *Nat Immunol* 2012;**13**:642−50.

66. Spence S, Fitzsimons A, Boyd CR, Kessler J, Fitzgerald D, Elliott J, et al. Suppressors of cytokine signaling 2 and 3 diametrically control macrophage polarization. *Immunity* 2013;**38**:66−78.

67. Schultze JL, Freeman T, Hume DA, Latz E. A transcriptional prespective on human macrophage biology. *Semin Immunol* 2015;**27**:44−50.

68. Lawrence T, Natoli G. Transcriptional regulation of macrophage polarization: enabling diversity with identity. *Nat Rev Immunol* 2011;**11**:750−61.

69. Hamilton TA, Zhao C, Pavicic Jr PG, Datta S. Myeloid colony-stimulating factors as regulators of macrophage polarization. *Front Immunol* 2014;**5**:554.

70. Bohlson SS, O'Conner SD, Hulsebus HJ, Ho M-M, Fraser DA. Complement, C1q, and C1q-related molecules regulate macrophage polarization. *Front Immunol* 2014;**5**:402.

71. Graff JW, Dickson AM, Clay G, McCaffrey AP, Wilson ME. Identifying functional microRNAs in macrophages with polarized phenotypes. *J Biol Chem* 2012;**287**: 21816−25.

72. Liu G, Abraham E. MicroRNAs in immune response and macrophage polarization. *Arterioscler Thromb Vasc Biol* 2013;**33**:170−7.

73. Carthew RW, Sontheimer EJ. Origins and mechanisms of miRNAs and siRNAs. *Cell* 2009;**136**:642−55.

74. Martinez-Nunez RT, Louafi F, Sanchez-Elsner T. The interleukin 13 (IL-13) pathway in human macrophages is modulated by microRNA-155 via direct targeting of interleukin 13 receptor alpha1 (IL13Ralpha1). *J Biol Chem* 2011;**286**:1786−94.

75. Cai X, Yin Y, Li N, Zhu D, Zhang J, Zhang CY, et al. Re-polarization of tumor-associated macrophages to pro-inflammatory M1 macrophages by microRNA-155. *J Mol Cell Biol* 2012;**4**:341−3.

76. Banerjee S, Xie N, Cui H, Tan Z, Yang S, Icyuz M, et al. MicroRNA let-7c regulates macrophage polarization. *J Immunol* 2013;**190**:6542−9.

77. Biswas SK, Mantovani A. Orchestration of metabolism by macrophages. *Cell Metab* 2012;**15**:432−7.

78. Kelly B, O'Neill LAJ. Metabolic reprogramming in macrophages and dendritic cells in innate immunity. *Cell Res* 2015;**25**:771−84.

79. Galván-Peña S, O'Neill LAJ. Metabolic reprogramming in macrophage polarization. *Front Immunol* 2014;**5**:420.

80. O' Neill LAJ. Succinate strikes. *Nature* 2014;**515**:350−1.

81. O'Neill LAJ. A broken Krebs cycle in macrophages. *Immunity* 2015;**42**:393−4.

82. Tannahill GM, Curtis AM, Adamik J, Palsson-McDermott EM, McGettrick AF, Goel G, et al. Succinate is an inflammatory signal that induces IL-1β through HIF-1α. *Nature* 2013;**496**:238−42.

83. Chouchani ET, Pell VR, Gaude E, Aksentijević D, Sundier SY, Robb EL, et al. Ischaemic accumulation of succinate controls reperfusion injury through mitochondrial ROS. *Nature* 2014;**515**:431−5.

84. Ivashkiv LB. Epigenetic regulation of macrophage polarization and function. *Trends Immunol* 2013;**34**:216−23.

85. Takeuch O, Akira S. Epigenetic control of macrophage polarization. *Eur J Immunol* 2011;**41**:2490−3.

86. Ishii M, Wen H, Corsa CA, Liu T, Coelho AL, Allen RM, et al. Epigenetic regulation of the alternatively activated macrophage phenotype. *Blood* 2009;**114**:3244−54.

87. Foster SL, Hargreaves DC, Medzhitov R. Gene-specific control of inflammation by TLR-induced chromatin modifications. *Nature* 2007;**447**:972−8.

88. Quintin J, Saeed S, Martens JH, Giamarellos-Bourboulis EJ, Ifrim DC, Logie C, et al. Candida albicans infection affords protection against reinfection via functional reprogramming of monocytes. *Cell Host Microbe* 2012;**12**:223−32.

89. Saeed S, Quintin J, Kerstens HH, Rao NA, Aghajanirefah A, Matarese F, et al. Epigenetic programming of monocyte-to-macrophage differentiation and trained innate immunity. *Science* 2014;**345**:1251086.

90. Covarrubias AJ, Aksoylar HI, Horng T. Control of macrophage metabolism and activation by mTOR and Akt signaling. *Semin Immunol* 2015. Available from: http://dx.doi.org/10.1016/j.smim.2015.08.001.

91. Murdoch C, Muthana M, Lewis CE. Hypoxia regulates macrophage functions in inflammation. *J Immunol* 2005;**175**:6257−63.

92. Laoui D, Van Overmeire E, Di Conza G, Aldeni C, Keirsse J, Morias Y, et al. Tumor hypoxia does not drive differentiation of tumor-associated macrophages but rather fine-tunes the M2-like macrophage population. *Cancer Res* 2014;**74**:24−30.

93. Casazza A, Laoui D, Wenes M, Rizzolio S, Bassani N, Mambretti M, et al. Impeding macrophage entry into hypoxic tumor areas by Sema3A/Nrp1 signaling blockade inhibits angiogenesis and restores antitumor immunity. *Cancer Cell* 2013;**24**:695−709.

94. Murdoch C, Lewis CE. Macrophage migration and gene expression in response to tumor hypoxia. *Int J Cancer* 2005;**117**:701−8.

95. Imtiyaz HZ, Simon MC. Hypoxia-inducible factors as essential regulators of inflammation. *Curr Top Microbiol Immunol* 2010;**345**:105−20.

96. Burke B, Giannoudis A, Corke KP, Gill D, Wells M, Ziegler-Heitbrock L, et al. Hypoxia-induced gene expression in human macrophages: implications for ischemic tissues and hypoxia-regulated gene therapy. *Am J Pathol* 2003;**163**:1233–43.

97. Denko NC. Hypoxia, HIF1 and glucose metabolism in the solid tumor. *Nat Rev Cancer* 2008;**8**:705–13.

98. Cramer T, Yamanishi Y, Clausen BE, Förster I, Pawlinski R, Mackman N, et al. HIF-1alpha is essential for myeloid cell-mediated inflammation. *Cell* 2003;**112**:645–57.

99. Takeda N, O'Dea EL, Doedens A, Kim J-W, Weidemann A, Stockmann C, et al. Differential activation and antagonistic function of HIF-{alpha} isoforms in macrophages are essential for NO homeostasis. *Genes Dev* 2010;**24**:491–501.

100. Byles V, Covarrubias AJ, Ben-Sahra I. The TSC-mTOR pathway regulates macrophage polarization. *Nat Commun* 2013;**4**:2834.

101. Weichhart T, Hengstschläger M, Linke M. Regulation of innate immune cell function by mTOR. *Nat Rev Immunol* 2015;**15**:599–614.

102. Dibble CC, Manning BD. Signal integration by mTORC1 coordinates nutrient input with biosynthetic output. *Nat Cell Biol* 2013;**15**:555–64.

103. Robey RB, Hay N. Is Akt the "Warburg kinase"?-Akt-energy metabolism interactions and oncogenesis. *Semin Cancer Biol* 2009;**19**:25–31.

104. Iwasaki A, Medzhitov R. Regulation of adaptive immunity by the innate immune system. *Science* 2010;**327**:291–5.

105. Uccelli A, Moretta L, Pistoia V. Mesenchymal stem cells in health and disease. *Nat Rev Immunol* 2008;**9**:726–36.

106. De Miguel MP, Fuentes-Juliàn S, Blazquez-Martinez A, Pascual CY, Aller MA, Aria J, et al. Immunosuppressive properties of mesenchymal stem cells: advances and applications. *Curr Mol Med* 2012;**12**:574–91.

107. Hoogduijn MJ, Popp F, Verbeek R, Masoodi M, Nicolaou A, Baan C, et al. The immuno-modulatory properties of mesenchymal stem cells and their use for immunotherapy. *Int Immunopharmacol* 2010;**10**:1496–500.

108. Chen L, Tredget EE, Wu PY, Wu Y. Paracrine factors of mesenchymal stem cells recruit macrophages and endothelial lineage cells and enhance wound healing. *PLoS One* 2008;**3**:e1886.

109. Prockop DJ. Concise review: two negative feedback loops place mesenchymal stem/stromal cells at the center of early regulators of inflammation. *Stem Cells* 2013;**31**:2042–6.

110. Kim J, Hematti P. Mesenchymal stem cell-educated macrophages: a novel type of alternatively activated macrophages. *Exp Hematol* 2009;**37**:1445–53.

111. Choi H, Lee RH, Bazhanov N, Oh JY, Prockop DJ. Anti-inflammatory protein TSG-6 secreted by activated MSCs attenuates zymosan-induced mouse peritonitis by decreasing TLR2/NF-kappaB signaling in resident macrophages. *Blood* 2011;**118**:330–8.

112. Eggenhofer E, Hoogduijn M. Mesenchymal stem cell-educated macrophages. *Transplant Res* 2012;**1**:1–5.

113. Zheng G, Ge M, Qiu G, Shu Q, Xu J. Mesenchymal stromal cells affect disease outcomes via macrophage polarization. *Stem Cells Int* 2015;**2015**:989473.

114. de Chaisermartin L, Goc J, Dannotte D, Validine P, Magdeleinat P, Alifano M, et al. Characterization of chemokines and adhesin molecules associated with T cell presence in terziary lymphoid structures in human lung cancer. *Cancer Res* 2011;**71**:6391–9.

115. Qian BZ, Pollard JW. Macrophage diversity enhances tumor progression and metastasis. *Cell* 2010;**141**:39–51.

116. Josephs DH, Bax JH, Karagiannis SN. Tumor-associated macrophages polarization and re-education with immunotherapy. *Front Biosci (Elite Ed)* 2015;7:334−51.

117. Mantovani A, Vecchi AP. Pharmacological modulation of monocytes and macrophages. *Curr Opinion Pharmacol* 2014;17:38−44.

118. Kalbasi A, June CH, Haas N, Vapiwala N. Radiation immunotherapy: a synergistic combination. *J Clin Invest* 2013;123:2756−63.

119. De Palma M, Lewis CE. Macrophage regulation of tumor responses to anticancer therapies. *Cancer Cell* 2013;23:277−86.

120. Garber K. First results for agents targeting cancer-related inflammation. *J Natl Cancer Inst* 2009;101:1110−12.

121. Pyonteck SM, Akkari L, Schuhmacher AJ, Bowman RL, Sevenich L, Quail DF, et al. CSF-1R inhibition alters macrophage polarization and blocks glioma progression. *Nat Med* 2013;19:1264−72.

122. Nagai T, Tanaka M, Tsuneyoshi Y, Xu B, Michie SA, Hasui K, et al. Targeting tumor-associated macrophages in an experimental glioma model with a recombinant immunotoxin to folate receptor beta. *Cancer Immunol Immunother* 2009;58:1577−86.

123. Luo Y, Zhou H, Krueger J, Kaplan C, Lee SH, Dolman C. Targeting tumor-associated macrophages as a novel strategy against breast cancer. *J Clin Invest* 2006;116:2132−41.

124. Beatty GL, Chiorean EG, Fishman MP, Saboury B, Teitelbaum UR, Sun W, et al. CD40 agonists alter tumor stroma and show efficacy against pancreatic carcinoma in mice and humans. *Science* 2011;331:1612−16.

125. Buhtoiarov IN, Sondel PM, Wigginton JM, Buhtoiarova TN, Yanke EM, Mahvi DA, et al. Anti-tumour synergy of cytotoxic chemotherapy and anti-CD40 plus CpG-ODN immunotherapy through repolarization of tumour-associated macrophages. *Immunology* 2011;132:226−39.

126. Chaudhuri AA, So AY, Sinha N, Gibson WS, Taganov KD, O'Connell RM. MicroRNA-125b potentiates macrophage activation. *J Immunol* 2011;187:5062−8.

127. O'Connell RM, Taganov KD, Boldin MP, Cheng G, Baltimore D. MicroRNA-155 is induced during the macrophage inflammatory response. *Proc Natl Acad Sci USA* 2007;104:1604−9.

128. Malas S, Harrasser M, Lacy KE, Karagiannis SN. Antibody therapies for melanoma: new and emerging opportunities to activate immunity (review). *Oncol Rep* 2014;32:875−86.

129. Grugan KD, McCabe FL, Kinder M, Greenplate AR, Harman BC, Ekert JE, et al. Tumor-associated macrophages promote invasion while retaining Fc-dependent anti-tumor function. *J Immunol* 2012;189:5457−66.

130. Minard-Colin V, Xiu Y, Poe JC, Horikawa M, Magro CM, Hamaguchi Y, et al. Lymphoma depletion during CD20 immunotherapy in mice is mediated by macrophage FcγRI, FcγRIII, and FcγRIV. *Blood* 2008;112:1205−13.

131. Oflazoglu E, Stone IJ, Gordon KA, Grewal IS, van Roijen N, Law CL, et al. Macrophages contribute to antitumor activity of the anti-CD30 antibody SGN-30. *Blood* 2007;110:4370−2.

CHAPTER 8

Modulating Inflammatory Cytokines: IL-1

Mark S. Gresnigt and Frank L. van de Veerdonk

Department of Internal Medicine, Radboud University Medical Center, Nijmegen, The Netherlands

8.1 INTRODUCTION

8.1.1 Classical IL-1 Family Members: IL-1α and IL-1β

Interleukin-1 (IL-1) was the first interleukin that was first cloned from human monocytes by Charles Dinarello in 1984.[1] Later two different cDNA clones of IL-1 were renamed to represent the two distinct cytokines IL-1α and IL-1β.[2] Although the IL-1 cytokine family consists today of 11 members that interact with 10 different receptors, decoy receptors, and coreceptors,[3] the first two pro-inflammatory cytokines discovered, IL-1α and IL-1β (collectively called IL-1), are the most extensively studied cytokines in immunology due to their prominent role in causing inflammation in a wide variety of diseases ranging from inflammatory syndromes to host defense against pathogens.

IL-1α is constitutively produced as a bioactive precursor in most types of cells and is especially produced in skin keratinocytes, epithelial cells of the mucosa, and in various organs such as the liver, lung, kidney, and heart.[4] IL-1α is not a typical interleukin and is secreted after activation of the cell. Upon apoptosis IL-1α becomes bound to chromatin thereby preventing release and subsequent stimulation of the host response.[5] However, during necrosis, such as caused by ischemia, the IL-1α precursor does not get bound to chromatin[5] and becomes released in the environment where it serves as an alarmin to signal to immune cells that cells are dying.[6] In addition, apoptotic bodies also contain the IL-1α precursor and can via IL-1α initiate neutrophil recruitment.[7] The IL-1α release by necrotic cells is a useful warning to alert leukocytes that a tissue is being damaged by, for example, an invading pathogen such as bacteria, fungi, or viruses. In addition, IL-1α plays an important role in sterile inflammation following tissue ischemia.

Immune Rebalancing. DOI: http://dx.doi.org/10.1016/B978-0-12-803302-9.00008-7

In contrast to IL-1α, IL-1β expression is restricted only to a few cells of the immune system, including monocytes, macrophages, and dendritic cells.[4] The precursor of IL-1β is biologically inactive and can be proteolytically activated by the protein complex called the inflammasome that activates an enzyme called caspase-1, which processes pro-IL-1β into bioactive IL-1β (Fig. 8.1). However, inflammasome independent cleavage of pro-IL-1β has also been described and can be done by serine proteases from neutrophils and proteases from other cells, and even by enzymes secreted by microorganisms (reviewed in[8]). In monocytes, caspase-1 is constitutively active leading to IL-1β release whenever IL-1β transcription is activated. However, in macrophages and dendritic cells a pure TLR agonist only activates *IL-1B* mRNA transcription and a secondary stimulus such as ATP is required as an inflammasome

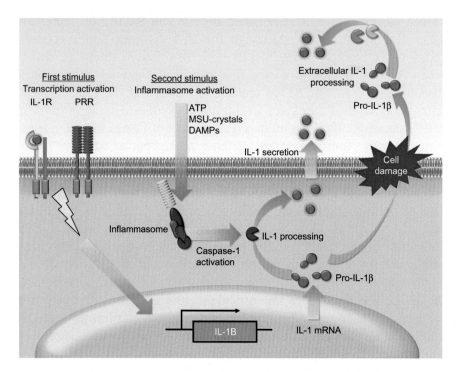

Figure 8.1 Induction and processing of IL-1β. Transcription of IL-1β can be induced by various signals from cytokine receptors, such as the IL-1R itself, but also by various classes of pattern recognition receptors. Since the IL-1B mRNA translates into an inactive precursor, pro-IL-1β, proteolytic processing of the protein is required. In monocytes caspase-1 is constitutively active and pro-IL-1β gets processed directly. However, in macrophages and dendritic cells a second stimulus to activate the inflammasome is required. Once IL-1β is truncated into its active form it becomes released extracellularly. In the event of cell death, the resulting pro-IL-1β will be released and proteases from all kind of sources, such as neutrophils, are able to alternatively process pro-IL-1β into its bioactive form. MSU, monosodiumurate crystals; DAMPs, danger associated molecular patterns.

activator.[9] IL-1β is secreted and can activate other immune cells by binding to the IL-1 receptor.

8.1.2 IL-1 Receptor Signaling

Both IL-1α and IL-1β trigger the inflammatory response by binding and activating the IL-1 receptor (IL-1R1), which consists of an extracellular immunoglobulin (Ig)-like domain and an intracellular signaling Toll/IL-1 receptor homology (TIR) domain that is shared between Toll-like receptors and the IL-1 receptor (Fig. 8.2). Upon ligand binding the coreceptor IL-1R3 (IL-1 receptor accessory protein; IL-1RAcP) becomes recruited to IL-1R1[10] and is crucial for mediating signal transduction.[11] MyD88 is the adapter molecule of the IL-1R and mediates downstream activation of

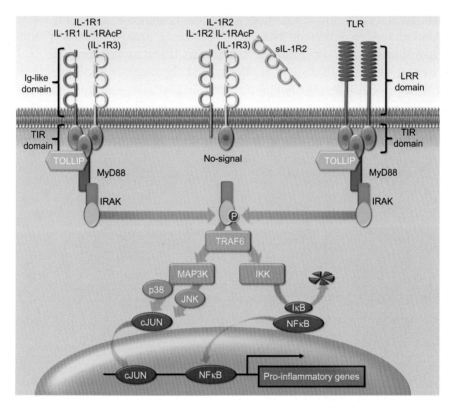

Figure 8.2 IL-1R signaling. The IL-1R consists of an Ig-like domain and an intracellular TIR-domain which is shared with Toll-like receptors resulting in the fact that TLRs and the IL-1R activate the same signaling cascade leading up to NFκB and cJUN activation. Following activation, a complex of MyD88, TOLLIP, and the IRAK proteins is formed. Ultimately leading to IRAK-phosphorylation and TRAF6 activation. TRAF6 regulates the degradation of the inhibitor complex of NFκB, IKK, and activates cJUN through the MAP3K:JNK and P38, leading to the activation of transcription of pro-inflammatory genes.

the transcription factor NFκB (Nuclear Factor Kappa Beta) after binding of IL-1 to its receptor.[12] Since this adapter molecule is also recruited to the TIR-domain of Toll-like receptors[13] downstream signaling of the IL-1R is similar to that of Toll-like receptors and results in subsequent activation of IRAK (IL-1-induced activation of interleukin-1 receptor-associated kinase), NFκB, and JNK (c-Jun N-terminal kinase) activation. The type 2 IL-1R (IL-1R2) lacks the intracellular TIR-domain and is therefore not able to activate downstream signaling, nevertheless it has affinity to bind IL-1, thereby serving as a decoy receptor. In addition, IL-1R2 can be secreted and thus can serves also as a soluble decoy receptor.[14,15]

8.2 BIOLOGICALS TARGETING IL-1

Anakinra is the most common agent used to block IL-1 (Fig. 8.3). Anakinra is recombinant human IL-1 receptor antagonist and inhibits IL-1 signaling by competitively binding to IL-1R, preventing the IL-1 receptor agonists, IL-1α and IL-1β, to bind the receptor and signal.[16–18] The short half-life of Anakinra requires daily injections to obtain an efficacious dose, and it has an excellent safety profile compared to other biologicals, with injection-site reactions as the most commonly reported adverse events.[19]

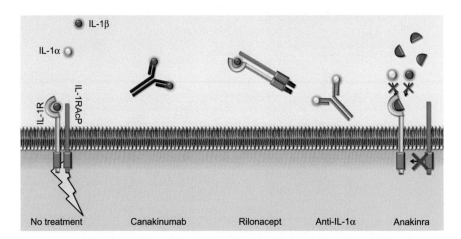

Figure 8.3 Treatment options in blocking IL-1. When IL-1α or IL-1β binds to IL-1R1 the coreceptor IL-1R3 (IL-1RAcP) becomes recruited which activates the signaling cascade. Several biologicals prevent IL-1 from signaling. Anakinra is recombinant human IL-1 Receptor antagonist. It binds the IL-1R, but prevents IL-1R3 from being recruited and activating signal transduction. Furthermore, it occupies the receptor thereby preventing both IL-1α and IL-1β from activating the IL-1R. Canakinumab, a monoclonal antibody against IL-1β, binds IL-1β and thereby prevents it from binding to the receptor. Rilonacept is a soluble IL-1 receptor with a FC-tail. Like Canakinumab it can sequester IL-1 before it can bind to the IL-1 receptor. Anti-IL-1α binds IL-1α and prevents it from activating the IL-1R1.

Other drugs that have been approved to target IL-1 signaling are Rilonacept, which is a soluble decoy receptor coupled to an antibody FC-fragment, and canakinumb, a monoclonal antibody against IL-1β. Targeting IL-1α can have a huge benefit over targeting the IL-1R pathway in general or only IL-1β. During stroke, mechanic ventilation, and heart attack sterile inflammation is induced by the release of IL-1α from dying cells. In these clinical circumstances targeting IL-1α specifically would be preferred over targeting the whole IL-1 axis. Although there is no approved IL-1α blocker on the market and there are no large trials or numerous studies that investigated blocking IL-1α in human disease, safety pilot studies in cancer show promising results.[20,21]

8.3 BLOCKING IL-1 IN DISEASE

IL-1 is crucial for regulating inflammatory responses and most human diseases are associated with a state of inflammation. It is therefore not surprising that targeting IL-1 can be a promising treatment option in many diseases, and indeed various trials and case reports have demonstrated beneficial responses of blocking IL-1 in human disease. The major classes of human diseases in which IL-1 has been described as playing a role in pathogenesis and could be targeted as a therapeutic option are: classical hereditary auto-inflammatory diseases, systemic inflammatory diseases, and rheumatic, cardiovascular, hematological, and metabolic diseases (Table 8.1).

8.3.1 Hereditary Auto-Inflammatory Diseases

This class of diseases is characterized by recurrent episodes of fever with systemic symptoms, such as arthralgias/arthritis, skin rashes and gastrointestinal symptoms. Most auto-inflammatory diseases have a clear association with dysregulated IL-1 responses, either due to mutations in regulatory mechanisms, such as the inflammasome, or due to mutations in the pathways regulating IL-1 signaling, such as deficiency of IL-1Ra.

Deficiency of Interleukin-1 Receptor Antagonist (DIRA) is caused by a mutation in the gene *IL-1RN* that encodes the protein IL-1Ra, and presents with neonatal onset of sterile multifocal osteomyelitis, periostosis, and pustulosis.[22] The condition is associated with increased IL-1 signaling and increased presence of Th17 cells at the site of inflammation, mainly the bones and skin. This disease highlights the importance of IL-1 in the pathology of skin and bone diseases, and

Table 8.1 Diseases Amendable to Blocking IL-1	
Hereditary Auto-inflammatory Diseases	
DIRA[22]	CAPS[23−33]
DITRA[34,35]	TRAPS[36−39]
FMF[40−42]	PAPA[43]
HIDS[44,45]	
Systemic Inflammatory Syndromes	
Behcet's disease[46,47]	SAPHO[48,49]
Still's disease[50−54]	PFAPA[55]
Rheumatic Diseases	
Rheumatoid arthritis[56−72]	Osteoarthritis[73,74]
Metabolic Disorders	
T2DM[75−79]	Gout[80−86]
Metabolic syndrome[87,88]	Pseudogout[89,90]
Cardiovascular Disease	
AMI[91−93]	Heart failure[94,95]
Hematological Disorders	
MM[96]	MAS[97−103]
Schnitzler syndrome[104,105]	

provides evidence of the role of IL-1 in driving pathological Th17 responses, that are associated with a wide variety of diseases. DIRA responds dramatically and rapidly to IL-1Ra, and it is important to recognize this life-threatening disease early because of its severity and good response to blocking IL-1.[22]

Deficiency of Interleukin-36 Receptor Antagonist (DITRA) is caused by mutations in the gene *IL-36RN*, which encodes IL-36Ra.[106] The disease is characterized by pustular psoriasis. It responds to anakinra, which demonstrates the link between IL-36 cytokines to IL-1 mediated responses.[34,35] This disease highlights the role of IL-36 in psoriasis and pustular skin diseases and paves the way for future therapeutic strategies based on blocking IL-36 cytokines by recombinant IL-36Ra. IL-36R signaling is linked to Th17 responses, again pointing to a crucial role of th17 cells in skin diseases.[107] Indeed recent studies have shown that blocking IL-17 in psoriasis also has beneficial effects.[108]

Familial Mediterranean fever (FMF) due to mutations in the *MEFV* gene lead to gain of function of pyrin, which results in inappropriate high IL-1β release.[109,110] FMF patients present with recurrent fever episodes, serositis, and systemic inflammation that is most often responsive to col-chicine. Most patients present with symptoms similar to an appendicitis and this is why these patients often undergo abdominal surgery before the diagnosis is made. FMF can predispose to vasculitis and inflammatory bowel disease. The pathogenesis of FMF is believed to be due to a hyper-activation of inflammasome-dependent IL-1β processing because of muta-tions in pyrin, and this inflammasome activation can be triggered by external triggers such as injury.[40,111] Anakinra has been documented to have beneficial effects in FMF and can be a first option in the treatment of these patients presenting with severe symptoms.[41,42]

Hyper IgD syndrome (HIDS) is characterized by recurrent episodes of fever, painful mouth ulcers, lymphadenopathy, skin rash, and high IgD levels.[112] It is caused by a mutation in the mevalonate kinase gene (*MVK*) resulting in a deficiency of this enzyme that plays a role in cholesterol synthesis.[113] The exact pathogenesis of the diseases remains unclear but it has been associated with increased IL-1β production, and blocking IL-1 signaling with anakinra results in relief of symptoms.[44,114] It is different from the classic mevalonate deficiency that results in an almost complete dysfunction of the mevalonate kinase enzyme that leads to a severe syndrome with fevers, developmental delay, hepatic damage, neurological symptoms and can result in early death. It is very rare, but important to recognize, since it also responds to blocking IL-1.[45]

Three cryopyrin associated periodic syndromes (CAPS) arise from mutations in a single gene, namely *NLRP3* that encodes a protein called cryopyrin, whose name is derived from the Greek words for cryo (cold) and pyro (fire). Cryopyrin is a crucial component for inflammasome activation. The three syndromes include Muckle-Wells syndrome (MWS), familial cold auto-inflammatory syndrome (FCAS), and neonatal-onset multisystem inflammatory disease (NOMID). The underlying pathogenesis in all diseases is related to increased inflammasome activation, and therefore these diseases are typically associated with IL-1β-driven pathology. MWS is characterized by intermittent episodes of fever, headache, urticarial rash, joint pain, progressive sensorineural hearing loss, and often later in the course of disease with secondary (AA) amyloidosis causing nephropathy. It is very similar to FCAS, formerly called familial cold urticarial, although FCAS is usually milder and is rarely associated with secondary amy-loidosis. The symptoms in FCAS are triggered by cold, which results in a systemic inflammatory response that is characterized by fever, urticarial rash, conjunctival injection, and arthralgias. The most severe CAPS syndrome is NOMID. This presents itself generally immediately at birth, and leads to fevers, erythematous rash resembling urticaria, and causes impaired growth. It is associated with characteristic abnormal facial morphology, with protruding eyes, frontal bossing, and a saddle-shaped nose. It can lead to premature death, and is associated with the development of secondary amyloidosis. Joint pains are common, which are due to proliferation of the cartilage at epiphyses that can resemble tumors. Although all three CAPS respond to blocking IL-1, it is often the fevers and skin problems that respond well and rapidly, while the bone disease is less responsive and more difficult to treat.[23–32,115] In addition, failure of blocking IL-1 in NOMID has been reported.[33] Given the known pathological mutation, a more targeted therapy, such as specific blocking of cryopyrin activity, could be an option that might be explored in the future.

Familial Hibernian fever, now known as tumor necrosis factor (TNF) receptor-1 associated periodic syndrome (TRAPS) is caused by mutations in *TNFRSF1* that encodes the 55-kD TNF receptor leading to intracellular receptor retention and impaired shedding of this receptor. The consequence is increased TNF signaling that results in recurrent fevers, rash, peri-orbital edema, arthritis, conjunctivitis, and myalgias. Although not common, a subset of patients will develop secondary amyloidosis primarily affecting the kidneys. Based on this knowledge therapy with a soluble TNF receptor, such as etanercept has been tried, however beneficial results have been reported to be partial or even absent in some patients. Moreover, other TNF blocking agents, such as infliximab have even been associated with worsening of the disease symptoms. In light of the known pathogenesis, namely increased TNF signaling, It is noteworthy that blocking IL-1 with anakinra or canakinumab has been reported to be highly effective,[36–39] suggesting that IL-1 plays a major role in TRAPS, and supports the concept that TNF can induce IL-1.[116]

PAPA syndrome, which is an acronym for pyogenic sterile arthritis, pyoderma gangrenosum, and acne, results from mutations in the gene *PSTPIP1* that affects both pyrin and protein tyrosine phosphatase that regulate innate and adaptive immune responses. These mutations increase the binding of the PSTPIP1 protein to pyrin, and probably interfere with the inhibitory effect of pyrin on the production of active IL-1β. Patients with PAPA particularly suffer from destructive arthritis and inflammatory skin rashes. Although glucocorticoids remain the standard of therapy, blocking IL-1 has been reported to be beneficial during flares of PAPA, and thus should be explored in the future as a therapeutic option in PAPA.[43]

8.3.2 Systemic Inflammatory Diseases Resembling Auto-Inflammatory Diseases

This group of diseases is characterized by multiorgan involvement without a known genetic cause and have symptoms that resemble classic hereditary auto-inflammatory diseases, such as recurrent episodes of fevers associated with skin and bone disease. Behçet's disease is a rare inflammatory disease in which the predominant features are recurrent oral and genital ulceration, and uveitis. Other characteristic symptoms include skin lesions, such as erythema nodosum-like lesions, and polyarthritis. Behçet's disease symptoms are amendable to anakinra, providing evidence that it there is an IL-1 mediated component in this disease.[46,47,117] The classical triad of daily spiking fever, a typical salmon-colored rash, and arthritis characterizes Still's disease. It is believed to be a polygenic disease and the pathogenesis seems to be driven by cytokines belonging to the IL-1 family, such as IL-1β and IL-18. Indeed blocking IL-1 with anakinra relieves symptoms, especially the fevers, almost immediately. The effects on arthritis are less clear, however, continued treatment of anakinra over a prolonged period of time results in symptom free intervals in almost every patient.[50-54] SAPHO syndrome—synovitis, acne, pustulosis, hyperostosis, and osteomyelitis collectively called the acronym SAPHO—is a disease that is classified under neutrophil dermatosis, and is typically associated with palmar and plantar pustulosis. It can present itself with aseptic osteoarticular lesions, and can been seen in the context of Behçet's disease, pustular psoriasis, and Sweet syndrome. The pathogenesis is not well understood, but the associated diseases have all been linked to IL-1 mediated pathology, and SAPHO has been reported to respond to anakinra.[48,49] One other systemic auto-inflammatory disease in which no causative mutation has been found is the periodic fever, aphthous stomatitis, pharyngitis, and adenopathy (PFAPA) syndrome. It usually presents in childhood, and pharyngitis, with aphtous ulcers in the mouth and high fevers should trigger the suspicion of this syndrome. The ulcers are not as large or painful as the ulcers of Behçet's syndrome. Based on the evidence that IL-1β activation is associated with PFAPA flares, five PFAPA patients were treated by blocking IL-1 with anakinra.[55] All patients showed a prompt clinical response suggesting that an activation of IL-1β during PFAPA flares is critical for disease pathology.

8.3.3 Rheumatic Diseases

Given the observation that IL-1 plays a crucial role in skin and bone diseases, it is not surprising that IL-1 blockade has been tried in rheumatic diseases. The classical rheumatic disease is rheumatoid arthritis (RA), which is characterized by a symmetric peripheral polyarthritis. The exact cause of the disease is unknown, but it is classified as an autoimmune disease, since it is associated with autoantibodies, such as anticitrullinated protein antibodies. The exact role of the autoantibodies is not clear in RA. The major issue in RA is that if it is untreated or unresponsive to treatment it can eventually lead to destruction of the joints with pain and loss of carrying out daily tasks. There is a vast body of reports that suggest that blocking IL-1 is beneficial in RA and more importantly has the capacity to prevent joint destruction.[56-71,118] The difficulty with the treatment of blocking IL-1 is that it does not have the relatively fast relief of pain and fatigue as can be seen with blocking TNF. However, after long-term use of anakinra with 24–48 weeks of treatment there is a clear beneficial effect on joint destruction when IL-1 is targeted.[61] Canakinumab has also been reported to reduce disease severity in patients failing on blocking TNF, although no studies have been conducted to demonstrate prevention of bone destruction on long-term treatment. This at least suggests that IL-1β might be an important mediator in the pathogenesis of RA.[119] The most common form of inflammatory arthritis is osteoarthritis, which can be localized, such as in the knee or wrist, or generalized where it includes more than three joints. It presents with joint pain and can eventually lead to destruction of the joints in a subset of patients. It is thought that repetitive physical force on the joint causes microtrauma, which activates chondrocytes that eventually leads to cartilage damage resulting in joint pain. IL-1 seems to play a role in a subset of patients with AO, since anakinra improved pain and swelling in an aggressive form of erosive osteoarthritis.[73] However, blocking IL-1 did not have such a dramatic effect in other patients with AO.[73,74,120,121]

8.3.4 Metabolic Diseases

The most common form of metabolic disease is type 2 diabetes mellitus (T2DM), which is characterized by hyperglycemia, insulin resistance, and is associated with obesity. The pathogenesis is due to destruction of the β-cells in the pancreas leading to insulin resistance. IL-1β has been shown to play a role in destruction of these β-cells, and glucose itself can induce IL-1β production, suggesting an auto-inflammatory loop leading to destruction of β-cells that is dependent on IL-1β secretion.[122,123] This hypothesis was tested in a double-blind, parallel-group trial involving 70 patients with T2DM, where 34 patients were assigned to receive anakinra for 13 weeks, and 36 patients received placebo. Blocking IL-1 improved glycemic control and β-cell secretory function, and also reduced markers of systemic inflammation.[75] Moreover, a 39-week follow-up study demonstrated that anankinra improved the proinsulin-to-insulin ratio and markers of systemic inflammation, such as CRP, which lasted 39 weeks after treatment withdrawal, suggesting that even a short course of IL-1 blockade therapy is able to restore β-cell function.[76] Other studies have confirmed the beneficial effects observed in T2D with various different approaches to block IL-1, including canakinumab, which provides evidence that indeed IL-1β is driving pathology in T2DM.[77−79] Since T2DM is associated with obesity and the metabolic syndrome that is characterized by insulin-resistance, blocking IL-1 was also investigated in a clinical trial in obese patients with insulin-resistance.[87] Although no effect was observed on insulin-resistance in these patients, anakinra improved the disposition index, which is the product of decreased insulin sensitivity and impaired insulin secretion, suggesting that anakinra improved β-cell function.[87] Indeed, it was shown that anakinra improved the first-phase insulin secretion in 16 patients with impaired glucose tolerance.[88] Another common metabolic disease that is associated with IL-1β driven pathology is gout. Gout is characterized by recurrent attacks of acute inflammatory arthritis and is associated with hyperuricemia. Interestingly, hyperuricemia alone is not sufficient for the development of gout. Moreover, urate crystals alone do not stimulate IL-1β, but will do this in the presence of free fatty acids (FFA), which is partially dependent on inflammasome activation[124,125] (Fig. 8.2). This also provides an explanation why gout attacks can be triggered by eating red meat and drinking alcohol, because these conditions are associated with an increase of FFA. Although the inflammasome will contribute to processing IL-1β, gout is characterized by neutrophilic infiltration, and these neutrophils can also contribute to cleaving IL-1β by secreting enzymes such as proteinase 3.[126] Blocking IL-1 has been successful in treating gout in many studies.[80–86] In addition, pseudogout that is caused by pyrophosphate deposition in the joints is also responsive to blocking IL-1.[89,90]

8.3.5 Cardiovascular

Acute myocardial infarction (AMI) will result in an inflammatory response that is characterized by an infiltration of neutrophils at the site of the injured myocardium and the local production of cytokines and chemokines that can eventually contribute to detrimental cardiac remodeling and heart failure.[127] IL-1 plays an important role in this process and is released by endothelial cells and at a later stage by infiltrating leukocytes.[128] A balanced IL-1 response during AMI is critical since IL-1 on the one hand leads to leukocyte recruitment that contributes to healing, while on the other hand IL-1 can promote cell death in cardiomyocytes.[128] In addition, IL-1 is able to suppress myocardial function.[129] Two clinical pilot trials with anakinra showed that in humans with AMI, blocking IL-1 contributed to the prevention of heart failure,[91,92] although a follow up study on these two trials, did not show an effect of anakinra on recurrent ischemic events.[93] Also, in patients with already established heart failure anakinra contributes to improvement of inflammatory markers and symptoms.[94,95] Currently a large trial called the Canakinumab Anti-Inflammatory Thrombosis Outcomes Study (CANTOS) is evaluating whether blocking IL-1β as compared with placebo can reduce rates of cardiovascular death, stroke, and recurrent myocardial infarction, among patients with stable coronary artery disease that are at high vascular risk despite currently available prevention strategies.[130]

8.3.6 Hematological Disorders

Multiple myeloma (MM) is a hematological malignancy that presents with osteolytic bone lesions and pathological fractures. It is caused by proliferation of malignant plasma cells that produce a monoclonal Ig. IL-1 can specifically induce osteoclast-activating factor production by multiple myeloma bone marrow cells, which contributes to increased bone resorption.[131] Therefore, blocking IL-1 has a clear rationale to be explored in the early phases of MM.[132] In patients with indolent myeloma that were at high risk to develop MM, treatment with anakinra was suggested to reduce the incidence of MM.[96] A rare disease associated with monoclonal gammopathy is Schnitzler syndrome.

It is characterized by urticarial rash, fever, and monoclonal gammopathy. Interestingly, Schnitzler syndrome is highly responsive to blocking IL-1, including canakinumab, underscoring the importance of IL-1β in this syndrome.[104,105]

A severe life-threatening disease associated with high mortality is macrophage activation syndrome (MAS), and it occurs specifically in the setting of severe Epstein Barr Virus (EBV) infection, Still's disease, or systemic lupus erythematosus. It is characterized by fever, lymphadenopathy, hepatosplenomegaly, cytopenias, and by high levels of circulating IL-18. MAS has been reported to respond to anakinra.[97–103] It is noteworthy that the current standard of therapy is initiated with drugs such as high dose glucocorticosteroids, cyclosporine, and etoposide. Anakinra has much fewer side effects and therefore it is important to realize that anakinra could be used as a first line treatment choice in diagnosed MAS. An additional argument for the importance of the IL-1 cytokines in MAS, is the finding that a gain of function mutation in *NLRC4*, a component of the inflammasome that can lead to activation of caspase-1, is associated with the development of MAS.[133]

8.4 CONCLUSIONS

IL-1 is a potent inflammatory cytokine involved in the pathogenesis of many human diseases. Rare disorders such as DIRA have provided unique insight in the role of this cytokine in disease and underscore the importance of IL-1 in regulating inflammatory responses in the bone and skin. The beneficial effects of blocking IL-1 in various classes of human disease ranging from autoimmune to metabolic disorders, underscores the importance of understanding IL-1-driven inflammatory responses and provides a rationale to further explore IL-1 targeted therapy in human disease.

REFERENCES

1. Auron PE, Webb AC, Rosenwasser LJ, Mucci SF, Rich A, Wolff SM, et al. Nucleotide sequence of human monocyte interleukin 1 precursor cDNA. *Proc Natl Acad Sci USA* 1984;**81**(24):7907–11.

2. March CJ, Mosley B, Larsen A, Cerretti DP, Braedt G, Price V, et al. Cloning, sequence and expression of two distinct human interleukin-1 complementary DNAs. *Nature* 1985;**315**(6021):641–7.

3. Garlanda C, Dinarello CA, Mantovani A. The interleukin-1 family: back to the future. *Immunity* 2013;**39**(6):1003–18.

4. Su AI, Cooke MP, Ching KA, Hakak Y, Walker JR, Wiltshire T, et al. Large-scale analysis of the human and mouse transcriptomes. *Proc Natl Acad Sci USA* 2002;**99**(7):4465–70.

5. Cohen I, Rider P, Carmi Y, Braiman A, Dotan S, White MR, et al. Differential release of chromatin-bound IL-1alpha discriminates between necrotic and apoptotic cell death by the ability to induce sterile inflammation. *Proc Natl Acad Sci USA* 2010;**107**(6):2574–9.

6. Kim B, Lee Y, Kim E, Kwak A, Ryoo S, Bae SH, et al. The interleukin-1alpha precursor is biologically active and is likely a key alarmin in the IL-1 family of cytokines. *Front Immunol* 2013;**4**:391.

7. Berda-Haddad Y, Robert S, Salers P, Zekraoui L, Farnarier C, Dinarello CA, et al. Sterile inflammation of endothelial cell-derived apoptotic bodies is mediated by interleukin-1alpha. *Proc Natl Acad Sci USA* 2011;**108**(51):20684–9.

8. Netea MG, van de Veerdonk FL, van der Meer JW, Dinarello CA, Joosten LA. Inflammasome-independent regulation of IL-1-family cytokines. *Annu Rev Immunol* 2015; **33**:49–77.

9. Netea MG, Nold-Petry CA, Nold MF, Joosten LA, Opitz B, van der Meer JH, et al. Differential requirement for the activation of the inflammasome for processing and release of IL-1beta in monocytes and macrophages. *Blood* 2009;**113**(10):2324–35.

10. Greenfeder SA, Nunes P, Kwee L, Labow M, Chizzonite RA, Ju G. Molecular cloning and characterization of a second subunit of the interleukin 1 receptor complex. *J Biol Chem* 1995;**270**(23):13757–65.

11. Wesche H, Korherr C, Kracht M, Falk W, Resch K, Martin MU. The interleukin-1 receptor accessory protein (IL-1RAcP) is essential for IL-1-induced activation of interleukin-1 receptor-associated kinase (IRAK) and stress-activated protein kinases (SAP kinases). *J Biol Chem* 1997;**272**(12):7727–31.

12. Burns K, Martinon F, Esslinger C, Pahl H, Schneider P, Bodmer JL, et al. MyD88, an adapter protein involved in interleukin-1 signaling. *J Biol Chem* 1998;**273**(20):12203–9.

13. Medzhitov R, Preston-Hurlburt P, Kopp E, Stadlen A, Chen C, Ghosh S, et al. MyD88 is an adaptor protein in the hToll/IL-1 receptor family signaling pathways. *Mol Cell* 1998;**2**(2): 253–8.

14. Kuhn PH, Marjaux E, Imhof A, De Strooper B, Haass C, Lichtenthaler SF. Regulated intramembrane proteolysis of the interleukin-1 receptor II by alpha-, beta-, and gamma-secretase. *J Biol Chem* 2007;**282**(16):11982–95.

15. Lorenzen I, Lokau J, Dusterhoft S, Trad A, Garbers C, Scheller J, et al. The membrane-proximal domain of A Disintegrin and Metalloprotease 17 (ADAM17) is responsible for recognition of the interleukin-6 receptor and interleukin-1 receptor II. *FEBS Lett* 2012;**586**(8): 1093–100.

16. Seckinger P, Williamson K, Balavoine JF, Mach B, Mazzei G, Shaw A, et al. A urine inhibitor of interleukin 1 activity affects both interleukin 1 alpha and 1 beta but not tumor necrosis factor alpha. *J Immunol* 1987;**139**(5):1541–5.

17. Seckinger P, Lowenthal JW, Williamson K, Dayer JM, MacDonald HR. A urine inhibitor of interleukin 1 activity that blocks ligand binding. *J Immunol* 1987;**139**(5):1546–9.

18. Carter DB, Deibel Jr MR, Dunn CJ, Tomich CS, Laborde AL, Slightom JL, et al. Purification, cloning, expression and biological characterization of an interleukin-1 receptor antagonist protein. *Nature* 1990;**344**(6267):633–8.

19. Kaiser C, Knight A, Nordstrom D, Pettersson T, Fransson J, Florin-Robertsson E, et al. Injection-site reactions upon Kineret (anakinra) administration: experiences and explanations. *Rheumatol Int* 2012;**32**(2):295–9.

20. Hong DS, Janku F, Naing A, Falchook GS, Piha-Paul S, Wheler JJ, et al. Xilonix, a novel true human antibody targeting the inflammatory cytokine interleukin-1 alpha, in non-small cell lung cancer. *Invest New Drugs* 2015;**33**(3):621–31.

21. Hong DS, Hui D, Bruera E, Janku F, Naing A, Falchook GS, et al. MABp1, a first-in-class true human antibody targeting interleukin-1alpha in refractory cancers: an open-label, phase 1 dose-escalation and expansion study. *Lancet Oncol* 2014;**15**(6):656–66.

22. Aksentijevich I, Masters SL, Ferguson PJ, Dancey P, Frenkel J, van Royen-Kerkhoff A, et al. An autoinflammatory disease with deficiency of the interleukin-1-receptor antagonist. *N Engl J Med* 2009;**360**(23):2426–37.

23. Hawkins PN, Lachmann HJ, McDermott MF. Interleukin-1-receptor antagonist in the Muckle-Wells syndrome. *N Engl J Med* 2003;**348**(25):2583–4.

24. Hoffman HM, Rosengren S, Boyle DL, Cho JY, Nayar J, Mueller JL, et al. Prevention of cold-associated acute inflammation in familial cold autoinflammatory syndrome by interleukin-1 receptor antagonist. *Lancet* 2004;**364**(9447):1779–85.

25. Lovell DJ, Bowyer SL, Solinger AM. Interleukin-1 blockade by anakinra improves clinical symptoms in patients with neonatal-onset multisystem inflammatory disease. *Arthritis Rheum* 2005;**52**(4):1283–6.

26. Metyas SK, Hoffman HM. Anakinra prevents symptoms of familial cold autoinflammatory syndrome and Raynaud's disease. *J Rheumatol* 2006;**33**(10):2085–7.

27. Ross JB, Finlayson LA, Klotz PJ, Langley RG, Gaudet R, Thompson K, et al. Use of anakinra (Kineret) in the treatment of familial cold autoinflammatory syndrome with a 16-month follow-up. *J Cutan Med Surg* 2008;**12**(1):8–16.

28. Leslie KS, Lachmann HJ, Bruning E, McGrath JA, Bybee A, Gallimore JR, et al. Phenotype, genotype, and sustained response to anakinra in 22 patients with autoinflammatory disease associated with CIAS-1/NALP3 mutations. *Arch Dermatol* 2006;**142**(12):1591–7.

29. Goldbach-Mansky R, Shroff SD, Wilson M, Snyder C, Plehn S, Barham B, et al. A pilot study to evaluate the safety and efficacy of the long-acting interleukin-1 inhibitor rilonacept (interleukin-1 Trap) in patients with familial cold autoinflammatory syndrome. *Arthritis Rheum* 2008;**58**(8):2432–42.

30. Hoffman HM, Throne ML, Amar NJ, Sebai M, Kivitz AJ, Kavanaugh A, et al. Efficacy and safety of rilonacept (interleukin-1 Trap) in patients with cryopyrin-associated periodic syndromes: results from two sequential placebo-controlled studies. *Arthritis Rheum* 2008;**58**(8):2443–52.

31. Lachmann HJ, Kone-Paut I, Kuemmerle-Deschner JB, Leslie KS, Hachulla E, Quartier P, et al. Use of canakinumab in the cryopyrin-associated periodic syndrome. *N Engl J Med* 2009;**360**(23):2416–25.

32. Sibley CH, Chioato A, Felix S, Colin L, Chakraborty A, Plass N, et al. A 24-month open-label study of canakinumab in neonatal-onset multisystem inflammatory disease. *Ann Rheum Dis* 2015;**74**(9):1714–19.

33. Matsubara T, Hasegawa M, Shiraishi M, Hoffman HM, Ichiyama T, Tanaka T, et al. A severe case of chronic infantile neurologic, cutaneous, articular syndrome treated with biologic agents. *Arthritis Rheum* 2006;**54**(7):2314–20.

34. Rossi-Semerano L, Piram M, Chiaverini C, De Ricaud D, Smahi A, Kone-Paut I. First clinical description of an infant with interleukin-36-receptor antagonist deficiency successfully treated with anakinra. *Pediatrics* 2013;**132**(4):e1043–7.

35. Tauber M, Viguier M, Alimova E, Petit A, Liote F, Smahi A, et al. Partial clinical response to anakinra in severe palmoplantar pustular psoriasis. *Br J Dermatol* 2014;**171**(3):646–9.

36. Gattorno M, Pelagatti MA, Meini A, Obici L, Barcellona R, Federici S, et al. Persistent efficacy of anakinra in patients with tumor necrosis factor receptor-associated periodic syndrome. *Arthritis Rheum* 2008;**58**(5):1516–20.

37. Sacre K, Brihaye B, Lidove O, Papo T, Pocidalo MA, Cuisset L, et al. Dramatic improvement following interleukin 1beta blockade in tumor necrosis factor receptor-1-associated syndrome (TRAPS) resistant to anti-TNF-alpha therapy. *J Rheumatol* 2008;**35**(2):357–8.

38. Simon A, Bodar EJ, van der Hilst JC, van der Meer JW, Fiselier TJ, Cuppen MP, et al. Beneficial response to interleukin 1 receptor antagonist in traps. *Am J Med* 2004;**117**(3):208–10.

39. Brizi MG, Galeazzi M, Lucherini OM, Cantarini L, Cimaz R. Successful treatment of tumor necrosis factor receptor-associated periodic syndrome with canakinumab. *Ann Intern Med* 2012;**156**(12):907–8.

40. Chae JJ, Aksentijevich I, Kastner DL. Advances in the understanding of familial Mediterranean fever and possibilities for targeted therapy. *Br J Haematol* 2009;**146**(5):467–78.

41. Basaran O, Uncu N, Celikel BA, Taktak A, Gur G, Cakar N. Interleukin-1 targeting treatment in familial Mediterranean fever: an experience of pediatric patients. *Mod Rheumatol* 2015;**25**(4):621–4.

42. Ozcakar ZB, Ozdel S, Yilmaz S, Kurt-Sukur ED, Ekim M, Yalcinkaya F. Anti-IL-1 treatment in familial Mediterranean fever and related amyloidosis. *Clin Rheumatol* 2014 [Epub ahead of print].

43. Dierselhuis MP, Frenkel J, Wulffraat NM, Boelens JJ. Anakinra for flares of pyogenic arthritis in PAPA syndrome. *Rheumatology* 2005;**44**(3):406–8.

44. Bodar EJ, Kuijk LM, Drenth JP, van der Meer JW, Simon A, Frenkel J. On-demand anakinra treatment is effective in mevalonate kinase deficiency. *Ann Rheum Dis* 2011;**70**(12):2155–8.

45. Ruiz Gomez A, Couce ML, Garcia-Villoria J, Torres A, Bana Souto A, Yague J, et al. Clinical, genetic, and therapeutic diversity in 2 patients with severe mevalonate kinase deficiency. *Pediatrics* 2012;**129**(2):e535–9.

46. Botsios C, Sfriso P, Furlan A, Punzi L, Dinarello CA. Resistant Behcet disease responsive to anakinra. *Ann Intern Med* 2008;**149**(4):284–6.

47. Caso F, Rigante D, Vitale A, Lucherini OM, Cantarini L. Efficacy of anakinra in refractory Behcet's disease sacroiliitis. *Clin Exp Rheumatol* 2014;**32**(4 Suppl. 84):S171.

48. Colina M, Pizzirani C, Khodeir M, Falzoni S, Bruschi M, Trotta F, et al. Dysregulation of P2X7 receptor-inflammasome axis in SAPHO syndrome: successful treatment with anakinra. *Rheumatology* 2010;**49**(7):1416–18.

49. Wendling D, Prati C, Aubin F. Anakinra treatment of SAPHO syndrome: short-term results of an open study. *Ann Rheum Dis* 2012;**71**(6):1098–100.

50. Nordstrom D, Knight A, Luukkainen R, van Vollenhoven R, Rantalaiho V, Kajalainen A, et al. Beneficial effect of interleukin 1 inhibition with anakinra in adult-onset Still's disease. An open, randomized, multicenter study. *J Rheumatol* 2012;**39**(10):2008–11.

51. Fitzgerald AA, Leclercq SA, Yan A, Homik JE, Dinarello CA. Rapid responses to anakinra in patients with refractory adult-onset Still's disease. *Arthritis Rheum* 2005;**52**(6):1794–803.

52. Kotter I, Wacker A, Koch S, Henes J, Richter C, Engel A, et al. Anakinra in patients with treatment-resistant adult-onset Still's disease: four case reports with serial cytokine measurements and a review of the literature. *Semin Arthritis Rheum* 2007;**37**(3):189–97.

53. Lequerre T, Quartier P, Rosellini D, Alaoui F, De Bandt M, Mejjad O, et al. Interleukin-1 receptor antagonist (anakinra) treatment in patients with systemic-onset juvenile idiopathic arthritis or adult onset Still disease: preliminary experience in France. *Ann Rheum Dis* 2008;**67**(3):302–8.

54. Giampietro C, Ridene M, Lequerre T, Costedoat Chalumeau N, Amoura Z, Sellam J, et al. Anakinra in adult-onset Still's disease: long-term treatment in patients resistant to conventional therapy. *Arthritis Care Res (Hoboken)* 2013;**65**(5):822−6.

55. Stojanov S, Lapidus S, Chitkara P, Feder H, Salazar JC, Fleisher TA, et al. Periodic fever, aphthous stomatitis, pharyngitis, and adenitis (PFAPA) is a disorder of innate immunity and Th1 activation responsive to IL-1 blockade. *Proc Natl Acad Sci USA* 2011;**108**(17): 7148−53.

56. Abramson SB, Amin A. Blocking the effects of IL-1 in rheumatoid arthritis protects bone and cartilage. *Rheumatology* 2002;**41**(9):972−80.

57. Bao J, Yue T, Liu W, Zhang Q, Zhou L, Xu HJ, et al. Secondary failure to treatment with recombinant human IL-1 receptor antagonist in Chinese patients with rheumatoid arthritis. *Clin Rheumatol* 2011;**30**(5):697−701.

58. Botsios C, Sfriso P, Furlan A, Ostuni P, Biscaro M, Fiocco U, et al. Anakinra, a recombinant human IL-1 receptor antagonist, in clinical practice. Outcome in 60 patients with severe rheumatoid arthritis. *Reumatismo* 2007;**59**(1):32−7.

59. Bresnihan B, Alvaro-Gracia JM, Cobby M, Doherty M, Domljan Z, Emery P, et al. Treatment of rheumatoid arthritis with recombinant human interleukin-1 receptor antagonist. *Arthritis Rheum* 1998;**41**(12):2196−204.

60. Bresnihan B, Cobby M. Clinical and radiological effects of anakinra in patients with rheumatoid arthritis. *Rheumatology* 2003;**42**(Suppl. 2):ii22−8.

61. Bresnihan B, Newmark R, Robbins S, Genant HK. Effects of anakinra monotherapy on joint damage in patients with rheumatoid arthritis. Extension of a 24-week randomized, placebo-controlled trial. *J Rheumatol* 2004;**31**(6):1103−11.

62. Cohen SB. The use of anakinra, an interleukin-1 receptor antagonist, in the treatment of rheumatoid arthritis. *Rheum Dis Clin North Am* 2004;**30**(2):365−80, vii.

63. Cohen SB, Moreland LW, Cush JJ, Greenwald MW, Block S, Shergy WJ, et al. A multicentre, double blind, randomised, placebo controlled trial of anakinra (Kineret), a recombinant interleukin 1 receptor antagonist, in patients with rheumatoid arthritis treated with background methotrexate. *Ann Rheum Dis* 2004;**63**(9):1062−8.

64. Cohen SB, Strand V, Aguilar D, Ofman JJ. Patient- versus physician-reported outcomes in rheumatoid arthritis patients treated with recombinant interleukin-1 receptor antagonist (anakinra) therapy. *Rheumatology* 2004;**43**(6):704−11.

65. Cohen SB, Woolley JM, Chan W. Anakinra 960180 study G. Interleukin 1 receptor antagonist anakinra improves functional status in patients with rheumatoid arthritis. *J Rheumatol* 2003;**30**(2):225−31.

66. Cunnane G, Madigan A, Murphy E, FitzGerald O, Bresnihan B. The effects of treatment with interleukin-1 receptor antagonist on the inflamed synovial membrane in rheumatoid arthritis. *Rheumatology* 2001;**40**(1):62−9.

67. Fleischmann RM, Schechtman J, Bennett R, Handel ML, Burmester GR, Tesser J, et al. Anakinra, a recombinant human interleukin-1 receptor antagonist (r-metHuIL-1ra), in patients with rheumatoid arthritis: a large, international, multicenter, placebo-controlled trial. *Arthritis Rheum* 2003;**48**(4):927−34.

68. Genant HK. Interleukin-1 receptor antagonist treatment of rheumatoid arthritis patients: radiologic progression and correlation of Genant/Sharp and Larsen scoring methods. *Semin Arthritis Rheum* 2001;**30**(5 Suppl. 2):26−32.

69. Jiang Y, Genant HK, Watt I, Cobby M, Bresnihan B, Aitchison R, et al. A multicenter, double-blind, dose-ranging, randomized, placebo-controlled study of recombinant human interleukin-1 receptor antagonist in patients with rheumatoid arthritis: radiologic progression and correlation of Genant and Larsen scores. *Arthritis Rheum* 2000;**43**(5):1001−9.

70. Kavanaugh A. Anakinra (interleukin-1 receptor antagonist) has positive effects on function and quality of life in patients with rheumatoid arthritis. *Adv Ther* 2006;**23**(2):208−17.

71. Nixon R, Bansback N, Brennan A. The efficacy of inhibiting tumour necrosis factor alpha and interleukin 1 in patients with rheumatoid arthritis: a meta-analysis and adjusted indirect comparisons. *Rheumatology* 2007;**46**(7):1140−7.

72. Monnet D, Kadi A, Izac B, Lebrun N, Letourneur F, Zinovieva E, et al. Association between the IL-1 family gene cluster and spondyloarthritis. *Ann Rheum Dis* 2012;**71**(6):885−90.

73. Bacconnier L, Jorgensen C, Fabre S. Erosive osteoarthritis of the hand: clinical experience with anakinra. *Ann Rheum Dis* 2009;**68**(6):1078−9.

74. Cohen SB, Proudman S, Kivitz AJ, Burch FX, Donohue JP, Burstein D, et al. A randomized, double-blind study of AMG 108 (a fully human monoclonal antibody to IL-1R1) in patients with osteoarthritis of the knee. *Arthritis Res Ther* 2011;**13**(4):R125.

75. Larsen CM, Faulenbach M, Vaag A, Volund A, Ehses JA, Seifert B, et al. Interleukin-1-receptor antagonist in type 2 diabetes mellitus. *N Engl J Med* 2007;**356**(15):1517−26.

76. Larsen CM, Faulenbach M, Vaag A, Ehses JA, Donath MY, Mandrup-Poulsen T. Sustained effects of interleukin-1 receptor antagonist treatment in type 2 diabetes. *Diabetes Care* 2009;**32**(9):1663−8.

77. Cavelti-Weder C, Babians-Brunner A, Keller C, Stahel MA, Kurz-Levin M, Zayed H, et al. Effects of gevokizumab on glycemia and inflammatory markers in type 2 diabetes. *Diabetes Care* 2012;**35**(8):1654−62.

78. Sloan-Lancaster J, Abu-Raddad E, Polzer J, Miller JW, Scherer JC, De Gaetano A, et al. Double-blind, randomized study evaluating the glycemic and anti-inflammatory effects of subcutaneous LY2189102, a neutralizing IL-1beta antibody, in patients with type 2 diabetes. *Diabetes Care* 2013;**36**(8):2239−46.

79. Rissanen A, Howard CP, Botha J, Thuren T, Global I. Effect of anti-IL-1beta antibody (canakinumab) on insulin secretion rates in impaired glucose tolerance or type 2 diabetes: results of a randomized, placebo-controlled trial. *Diabetes Obes Metab* 2012;**14**(12):1088−96.

80. Cronstein BN, Sunkureddi P. Mechanistic aspects of inflammation and clinical management of inflammation in acute gouty arthritis. *J Clin Rheumatol* 2013;**19**(1):19−29.

81. Ghosh P, Cho M, Rawat G, Simkin PA, Gardner GC. Treatment of acute gouty arthritis in complex hospitalized patients with anakinra. *Arthritis Care Res (Hoboken)* 2013;**65**(8): 1381−4.

82. Gratton SB, Scalapino KJ, Fye KH. Case of anakinra as a steroid-sparing agent for gout inflammation. *Arthritis Rheum* 2009;**61**(9):1268−70.

83. McGonagle D, Tan AL, Shankaranarayana S, Madden J, Emery P, McDermott MF. Management of treatment resistant inflammation of acute on chronic tophaceous gout with anakinra. *Ann Rheum Dis* 2007;**66**(12):1683−4.

84. Schumacher Jr HR, Evans RR, Saag KG, Clower J, Jennings W, Weinstein SP, et al. Rilonacept (interleukin-1 trap) for prevention of gout flares during initiation of uric acid-lowering therapy: results from a phase III randomized, double-blind, placebo-controlled, confirmatory efficacy study. *Arthritis Care Res (Hoboken)* 2012;**64**(10):1462−70.

85. Singh D, Huston KK. IL-1 inhibition with anakinra in a patient with refractory gout. *J Clin Rheumatol* 2009;**15**(7):366.

86. So A, De Smedt T, Revaz S, Tschopp J. A pilot study of IL-1 inhibition by anakinra in acute gout. *Arthritis Res Ther* 2007;**9**(2):R28.

87. van Asseldonk EJ, Stienstra R, Koenen TB, Joosten LA, Netea MG, Tack CJ. Treatment with Anakinra improves disposition index but not insulin sensitivity in nondiabetic subjects with the metabolic syndrome: a randomized, double-blind, placebo-controlled study. *J Clin Endocrinol Metab* 2011;**96**(7):2119−26.

88. van Poppel PC, van Asseldonk EJ, Holst JJ, Vilsboll T, Netea MG, Tack CJ. The interleukin-1 receptor antagonist anakinra improves first-phase insulin secretion and insulinogenic index in subjects with impaired glucose tolerance. *Diabetes Obes Metab* 2014;**16**(12):1269–73.

89. Announ N, Palmer G, Guerne PA, Gabay C. Anakinra is a possible alternative in the treatment and prevention of acute attacks of pseudogout in end-stage renal failure. *Joint Bone Spine* 2009;**76**(4):424–6.

90. McGonagle D, Tan AL, Madden J, Emery P, McDermott MF. Successful treatment of resistant pseudogout with anakinra. *Arthritis Rheum* 2008;**58**(2):631–3.

91. Abbate A, Kontos MC, Grizzard JD, Biondi-Zoccai GG, Van Tassell BW, Robati R, et al. Interleukin-1 blockade with anakinra to prevent adverse cardiac remodeling after acute myocardial infarction (Virginia Commonwealth University Anakinra Remodeling Trial [VCU-ART] Pilot study). *Am J Cardiol* 2010;**105**(10):1371–7.e1.

92. Abbate A, Van Tassell BW, Biondi-Zoccai G, Kontos MC, Grizzard JD, Spillman DW, et al. Effects of interleukin-1 blockade with anakinra on adverse cardiac remodeling and heart failure after acute myocardial infarction [from the Virginia Commonwealth University-Anakinra Remodeling Trial (2) (VCU-ART2) pilot study]. *Am J Cardiol* 2013;**111**(10):1394–400.

93. Abbate A, Kontos MC, Abouzaki NA, Melchior RD, Thomas C, Van Tassell BW, et al. Comparative safety of interleukin-1 blockade with anakinra in patients with ST-segment elevation acute myocardial infarction (from the VCU-ART and VCU-ART2 pilot studies). *Am J Cardiol* 2015;**115**(3):288–92.

94. Van Tassell BW, Arena RA, Toldo S, Mezzaroma E, Azam T, Seropian IM, et al. Enhanced interleukin-1 activity contributes to exercise intolerance in patients with systolic heart failure. *PLoS One* 2012;**7**(3):e33438.

95. Van Tassell BW, Arena R, Biondi-Zoccai G, McNair Canada J, Oddi C, Abouzaki NA, et al. Effects of interleukin-1 blockade with anakinra on aerobic exercise capacity in patients with heart failure and preserved ejection fraction (from the D-HART pilot study). *Am J Cardiol* 2014;**113**(2):321–7.

96. Lust JA, Lacy MQ, Zeldenrust SR, Dispenzieri A, Gertz MA, Witzig TE, et al. Induction of a chronic disease state in patients with smoldering or indolent multiple myeloma by targeting interleukin 1{beta}-induced interleukin 6 production and the myeloma proliferative component. *Mayo Clin Proc* 2009;**84**(2):114–22.

97. Bruck N, Suttorp M, Kabus M, Heubner G, Gahr M, Pessler F. Rapid and sustained remission of systemic juvenile idiopathic arthritis-associated macrophage activation syndrome through treatment with anakinra and corticosteroids. *J Clin Rheumatol* 2011;**17**(1):23–7.

98. Durand M, Troyanov Y, Laflamme P, Gregoire G. Macrophage activation syndrome treated with anakinra. *J Rheumatol* 2010;**37**(4):879–80.

99. Kahn PJ, Cron RQ. Higher-dose Anakinra is effective in a case of medically refractory macrophage activation syndrome. *J Rheumatol* 2013;**40**(5):743–4.

100. Kelly A, Ramanan AV. A case of macrophage activation syndrome successfully treated with anakinra. *Nat Clin Prac Rheumatol* 2008;**4**(11):615–20.

101. Loh NK, Lucas M, Fernandez S, Prentice D. Successful treatment of macrophage activation syndrome complicating adult Still disease with anakinra. *Intern Med J* 2012;**42**(12):1358–62.

102. Rajasekaran S, Kruse K, Kovey K, Davis AT, Hassan NE, Ndika AN, et al. Therapeutic role of anakinra, an interleukin-1 receptor antagonist, in the management of secondary hemophagocytic lymphohistiocytosis/sepsis/multiple organ dysfunction/macrophage activating syndrome in critically ill children*. *Pediatr Crit Care Med* 2014;**15**(5):401–8.

103. Tayer-Shifman OE, Ben-Chetrit E. Refractory macrophage activation syndrome in a patient with SLE and APLA syndrome—successful use of PET- CT and Anakinra in its diagnosis and treatment. *Mod Rheumatol* 2015;**25**(6):954−7.

104. de Koning HD, Schalkwijk J, van der Ven-Jongekrijg J, Stoffels M, van der Meer JW, Simon A. Sustained efficacy of the monoclonal anti-interleukin-1 beta antibody canakinumab in a 9-month trial in Schnitzler's syndrome. *Ann Rheum Dis* 2013;**72**(10):1634−8.

105. de Koning HD, Bodar EJ, Simon A, van der Hilst JC, Netea MG, van der Meer JW. Beneficial response to anakinra and thalidomide in Schnitzler's syndrome. *Ann Rheum Dis* 2006;**65**(4):542−4.

106. Marrakchi S, Guigue P, Renshaw BR, Puel A, Pei XY, Fraitag S, et al. Interleukin-36-receptor antagonist deficiency and generalized pustular psoriasis. *N Engl J Med* 2011;**365**(7):620−8.

107. van de Veerdonk FL, Stoeckman AK, Wu G, Boeckermann AN, Azam T, Netea MG, et al. IL-38 binds to the IL-36 receptor and has biological effects on immune cells similar to IL-36 receptor antagonist. *Proc Natl Acad Sci USA* 2012;**109**(8):3001−5.

108. Langley RG, Elewski BE, Lebwohl M, Reich K, Griffiths CE, Papp K, et al. Secukinumab in plaque psoriasis—results of two phase 3 trials. *N Engl J Med* 2014;**371**(4):326−38.

109. Bernot A, da Silva C, Petit JL, Cruaud C, Caloustian C, Castet V, et al. Non-founder mutations in the MEFV gene establish this gene as the cause of familial Mediterranean fever (FMF). *Hum Mol Genet* 1998;**7**(8):1317−25.

110. French FMFC. A candidate gene for familial Mediterranean fever. *Nat Genet* 1997;**17**(1):25−31.

111. Srinivasula SM, Poyet JL, Razmara M, Datta P, Zhang Z, Alnemri ES. The PYRIN-CARD protein ASC is an activating adaptor for caspase-1. *J Biol Chem* 2002;**277**(24):21119−22.

112. van der Meer JW, Vossen JM, Radl J, van Nieuwkoop JA, Meyer CJ, Lobatto S, et al. Hyperimmunoglobulinaemia D and periodic fever: a new syndrome. *Lancet* 1984;**1**(8386):1087−90.

113. Drenth JP, Cuisset L, Grateau G, Vasseur C, van de Velde-Visser SD, de Jong JG, et al. Mutations in the gene encoding mevalonate kinase cause hyper-IgD and periodic fever syndrome. International Hyper-IgD Study Group. *Nat Genet* 1999;**22**(2):178−81.

114. van der Hilst JC, Bodar EJ, Barron KS, Frenkel J, Drenth JP, van der Meer JW, et al. Long-term follow-up, clinical features, and quality of life in a series of 103 patients with hyperimmunoglobulinemia D syndrome. *Medicine* 2008;**87**(6):301−10.

115. Gattorno M, Tassi S, Carta S, Delfino L, Ferlito F, Pelagatti MA, et al. Pattern of interleukin-1beta secretion in response to lipopolysaccharide and ATP before and after interleukin-1 blockade in patients with CIAS1 mutations. *Arthritis Rheum* 2007;**56**(9):3138−48.

116. Dinarello CA, Cannon JG, Wolff SM, Bernheim HA, Beutler B, Cerami A, et al. Tumor necrosis factor (cachectin) is an endogenous pyrogen and induces production of interleukin 1. *J Exp Med* 1986;**163**(6):1433−50.

117. Mesquida M, Molins B, Llorenc V, Hernandez MV, Espinosa G, Dick AD, et al. Current and future treatments for Behcet's uveitis: road to remission. *Int Ophthalmol* 2014;**34**(2):365−81.

118. Singh JA, Christensen R, Wells GA, Suarez-Almazor ME, Buchbinder R, Lopez-Olivo MA, et al. Biologics for rheumatoid arthritis: an overview of Cochrane reviews. *Sao Paulo Med J* 2010;**128**(5):309−10.

119. Alten R, Gomez-Reino J, Durez P, Beaulieu A, Sebba A, Krammer G, et al. Efficacy and safety of the human anti-IL-1beta monoclonal antibody canakinumab in rheumatoid arthritis: results of a 12-week, Phase II, dose-finding study. *BMC Musculoskelet Disord* 2011;**12**:153.

120. Chevalier X, Goupille P, Beaulieu AD, Burch FX, Bensen WG, Conrozier T, et al. Intraarticular injection of anakinra in osteoarthritis of the knee: a multicenter, randomized, double-blind, placebo-controlled study. *Arthritis Rheum* 2009;**61**(3):344−52.

121. Chevalier X, Giraudeau B, Conrozier T, Marliere J, Kiefer P, Goupille P. Safety study of intraarticular injection of interleukin 1 receptor antagonist in patients with painful knee osteoarthritis: a multicenter study. *J Rheumatol* 2005;**32**(7):1317−23.

122. Maedler K, Sergeev P, Ris F, Oberholzer J, Joller-Jemelka HI, Spinas GA, et al. Glucose-induced beta cell production of IL-1beta contributes to glucotoxicity in human pancreatic islets. *J Clin Invest* 2002;**110**(6):851−60.

123. Donath MY, Shoelson SE. Type 2 diabetes as an inflammatory disease. *Nat Rev Immunol* 2011;**11**(2):98−107.

124. Joosten LA, Netea MG, Mylona E, Koenders MI, Malireddi RK, Oosting M, et al. Engagement of fatty acids with Toll-like receptor 2 drives interleukin-1beta production via the ASC/caspase 1 pathway in monosodium urate monohydrate crystal-induced gouty arthritis. *Arthritis Rheum* 2010;**62**(11):3237−48.

125. Mylona EE, Mouktaroudi M, Crisan TO, Makri S, Pistiki A, Georgitsi M, et al. Enhanced interleukin-1beta production of PBMCs from patients with gout after stimulation with Toll-like receptor-2 ligands and urate crystals. *Arthritis Res Ther* 2012;**14**(4):R158.

126. Joosten LA, Netea MG, Fantuzzi G, Koenders MI, Helsen MM, Sparrer H, et al. Inflammatory arthritis in caspase 1 gene-deficient mice: contribution of proteinase 3 to caspase 1-independent production of bioactive interleukin-1beta. *Arthritis Rheum* 2009;**60**(12):3651−62.

127. Abbate A, Van Tassell BW, Biondi-Zoccai GG. Blocking interleukin-1 as a novel therapeutic strategy for secondary prevention of cardiovascular events. *BioDrugs* 2012;**26**(4):217−33.

128. Abbate A, Salloum FN, Vecile E, Das A, Hoke NN, Straino S, et al. Anakinra, a recombinant human interleukin-1 receptor antagonist, inhibits apoptosis in experimental acute myocardial infarction. *Circulation* 2008;**117**(20):2670−83.

129. Pomerantz BJ, Reznikov LL, Harken AH, Dinarello CA. Inhibition of caspase 1 reduces human myocardial ischemic dysfunction via inhibition of IL-18 and IL-1beta. *Proc Natl Acad Sci USA* 2001;**98**(5):2871−6.

130. Ridker PM, Thuren T, Zalewski A, Libby P. Interleukin-1beta inhibition and the prevention of recurrent cardiovascular events: rationale and design of the Canakinumab Anti-inflammatory Thrombosis Outcomes Study (CANTOS). *Am Heart J* 2011;**162**(4):597−605.

131. Torcia M, Lucibello M, Vannier E, Fabiani S, Miliani A, Guidi G, et al. Modulation of osteoclast-activating factor activity of multiple myeloma bone marrow cells by different interleukin-1 inhibitors. *Exp Hematol* 1996;**24**(8):868−74.

132. Lust JA, Donovan KA. The role of interleukin-1 beta in the pathogenesis of multiple myeloma. *Hematol Oncol Clin North Am* 1999;**13**(6):1117−25.

133. Canna SW, de Jesus AA, Gouni S, Brooks SR, Marrero B, Liu Y, et al. An activating NLRC4 inflammasome mutation causes autoinflammation with recurrent macrophage activation syndrome. *Nat Genet* 2014;**46**(10):1140−6.

Systems Medicine of Autoimmune Diseases: From Understanding Complexity to Precision Treatments

Julio Raúl Fernández Massó

Department of Systems Biology, Center for Genetic Engineering and Biotechnology, Cubanacan, Havana, Cuba

9.1 INTRODUCTION

Recent years have seen the rapid emergence of Systems Medicine as a new discipline.[1] In the biomedical sciences research has moved from a reductionist approach to a "Systems Medicine" paradigm that attempts to understand biology and pathophysiology in an integrative manner. This approach is driven by systems strategies and new technological advancements for disease diagnostics, prevention, and therapeutics, together with the increasing digitization of medicine.[2] Key to Systems Medicine is the transformation of medicine from a discipline that assesses diseases as simplified independent symptoms in organs and tissues to the challenge of dealing with disease in its complexity.

The fundamental principle of a systems approach to medicine is that disease arises as a consequence of one or more disease-perturbed networks in cells of the relevant organ. Because diseases result from perturbed networks there are early signals that can be tracked, even presymptomatically, as we come to a deep understanding of their functioning.[3] Systems Medicine deals with this complexity by generating billions of data points of individual patient. Systems Biology tools are used to reduce this huge data dimensionality to simple hypotheses about health and disease network.[4] A key challenge for Systems Medicine relates to the appreciation of disease complexity, reflected in these perturbed molecular networks as revealed through sophisticated analysis of ever increasing "omics" data.[5,6]

Immune Rebalancing. DOI: http://dx.doi.org/10.1016/B978-0-12-803302-9.00009-9

Autoimmune diseases are perhaps among the most complex diseases, and pose significant challenges for treatment. The challenge of autoimmune diseases has been both theoretical and practical. Autoimmune diseases are disorders characterized by an inappropriate immune response against constituents normally present in the human body. The causes of autoimmune conditions are largely unknown, but it appears that there is an inherited genetic predisposition in many cases. Autoimmune diseases are typically multifactorial polygenic diseases and affect approximately 3–5% of the world population.[7] More than 100 different types have been recognized, and the majority of autoimmune problems are associated with nine disorders: rheumatoid arthritis (RA), type I diabetes mellitus (T1DM), multiple sclerosis (MS), psoriasis (PS), systemic lupus erythematosus (SLE), ulcerative colitis (UC), Crohn's disease (CD), celiac disease (CeD), and scleroderma.

Autoimmune diseases arise from interactions between environmental, epigenetic, and genetic factors that result in persistent activation of immune responses and their biological networks.[8,9] It is assumed that the onset of these diseases in predisposed individuals may also reflect random processes during immune cell development such as immunoglobulin or T cell receptor gene recombination and mutation.[10] Common genes are likely to be involved in autoimmune diseases, as the chromosomal regions that contain susceptibility genes coincide.[11] Our incomplete understanding of autoreactive inflammatory processes, the clinical heterogeneity of the diseases, and their complex pathogeneses are among the factors that render a specific treatment challenging.[12]

Translating the knowledge about autoimmune disease biology into clinical practice is of the greatest importance and remains a daunting task. Prior to the genomic era, immunologists relied on very limited molecular testing in addition to conventional clinical presentation and immunological analyses to guide practice.[8] Dramatic advances in genomics and proteomics over the last decade have enabled innovative strategies for interrogating autoimmune diseases through detailed molecular analyses.[13,14] One of the challenges in Systems Medicine is to develop tools and strategies to stratify patients properly to identify the appropriate treatment.[15] This would protect the patients against unnecessary drug exposure, loss of time and side effects improving compliance and probably reducing health care expenditures.

This chapter seeks to provide an overview on the applications of Systems Medicine in the study of autoimmune diseases. Examples of various applications of Systems Medicine will be described and some challenges for future work will be identified.

9.2 FROM SYSTEMS BIOLOGY TO SYSTEMS MEDICINE

When the concept of Systems Biology is applied to the field of health sciences, it is called Systems Medicine. Systems Biology and Systems Medicine are practically identical concepts, except that the former is general and the latter is particularly focused on medicine. Systems Medicine is an adaptation and extension of Systems Biology, embracing the paradigm from recent years that have shifted Life Sciences "from a fragmented to a systems approach, linear to non-linear methodology and from genome to physiome based analysis."[2,16,17]

Systems Biology is hypothesis-driven, where a structured and precise model is formulated from existing data. The data used in the models is based on high throughput experiments that should be global, generated from different experimental platforms and able to be integrated. The data should be able to monitor networks dynamically and provide deep insight into biology of disease and should be able to capture the heterogeneity of phenotypes. To handle the enormous amount of data and manage the signal to noise problems, proper statistics and bioinformatics solutions should be used. Once the data is generated a descriptive model should be evaluated for its capacity to predict a therapeutic outcome (Fig. 9.1).[18−20]

9.3 SYSTEMS BIOLOGY AND THE EMERGING TECHNOLOGIES

The basic purpose of Systems Biology is the systems-level understanding of a cell or an organism,[6] which can be summarized in the context of molecular networks as the ability to:

1. Understand the structure of all the components of a cell/organism up to molecular level,
2. Predict the future state of the cell/organism under a normal environment,

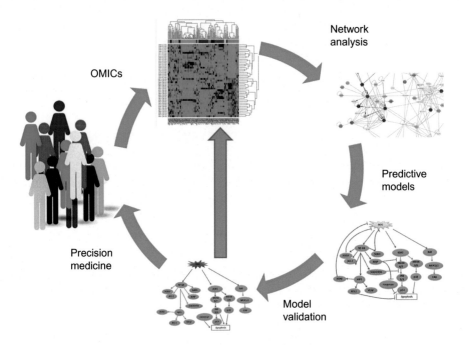

OMICs

Network
analysis

Predictive
models

Model
validation

Precision
medicine

Figure 9.1 The key steps in Systems Medicine.

3. Predict the output responses for a given input stimulus, and
4. Estimate the changes in system behavior upon perturbation of the components or the environment.

The key to understanding the complexity of autoimmunity as a disease is to effectively utilize systems approaches to deeply and correctly interpret data streams made possible by the emerging technologies of contemporary biology. The complex interactions within the immune system that result in effective host defense under normal conditions and inflammatory disease when perturbed can only be dissected in a comprehensive way by systems biology approaches.[21,22]

9.4 APPLICATION OF EMERGING TECHNOLOGIES IN AUTOIMMUNE RESEARCH

Emerging technologies in genomics, transcriptomics, proteomics, microfluidics, and single-cell analysis are transforming research and in the past several years have started to make an impact in the medical practice (Table 9.1). Systems Biology in autoimmune diseases has

Table 9.1 Omics Data Types Used to Build and Test Human Pathway and Disease Networks

Omics Type	Description	Number of Components	Tools
Genomics	The entire DNA sequence in a cell or sample	3 billion bases	Sequencing
Transcriptomics	RNA transcripts, including alternatively spliced variants of protein-encoding messenger RNA and noncoding RNA molecules (miRNA and lncRNA) that regulate transcription via gene silencing	30,000	Microarray, PCR and RNA-Seq
Epigenetics	Nongenomic-encoded DNA modifications, including methylated CpG genomic sequences	20–30 million	MethylCap-Seq and Next-Generation Sequencing
Proteomics	Proteins, enzymes, receptors and structural units of the cell, including modifications as phosphorylation	200,000	Mass spectrometry, protein array, immuno-based methods, yeast two hybrid
Metabolomics	Small biomolecules in the cell, including lipids, nucleotides, dipeptides and hormones	Approximately 40,000	Mass spectrometry

included genomics, expression profiling and functional analysis of DNA, RNA, protein, and metabolites of specific cell subsets in each stage of disease.[1,23] Moreover it has been successfully used to explain the mechanism of action of different drugs used in preclinical and clinical studies.[24]

9.4.1 Genomics

In genome-wide association studies, several inherited polymorphisms that cause autoimmune diseases have been identified. The strongest genetic associations, for most autoimmune diseases, are with the HLA locus. HLA haplotype linkages are shared between autoimmune diseases, and most HLA associations seem to be disease-specific.[25] Additionally, other loci are also shared between different autoimmune diseases. For example, variants in the tumor necrosis factor alpha-inducible protein 3 gene have been associated to SLE, RA, CD, UC, CeD, and alopecia areata,[26] with varying degrees of risk.

A number of single nucleotide polymorphism (SNP) is estimated to share pathogenic pathways in the development of autoimmune diseases.

More than 100 disease-risk SNPs have been identified in CeD,[27] CD,[28] MS,[29,30] PS,[31] RA,[32–34] SLE,[35,36] and T1DM.[37,38] Interestingly, Hu et al.[39] found that 47 of 107 immune-mediated disease risk SNPs are associated with multiple autoimmune diseases, leading to the proposal that distinct groups of interacting molecules that share a disease risk are encoded close to SNPs that influence the same subsets of diseases. According to this finding, the stratification of autoimmune disease patients by genotype, instead of phenotype, could be more effective in treating patients. This strategy of stratification, not by tumor localization but by tumor genotype, already has been proposed for the treatment of cancer patients.[40–43]

The most striking evidence of environmental effects on the development of autoimmune diseases is the high discordance rate observed in monozygotic twins.[44–46] Discordance enables the study of epigenetic changes that could lead to the development of autoimmunity. In an individual with a susceptible genotype, exposure to environmental factors, not only triggers downstream signaling of the susceptible genes but also could initiate epigenetic changes during the development of autoimmune responses.[47–49]

Contradictory results on the role of epigenetics in the development of autoimmune diseases in monozygotic twins have been described. Baranzini et al.[44] sequences the genome of one MS discordant monozygotic twin pair, as well as messenger RNA transcriptome and epigenome sequences of CD41 lymphocytes from three MS-discordant, monozygotic twin pairs. In this first systematic effort to estimate sequence variation among monozygotic cotwins, the authors did not find evidence for genetic, epigenetic, or transcriptome differences that could explain disease discordance.

On the contrary, candidate gene studies of autoimmune diseases have identified a small set of genes that undergo epigenetic changes, such as aberrant DNA demethylation, histone modification, and micro-RNAs (miRNAs), in rheumatic diseases. T cells from patients with SLE or RA, as well as synovial fibroblasts from individuals with RA,[50,51] contain hypomethylated DNA sequences and/or histone modifications in particular cell types. The identification of target sequences for epigenetic deregulation will provide clinical markers for diagnosis, disease progression, and therapies for autoimmune diseases.

9.4.2 Transcriptomic Profiling and Disease Stratification

Transcriptomic research in patients with autoimmune diseases can be used to guide other biologic approaches, including proteomics or genomic studies, and can also provide the basis for early translational and clinical applications. The applications of transcriptomics in autoimmune diseases include the following:

1. To identify transcriptional differences between autoimmune disease patients and healthy controls and patients with other autoimmune disorders, or between different clinical forms or activity phases of the disease.[52,53]
2. To identify molecular pathways involved in the inflammatory processes taking place in the course of disease.[54,55]
3. To investigate the transcriptional changes associated with the effects of therapies used in the treatment of patient.[56–58]

Another area of study in transcriptomics is the differential expression of miRNAs, a class of small noncoding RNAs that regulate gene expression by pairing with their target mRNAs and are often deregulated in autoimmune diseases.[59] miRNAs have been suspected to play an important role in the immune system based on their high expression in immune cells.[60] Moreover, miRNAs had been shown to play an important role in autoimmune processes.[61–63] For example, several miRNAs have been associated with MS, MS relapses, and/or MS pathogenesis.[64] Although the studies published so far are very promising, a consensus regarding which miRNAS can be used as biomarkers needs to be reached.

Blood transcriptome studies to determine the expression levels of mRNAs of a given cell population are essential for autoimmunity-related translational research.[65–68] Such transcriptome studies measure the levels of RNA transcripts in patient samples, which have been influenced by environmental factors or pathologic conditions. Well-known examples of successful blood transcriptome analyses have been reported in the case of SLE. In 2003, two independent teams identified a strong interferon (IFN) signature in pediatric and adult SLE patients, with a central role for dendritic cells and IFNα in the disease.[69]

9.4.3 Proteomics Approach

Proteomics, the study of the function as well as the primary structure of proteins, allows for the large scale study of protein profiles in complex biological samples. It is anticipated that a future merger of proteomics with cell biology will yield a better understanding of regulation of cellular processes, both in healthy and diseased states.[23,70] The evolution of mass spectrometry techniques towards high resolution and higher throughput machinery has been essential for the advancement of the field.[23] Another key element in proteomics is protein identification. This is typically done by one of two methods: database searching and de novo sequencing. A combination of database searching and de novo sequencing is a powerful method to increase the number of identified peptides in a proteomics setting.[71,72]

New insights in MS have been described using proteomics. A focused proteomic analysis of well-characterized human MS brain lesions, acute plaque, chronic active plaque, and chronic plaque, have been enriched by laser-capture microdissection and analyzed by mass spectrometry. The lesion-specific proteome allows to reveal the unique proteins identified in all three MS lesions possessing functions currently unknown. In addition, the analysis reveals the extensive interface between the coagulation system and brain inflammation, providing new functional insights into the pathogenesis of MS.[73]

Protein−protein interaction (PPI) identification is another important application of the proteomics studies.[74] The current estimates suggest that the human interactome comprises approximately 130,000−650,000 protein interactions.[75,76] However, only a subset of these interactions has been experimentally identified.[4,77] The study of Gao and Wang[78] illustrates the potential of the PPI information in prioritizing positional candidate genes for T1DM. Such systemic approaches lead to 68 novel candidate genes for T1DM that should require further validation.

9.4.4 Network Biology

As our theories of Systems Biology grow more sophisticated, the models we use to represent them become larger and more complex.[79] In recent years, network biology has emerged as a powerful paradigm to visualize and analyze large data ensembles in novel ways with unparalleled flexibility.[3,80−82] Biological networks are conveniently and effectively represented in computers by graph data structures, which formally comprise a set of relations (edges) between biological entities or processes (nodes). Most often the edges in such abstractions have specific directionality, and can accurately represent the semantics of the relationship between the entities being connected.[79,83]

There are many repositories of pathway data available to researchers today. They are generally organized around molecular interactions, gene regulatory networks, signal transduction pathways, or metabolic pathways. Pathguide (http://www.pathguide.org) currently lists some 547 pathway and molecular interaction related resources, the majority of which are available at no cost to the user.[84] Unfortunately, although typically for databases of any kind, each of these pathway resources uses its own data format and data model. These data formats and models are most often inconsistent with one another, and so typically the data are not interchangeable across resources.[85]

A network of disorders and disease genes linked by known disorder gene associations offers a platform to explore in a single graph theoretic framework all known phenotype and disease gene associations, indicating the common genetic origin of many diseases. Genes associated with similar disorders show both higher likelihoods of physical interactions between their products and higher expression profiling similarities for their transcripts, supporting the existence of distinct disease-specific functional modules.[3,86,87]

Using the network information available in databases in combination with experimental data derived from genomics, transcriptomics, or proteomics experiments have enabled a detailed look at the genetic landscape of complex human phenotypes.[87–90] For example, identification of genetic similarities among complex diseases, particularly autoimmune diseases, is a topic of intense research in network biology.[91,92]

Baranzini et al.,[87] based on the information of two GWAS in MS that takes into account all SNPs with evidence of association, conducted a pathway-oriented analysis. In the MS datasets were identified subnetworks of genes from immunological pathways previously known as related to MS. This analysis also identified for the first time neural pathways, as axon-guidance and synaptic potentiation as overrepresented in MS. Another example of network analysis is the work conducted by Lee et al.[90] The authors showed that bone marrow cells from patients with RA had abnormal functional networks in immune response and cell cycle when compared with the bone marrow cells from osteoarthritis patients. Their results suggest that the over-expression of genes that take part in the antigen presentation pathway and IFN signaling contribute to the pathogenesis of RA.

Other networks analysis has been conducted on problems in pharmacology, to allow systems level descriptions of drug action, rapid identification of novel therapeutic strategies, and potentially safer and more effective drugs development and prescription.[93]

9.4.5 Big-Data Information and Computation Technology

Biology has recently become a "big-data science" supported by the advances in high-throughput experimental technologies. Data-intensive science consists of three basic activities: capture, curation, and data mining.[6] All three of these phases of handling big data raise many new research challenges to pursue in systems medicine. The most significant challenge in systems medicine is computation; the data have to be stored in databases, annotated, analyzed, and finally correctly interpreted by large multidisciplinary research teams. An astonishing number of databases, analysis tools, and algorithms for computational systems biology analysis are published each year and deciding which is the best solution for each specific problem is difficult.

Systems modeling approaches may have an important role in the personalization of medicine. It has been established that mechanistic systems models can be used to identify biomarkers of responding subpopulations.[94] Systems modeling approaches already have demonstrated promise informing therapeutic decisions with statistical calibration of population clinical measures, reflecting the underlying mechanistic heterogeneity.[95]

At the same time, systems medicine poses many challenges for generating sufficient data to deal with the enormous signal to noise problems. It would need a large patient population to deal with the extensive disease stratification that will, for example, divide MS patients into different subtypes of disease. In the future the human genome will be a routine portion of each individual patient's medical record. The average patient will be surrounded by billions of data points in the future. In addition, we would deal with the enormous amounts of data that will be generated with the extensive use of single-cell analyses, as well as the data generated by the new in vivo imaging technologies. New computational tools would be required to reduce this enormous dimensionality into simple hypotheses about health and disease. The opportunities are overwhelming; the informational technology challenges are outstanding.[96]

9.5 FROM SYSTEMS MEDICINE TO PRECISION MEDICINE

The final goal of Systems Medicine approaches could be defined as Precision Medicine. Precision medicine has been defined as the tailoring of medical treatment to the characteristics of an individual patient. Knowing an individual's genomics has created a remarkable and unprecedented opportunity to improve medical treatment and develop preventative strategies to preserve health.[96-98] For the moment the proposed benefits of precision medicine to the patient include:

1. Detecting disease at an earlier stage, when it is easier and less expensive to treat effectively
2. Stratifying patients into groups that enable the selection of optimal therapy
3. Reducing adverse drug reactions by more effective early assessment of individual drug responses
4. Improving the selection of new biochemical targets for drug discovery
5. Reducing the time, cost, and failure rate of clinical trials for new therapies
6. Shifting the emphasis in medicine from reaction to prevention and from disease to wellness

In summary, systems medicine provides tools to investigate and characterize disease heterogeneity. To this end the analyses follow a general three-step procedure: (i) the need to identify the relevant biomarkers for each case of heterogeneity; (ii) develop predictive and validated statistically models with the potential to be applied in the clinic; and (iii) the usefulness of the models in a clinical scenario has to be validated. From a Systems Medicine perspective predictions made must be personalized and useful for treating patients.

REFERENCES

1. Wang RS, Maron BA, Loscalzo J. Systems medicine: evolution of systems biology from bench to bedside. *Wiley Interdiscip Rev Syst Biol Med* 2015;7(4):141–61. Available from: http://dx.doi.org/10.1002/wsbm.1297.

2. Tillmann T, Gibson AR, Scott G, Harrison O, Dominiczak A, Hanlon P. Systems Medicine 2.0: potential benefits of combining electronic health care records with systems science models. *J Med Internet Res* 2015;17(3):e64. Available from: http://dx.doi.org/10.2196/jmir.3082.

3. Zhou X, Menche J, Barabasi AL, Sharma A. Human symptoms-disease network. *Nat Commun* 2014;5:4212. Available from: http://dx.doi.org/10.1038/ncomms5212.

4. Furlong LI. Human diseases through the lens of network biology. *Trends Genet* 2013; **29**(3):150−9. Available from: http://dx.doi.org/10.1016/j.tig.2012.11.004.

5. Ndiaye NC. Systems Medicine in the era of "Big Data": a game-changer for Personalized Medicine? *Drug Metabol Drug Interact* 2014;**29**(3):127. Available from: http://dx.doi.org/ 10.1515/dmdi-2014-0022.

6. Altaf-Ul-Amin M, Afendi FM, Kiboi SK, Kanaya S. Systems biology in the context of big data and networks. *Biomed Res Int* 2014;**2014**:428570. Available from: http://dx.doi.org/ 10.1155/2014/428570.

7. Wang L, Wang FS, Gershwin ME. Human autoimmune diseases: a comprehensive update. *J Intern Med* 2015. Available from: http://dx.doi.org/10.1111/joim.12395.

8. Blumberg RS, Dittel B, Hafler D, von Herrath M, Nestle FO. Unraveling the autoimmune translational research process layer by layer. *Nat Med* 2012;**18**(1):35−41. Available from: http://dx.doi.org/10.1038/nm.2632.

9. Goldblatt F, O'Neill SG. Clinical aspects of autoimmune rheumatic diseases. *Lancet* 2013;**382**(9894):797−808. Available from: http://dx.doi.org/10.1016/S0140-6736(13)61499-3.

10. Yu X, Almeida JR, Darko S, van der Burg M, DeRavin SS, Malech H, et al. Human syndromes of immunodeficiency and dysregulation are characterized by distinct defects in T-cell receptor repertoire development. *J Allergy Clin Immunol* 2014;**133**(4):1109−15. Available from: http://dx.doi.org/10.1016/j.jaci.2013.11.018.

11. Diaz-Gallo LM, Martin J. Common genes in autoimmune diseases: a link between immune-mediated diseases. *Expert Rev Clin Immunol* 2012;**8**(2):107−9. Available from: http://dx.doi. org/10.1586/eci.11.90.

12. Cho JH, Feldman M. Heterogeneity of autoimmune diseases: pathophysiologic insights from genetics and implications for new therapies. *Nat Med* 2015;**21**(7):730−8. Available from: http://dx.doi.org/10.1038/nm.3897.

13. Johar AS, Mastronardi C, Rojas-Villarraga A, Patel HR, Chuah A, Peng K, et al. Novel and rare functional genomic variants in multiple autoimmune syndrome and Sjogren's syndrome. *J Transl Med* 2015;**13**:173. Available from: http://dx.doi.org/10.1186/s12967-015-0525-x.

14. Ohyama K, Baba M, Tamai M, Aibara N, Ichinose K, Kishikawa N, et al. Proteomic profiling of antigens in circulating immune complexes associated with each of seven autoimmune diseases. *Clin Biochem* 2015;**48**(3):181−5. Available from: http://dx.doi.org/10.1016/ j.clinbiochem.2014.11.008.

15. Critchley-Thorne RJ, Miller SM, Taylor DL, Lingle WL. Applications of cellular systems biology in breast cancer patient stratification and diagnostics. *Comb Chem High Throughput Screen* 2009;**12**(9):860−9.

16. Gomez-Cabrero D, Menche J, Cano I, Abugessaisa I, Huertas-Miguelanez M, Tenyi A, et al. Systems medicine: from molecular features and models to the clinic in COPD. *J Transl Med* 2014;**12**(Suppl. 2):S4. Available from: http://dx.doi.org/10.1186/1479-5876-12-S2-S4.

17. Majumder D, Mukherjee A. A passage through systems biology to systems medicine: adoption of middle-out rational approaches towards the understanding of therapeutic outcomes in cancer. *Analyst* 2011;**136**(4):663−78. Available from: http://dx.doi.org/10.1039/C0AN00746C.

18. Root-Bernstein R. Towards an integration of mathematical models, theories and observations concerning autoimmune diseases. *J Theor Biol* 2015;**375**:1−3. Available from: http://dx. doi.org/10.1016/j.jtbi.2015.04.003.

19. Serra R. Complex systems models in biology and medicine: generic properties and applications. *Comput Math Methods Med* 2014;**2014**:580509. Available from: http://dx.doi.org/ 10.1155/2014/580509.

20. Wolkenhauer O, Auffray C, Brass O, Clairambault J, Deutsch A, Drasdo D, et al. Enabling multiscale modeling in systems medicine. *Genome Med* 2014;**6**(3):21. Available from: http:// dx.doi.org/10.1186/gm538.

21. Kim HY, Kim HR, Lee SH. Advances in systems biology approaches for autoimmune diseases. *Immune Netw* 2014;**14**(2):73−80. Available from: http://dx.doi.org/10.4110/in.2014.14.2.73.

22. Zak DE, Aderem A. Systems biology of innate immunity. *Immunol Rev* 2009;**227**(1):264−82. Available from: http://dx.doi.org/10.1111/j.1600-065X.2008.00721.x.

23. Ebhardt HA, Root A, Sander C, Aebersold R. Applications of targeted proteomics in systems biology and translational medicine. *Proteomics* 2015. Available from: http://dx.doi.org/10.1002/pmic.201500004.

24. Gottlieb A, Altman RB. Integrating systems biology sources illuminates drug action. *Clin Pharmacol Ther* 2014;**95**(6):663−9. Available from: http://dx.doi.org/10.1038/clpt.2014.51.

25. Trowsdale J. The MHC, disease and selection. *Immunol Lett* 2011;**137**(1−2):1−8. Available from: http://dx.doi.org/10.1016/j.imlet.2011.01.002.

26. Ramos PS, Criswell LA, Moser KL, Comeau ME, Williams AH, Pajewski NM, et al. A comprehensive analysis of shared loci between systemic lupus erythematosus (SLE) and sixteen autoimmune diseases reveals limited genetic overlap. *PLoS Genet* 2011;**7**(12):e1002406. Available from: http://dx.doi.org/10.1371/journal.pgen.1002406.

27. Kumar V, Wijmenga C, Withoff S. From genome-wide association studies to disease mechanisms: celiac disease as a model for autoimmune diseases. *Semin Immunopathol* 2012;**34**(4):567−80. Available from: http://dx.doi.org/10.1007/s00281-012-0312-1.

28. Franke A, McGovern DP, Barrett JC, Wang K, Radford-Smith GL, Ahmad T, et al. Genome-wide meta-analysis increases to 71 the number of confirmed Crohn's disease susceptibility loci. *Nat Genet* 2010;**42**(12):1118−25. Available from: http://dx.doi.org/10.1038/ng.717.

29. Oksenberg JR, Baranzini SE, Sawcer S, Hauser SL. The genetics of multiple sclerosis: SNPs to pathways to pathogenesis. *Nat Rev Genet* 2008;**9**(7):516−26. Available from: http://dx.doi.org/10.1038/nrg2395.

30. Gourraud PA, Harbo HF, Hauser SL, Baranzini SE. The genetics of multiple sclerosis: an up-to-date review. *Immunol Rev* 2012;**248**(1):87−103. Available from: http://dx.doi.org/10.1111/j.1600-065X.2012.01134.x.

31. Duffin KC, Chandran V, Gladman DD, Krueger GG, Elder JT, Rahman P. Genetics of psoriasis and psoriatic arthritis: update and future direction. *J Rheumatol* 2008;**35**(7):1449−53.

32. Stahl EA, Raychaudhuri S, Remmers EF, Xie G, Eyre S, Thomson BP, et al. Genome-wide association study meta-analysis identifies seven new rheumatoid arthritis risk loci. *Nat Genet* 2010;**42**(6):508−14. Available from: http://dx.doi.org/10.1038/ng.582.

33. Govind N, Choudhury A, Hodkinson B, Ickinger C, Frost J, Lee A, et al. Immunochip identifies novel, and replicates known, genetic risk loci for rheumatoid arthritis in black South Africans. *Mol Med* 2014;**20**:341−9. Available from: http://dx.doi.org/10.2119/molmed.2014.00097.

34. Jiang L, Yin J, Ye L, Yang J, Hemani G, Liu AJ, et al. Novel risk loci for rheumatoid arthritis in Han Chinese and congruence with risk variants in Europeans. *Arthritis Rheumatol* 2014;**66**(5):1121−32. Available from: http://dx.doi.org/10.1002/art.38353.

35. You Y, Zhai ZF, Chen FR, Chen W, Hao F. Autoimmune risk loci of IL12RB2, IKZF1, XKR6, TMEM39A and CSK in Chinese patients with systemic lupus erythematosus. *Tissue Antigens* 2015;**85**(3):200−3. Available from: http://dx.doi.org/10.1111/tan.12522.

36. Gateva V, Sandling JK, Hom G, Taylor KE, Chung SA, Sun X, et al. A large-scale replication study identifies TNIP1, PRDM1, JAZF1, UHRF1BP1 and IL10 as risk loci for systemic lupus erythematosus. *Nat Genet* 2009;**41**(11):1228−33. Available from: http://dx.doi.org/10.1038/ng.468.

37. Barrett JC, Clayton DG, Concannon P, Akolkar B, Cooper JD, Erlich HA, et al. Genome-wide association study and meta-analysis find that over 40 loci affect risk of type 1 diabetes. *Nat Genet* 2009;**41**(6):703−7. Available from: http://dx.doi.org/10.1038/ng.381.

38. Cooper JD, Smyth DJ, Smiles AM, Plagnol V, Walker NM, Allen JE, et al. Meta-analysis of genome-wide association study data identifies additional type 1 diabetes risk loci. *Nat Genet* 2008;**40**(12):1399−401. Available from: http://dx.doi.org/10.1038/ng.249.

39. Hu X, Kim H, Stahl E, Plenge R, Daly M, Raychaudhuri S. Integrating autoimmune risk loci with gene-expression data identifies specific pathogenic immune cell subsets. *Am J Hum Genet* 2011;**89**(4):496−506. Available from: http://dx.doi.org/10.1016/j.ajhg.2011.09.002.

40. Cooperberg MR, Davicioni E, Crisan A, Jenkins RB, Ghadessi M, Karnes RJ. Combined value of validated clinical and genomic risk stratification tools for predicting prostate cancer mortality in a high-risk prostatectomy cohort. *Eur Urol* 2015;**67**(2):326−33. Available from: http://dx.doi.org/10.1016/j.eururo.2014.05.039.

41. Ding H, Wang C, Huang K, Machiraju R. iGPSe: a visual analytic system for integrative genomic based cancer patient stratification. *BMC Bioinformatics* 2014;**15**:203. Available from: http://dx.doi.org/10.1186/1471-2105-15-203.

42. Moschos SA. Genomic biomarkers for patient selection and stratification: the cancer paradigm. *Bioanalysis* 2012;**4**(20):2499−511. Available from: http://dx.doi.org/10.4155/bio.12.241.

43. Schoenborn JR, Nelson P, Fang M. Genomic profiling defines subtypes of prostate cancer with the potential for therapeutic stratification. *Clin Cancer Res* 2013;**19**(15):4058−66. Available from: http://dx.doi.org/10.1158/1078-0432.CCR-12-3606.

44. Baranzini SE, Mudge J, van Velkinburgh JC, Khankhanian P, Khrebtukova I, Miller NA, et al. Genome, epigenome and RNA sequences of monozygotic twins discordant for multiple sclerosis. *Nature* 2010;**464**(7293):1351−6. Available from: http://dx.doi.org/10.1038/nature08990.

45. Hansen T, Skytthe A, Stenager E, Petersen HC, Kyvik KO, Bronnum-Hansen H. Risk for multiple sclerosis in dizygotic and monozygotic twins. *Mult Scler* 2005;**11**(5):500−3.

46. O'Hanlon TP, Rider LG, Gan L, Fannin R, Paules RS, Umbach DM, et al. Gene expression profiles from discordant monozygotic twins suggest that molecular pathways are shared among multiple systemic autoimmune diseases. *Arthritis Res Ther* 2011;**13**(2):R69. Available from: http://dx.doi.org/10.1186/ar3330.

47. Gupta B, Hawkins RD. Epigenomics of autoimmune diseases. *Immunol Cell Biol* 2015; **93**(3):271−6. Available from: http://dx.doi.org/10.1038/icb.2015.18.

48. Picascia A, Grimaldi V, Pignalosa O, De Pascale MR, Schiano C, Napoli C. Epigenetic control of autoimmune diseases: from bench to bedside. *Clin Immunol* 2015;**157**(1):1−15. Available from: http://dx.doi.org/10.1016/j.clim.2014.12.013.

49. Zhang Z, Zhang R. Epigenetics in autoimmune diseases: pathogenesis and prospects for therapy. *Autoimmun Rev* 2015;**4**(10):854−63. Available from: http://dx.doi.org/10.1016/j.autrev.2015.05.008.

50. Viatte S, Plant D, Raychaudhuri S. Genetics and epigenetics of rheumatoid arthritis. *Nat Rev Rheumatol* 2013;**9**(3):141−53. Available from: http://dx.doi.org/10.1038/nrrheum.2012.237.

51. Quintero-Ronderos P, Montoya-Ortiz G. Epigenetics and autoimmune diseases. *Autoimmune Dis* 2012;**2012**:593720. Available from: http://dx.doi.org/10.1155/2012/593720.

52. Achiron A, Grotto I, Balicer R, Magalashvili D, Feldman A, Gurevich M. Microarray analysis identifies altered regulation of nuclear receptor family members in the pre-disease state of multiple sclerosis. *Neurobiol Dis* 2010;**38**(2):201−9. Available from: http://dx.doi.org/10.1016/j.nbd.2009.12.029.

53. van der Pouw Kraan TC, van Gaalen FA, Kasperkovitz PV, Verbeet NL, Smeets TJ, Kraan MC, et al. Rheumatoid arthritis is a heterogeneous disease: evidence for differences in the activation of

the STAT-1 pathway between rheumatoid tissues. *Arthritis Rheum* 2003;**48**(8):2132−45. Available from: http://dx.doi.org/10.1002/art.11096.

54. Iglesias AH, Camelo S, Hwang D, Villanueva R, Stephanopoulos G, Dangond F. Microarray detection of E2F pathway activation and other targets in multiple sclerosis peripheral blood mononuclear cells. *J Neuroimmunol* 2004;**150**(1−2):163−77. Available from: http://dx.doi.org/10.1016/j.jneuroim.2004.01.017.

55. Asquith DL, Ballantine LE, Nijjar JS, Makdasy MK, Patel S, Wright PB, et al. The liver X receptor pathway is highly upregulated in rheumatoid arthritis synovial macrophages and potentiates TLR-driven cytokine release. *Ann Rheum Dis* 2013;**72**(12):2024−31. Available from: http://dx.doi.org/10.1136/annrheumdis-2012-202872.

56. Satoh J, Nanri Y, Tabunoki H, Yamamura T. Microarray analysis identifies a set of CXCR3 and CCR2 ligand chemokines as early IFNbeta-responsive genes in peripheral blood lymphocytes in vitro: an implication for IFNbeta-related adverse effects in multiple sclerosis. *BMC Neurol* 2006;**6**:18. Available from: http://dx.doi.org/10.1186/1471-2377-6-18.

57. Koike F, Satoh J, Miyake S, Yamamoto T, Kawai M, Kikuchi S, et al. Microarray analysis identifies interferon beta-regulated genes in multiple sclerosis. *J Neuroimmunol* 2003;**139**(1−2):109−18.

58. Ben-Chetrit E, Bergmann S, Sood R. Mechanism of the anti-inflammatory effect of colchicine in rheumatic diseases: a possible new outlook through microarray analysis. *Rheumatology (Oxford)* 2006;**45**(3):274−82. Available from: http://dx.doi.org/10.1093/rheumatology/kei140.

59. Pauley KM, Cha S, Chan EK. MicroRNA in autoimmunity and autoimmune diseases. *J Autoimmun* 2009;**32**(3−4):189−94. Available from: http://dx.doi.org/10.1016/j.jaut.2009.02.012.

60. Chen CZ, Li L, Lodish HF, Bartel DP. MicroRNAs modulate hematopoietic lineage differentiation. *Science* 2004;**303**(5654):83−6. Available from: http://dx.doi.org/10.1126/science.1091903.

61. Xiao C, Srinivasan L, Calado DP, Patterson HC, Zhang B, Wang J, et al. Lymphoproliferative disease and autoimmunity in mice with increased miR-17-92 expression in lymphocytes. *Nat Immunol* 2008;**9**(4):405−14. Available from: http://dx.doi.org/10.1038/ni1575.

62. Zhou X, Jeker LT, Fife BT, Zhu S, Anderson MS, McManus MT, et al. Selective miRNA disruption in T reg cells leads to uncontrolled autoimmunity. *J Exp Med* 2008;**205**(9):1983−91. Available from: http://dx.doi.org/10.1084/jem.20080707.

63. Yang Y, Zhang K, Zhou R. Meta-analysis of pre-miRNA polymorphisms association with susceptibility to autoimmune diseases. *Immunol Invest* 2014;**43**(1):13−27. Available from: http://dx.doi.org/10.3109/08820139.2013.822389.

64. Guerau-de-Arellano M, Alder H, Ozer HG, Lovett-Racke A, Racke MK. miRNA profiling for biomarker discovery in multiple sclerosis: from microarray to deep sequencing. *J Neuroimmunol* 2012;**248**(1−2):32−9. Available from: http://dx.doi.org/10.1016/j.jneuroim.2011.10.006.

65. Croze E. Differential gene expression and translational approaches to identify biomarkers of interferon beta activity in multiple sclerosis. *J Interferon Cytokine Res* 2010;**30**(10):743−9. Available from: http://dx.doi.org/10.1089/jir.2010.0022.

66. Liew CC, Ma J, Tang HC, Zheng R, Dempsey AA. The peripheral blood transcriptome dynamically reflects system wide biology: a potential diagnostic tool. *J Lab Clin Med* 2006;**147**(3):126−32. Available from: http://dx.doi.org/10.1016/j.lab.2005.10.005.

67. Mohr S, Liew CC. The peripheral-blood transcriptome: new insights into disease and risk assessment. *Trends Mol Med* 2007;**13**(10):422−32. Available from: http://dx.doi.org/10.1016/j.molmed.2007.08.003.

68. Teixeira VH, Olaso R, Martin-Magniette ML, Lasbleiz S, Jacq L, Oliveira CR, et al. Transcriptome analysis describing new immunity and defense genes in peripheral blood

mononuclear cells of rheumatoid arthritis patients. *PLoS One* 2009;**4**(8):e6803. Available from: http://dx.doi.org/10.1371/journal.pone.0006803.

69. Pascual V, Banchereau J, Palucka AK. The central role of dendritic cells and interferon-alpha in SLE. *Curr Opin Rheumatol* 2003;**15**(5):548−56.

70. Rust S, Guillard S, Sachsenmeier K, Hay C, Davidson M, Karlsson A, et al. Combining phenotypic and proteomic approaches to identify membrane targets in a "triple negative" breast cancer cell type. *Mol Cancer* 2013;**12**:11. Available from: http://dx.doi.org/10.1186/1476-4598-12-11.

71. Wang X, Zhang B. Integrating genomic, transcriptomic, and interactome data to improve peptide and protein identification in shotgun proteomics. *J Proteome Res* 2014;**13**(6):2715−23. Available from: http://dx.doi.org/10.1021/pr500194t.

72. Hoopmann MR, Moritz RL. Current algorithmic solutions for peptide-based proteomics data generation and identification. *Curr Opin Biotechnol* 2013;**24**(1):31−8. Available from: http://dx.doi.org/10.1016/j.copbio.2012.10.013.

73. Han MH, Hwang SI, Roy DB, Lundgren DH, Price JV, Ousman SS, et al. Proteomic analysis of active multiple sclerosis lesions reveals therapeutic targets. *Nature* 2008;**451**(7182):1076−81. Available from: http://dx.doi.org/10.1038/nature06559.

74. Sevimoglu T, Arga KY. The role of protein interaction networks in systems biomedicine. *Comput Struct Biotechnol J* 2014;**11**(18):22−7. Available from: http://dx.doi.org/10.1016/j.csbj.2014.08.008.

75. Sambourg L, Thierry-Mieg N. New insights into protein-protein interaction data lead to increased estimates of the *S. cerevisiae* interactome size. *BMC Bioinformatics* 2010;**11**:605. Available from: http://dx.doi.org/10.1186/1471-2105-11-605.

76. Stumpf MP, Thorne T, de Silva E, Stewart R, An HJ, Lappe M, et al. Estimating the size of the human interactome. *Proc Natl Acad Sci USA* 2008;**105**(19):6959−64. Available from: http://dx.doi.org/10.1073/pnas.0708078105.

77. de Souza N. Systems biology: an expanded human interactome. *Nat Methods* 2015;**12**(2):107.

78. Gao S, Wang X. Predicting type 1 diabetes candidate genes using human protein−protein interaction networks. *J Comput Sci Syst Biol* 2009;**2**:133. Available from: http://dx.doi.org/10.4172/jcsb.1000025.

79. Slater T. Recent advances in modeling languages for pathway maps and computable biological networks. *Drug Discov Today* 2014;**19**(2):193−8. Available from: http://dx.doi.org/10.1016/j.drudis.2013.12.011.

80. Yildirim MA, Goh KI, Cusick ME, Barabasi AL, Vidal M. Drug-target network. *Nat Biotechnol* 2007;**25**(10):1119−26. Available from: http://dx.doi.org/10.1038/nbt1338.

81. Goh KI, Cusick ME, Valle D, Childs B, Vidal M, Barabasi AL. The human disease network. *Proc Natl Acad Sci USA* 2007;**104**(21):8685−90. Available from: http://dx.doi.org/10.1073/pnas.0701361104.

82. Barabasi AL, Oltvai ZN. Network biology: understanding the cell's functional organization. *Nat Rev Genet* 2004;**5**(2):101−13. Available from: http://dx.doi.org/10.1038/nrg1272.

83. Barabasi AL. Network science. *Philos Trans A Math Phys Eng Sci* 2013;**371**(1987):20120375. Available from: http://dx.doi.org/10.1098/rsta.2012.0375.

84. Bader GD, Cary MP, Sander C. Pathguide: a pathway resource list. *Nucleic Acids Res* 2006;**34**(Database issue):D504−6. Available from: http://dx.doi.org/10.1093/nar/gkj126.

85. Luciano JS. PAX of mind for pathway researchers. *Drug Discov Today* 2005;**10**(13):937−42. Available from: http://dx.doi.org/10.1016/S1359-6446(05)03501-4.

86. Hidalgo CA, Blumm N, Barabasi AL, Christakis NA. A dynamic network approach for the study of human phenotypes. *PLoS Comput Biol* 2009;**5**(4):e1000353. Available from: http://dx.doi.org/10.1371/journal.pcbi.1000353.

87. Baranzini SE, Galwey NW, Wang J, Khankhanian P, Lindberg R, Pelletier D, et al. Pathway and network-based analysis of genome-wide association studies in multiple sclerosis. *Hum Mol Genet* 2009;**18**(11):2078−90. Available from: http://dx.doi.org/10.1093/hmg/ddp120.

88. Sharma A, Gulbahce N, Pevzner SJ, Menche J, Ladenvall C, Folkersen L, et al. Network-based analysis of genome wide association data provides novel candidate genes for lipid and lipoprotein traits. *Mol Cell Proteomics* 2013;**12**(11):3398−408. Available from: http://dx.doi.org/10.1074/mcp.M112.024851.

89. Rozenblatt-Rosen O, Deo RC, Padi M, Adelmant G, Calderwood MA, Rolland T, et al. Interpreting cancer genomes using systematic host network perturbations by tumour virus proteins. *Nature* 2012;**487**(7408):491−5. Available from: http://dx.doi.org/10.1038/nature11288.

90. Lee HM, Sugino H, Aoki C, Shimaoka Y, Suzuki R, Ochi K, et al. Abnormal networks of immune response-related molecules in bone marrow cells from patients with rheumatoid arthritis as revealed by DNA microarray analysis. *Arthritis Res Ther* 2011;**13**(3):R89. Available from: http://dx.doi.org/10.1186/ar3364.

91. Zhernakova A, Withoff S, Wijmenga C. Clinical implications of shared genetics and pathogenesis in autoimmune diseases. *Nat Rev Endocrinol* 2013;**9**(11):646−59. Available from: http://dx.doi.org/10.1038/nrendo.2013.161.

92. Gutierrez-Achury J, Coutinho de Almeida R, Wijmenga C. Shared genetics in coeliac disease and other immune-mediated diseases. *J Intern Med* 2011;**269**(6):591−603. Available from: http://dx.doi.org/10.1111/j.1365-2796.2011.02375.x.

93. Berger SI, Iyengar R. Network analyses in systems pharmacology. *Bioinformatics* 2009;**25**(19):2466−72. Available from: http://dx.doi.org/10.1093/bioinformatics/btp465.

94. Qiu P, Wang ZJ, Liu KJ, Hu ZZ, Wu CH. Dependence network modeling for biomarker identification. *Bioinformatics* 2007;**23**(2):198−206. Available from: http://dx.doi.org/10.1093/bioinformatics/btl553.

95. Bordbar A, Palsson BO. Using the reconstructed genome-scale human metabolic network to study physiology and pathology. *J Intern Med* 2012;**271**(2):131−41. Available from: http://dx.doi.org/10.1111/j.1365-2796.2011.02494.x.

96. Hess GP, Fonseca E, Scott R, Fagerness J. Pharmacogenomic and pharmacogenetic-guided therapy as a tool in precision medicine: current state and factors impacting acceptance by stakeholders. *Genet Res (Camb)* 2015;**97**:e13. Available from: http://dx.doi.org/10.1017/S0016672315000099.

97. Robinson PN. Deep phenotyping for precision medicine. *Hum Mutat* 2012;**33**(5):777−80. Available from: http://dx.doi.org/10.1002/humu.22080.

98. Siest G. Systems medicine, stratified medicine, personalized medicine but not precision medicine. *Drug Metabol Drug Interact* 2014;**29**(1):1−2. Available from: http://dx.doi.org/10.1515/dmdi-2013-0068.

CHAPTER *10*

The Microbiota and Its Modulation in Immune-Mediated Disorders

Meirav Pevsner-Fischer, Chagai Rot, Timur Tuganbaev and Eran Elinav
Department of Immunology, Weizmann Institute of Science, Rehovot, Israel

10.1 INTRODUCTION

Bacteria, viruses, archaea, and fungi inhabiting the mucosal surfaces of the human body are collectively termed the microbiota, and have coevolved with the human body for millions of years. This has resulted in the development of diverse and extensive host−microbiota interactions, influencing multiple physiological processes, including metabolism and the normal development and function of the immune system.[1] The densest microbiota resides in the mammalian gastrointestinal (GI) tract, where it forms a diverse community of trillions of microorganisms, now believed to be an integral part of the human holobiome. While comprising only 1−3% of the total body mass, an individual's gut microbiota cells and genes outnumber those of the human body's cells by a ratio of up to 10:1 and 100:1, respectively.[1] Bacterial composition varies along the GI tract, as each species colonizes a specific niche. Disruption of the microbial community, termed dysbiosis, is suggested to constitute a major risk factor for an increasing array of diseases, including susceptibility to common multifactorial disorders, such as obesity and its complications, infection, auto-inflammation, metabolic homeostasis, and even cancer.[2] In this chapter we will provide an overview of the establishment of the gut microbiota during human development, describe how it influences the establishment and normal functions of the host immune system, and the means by which we can control and alter its composition and function. We will then focus on a few examples demonstrating how dysbiotic microbiota composition and function may affect the pathogenesis of various immune-mediated disorders. Throughout this review, we will describe works utilizing next generation-based strategies for classification of

Immune Rebalancing. DOI: http://dx.doi.org/10.1016/B978-0-12-803302-9.00010-5

microbiota composition and function. The most widely used technique is 16S rRNA sequencing. Amplification and sequencing of the bacterial 16S ribosomal RNA, a component of the 30S small subunit of prokaryotic ribosomes,[3] enables one to assign operational taxonomic unit and to describe the relative abundances of microbiota genus-level members. More advanced sequencing methods are termed shotgun metagenomic sequencing, and allows defining the entire gene, pathway, and module contents of given microbiota configurations, enabling characterization at the functional level. In recent years, metabolomics and proteomic platforms now enable to also characterize the microbiota secretome, allowing the deciphering of thousands of molecules produced or modulated by the microbiota, which participate in host-microbial cross-talk in health and disease. An additional important tool in microbiota research, and described throughout this review, involves the use of germ-free (GF) mice. These are sterile mice housed in positive pressure isolators, which are free from microbial exposure. Their use allows the study of biological processes occurring in the absence of microbial colonization, as well as the transfer of defined disease-associated bacteria or whole microbiota configurations and the study of their roles in health and disease. In all, the emerging data presented in this review suggests that interventions affecting microbiota functions and interactions with the host may be manipulated as future therapeutics targeting common immune-related disorders.

10.2 DEVELOPMENT OF THE GUT MICROBIOTA

The microbial colonization of the infant GI tract is an integral process of the normal human lifecycle. The in utero environment has been traditionally considered to be sterile, with microbial colonization of the gut beginning at birth. The neonate is exposed and rapidly colonized by microbes, starting with those normally inhabiting the maternal vagina and GI tract.[4] Recently, live bacteria were suggested to be found in human meconium, the newborn's first intestinal stools, composed of material that has been ingested or secreted in the gut during fetal life[5,6] suggesting that the fetal environment may not be entirely sterile. The maternal GI tract was suggested to be the origin of this efflux of microorganisms toward the fetus. A recent study showed that oral administration of a labeled *Enterococcus faecium* to pregnant female mice resulted in the detection of the labeled strain in the offspring's meconium.[5] Acquisition of the microbiota composition in early life is suggested to depend on exposure to external conditions, such as mode of delivery, breast feeding, early-life exposure to antibiotics, and more.[7] For example, vaginally-delivered infants feature a gut microbiome that resembles their own mother's vaginal microbiota, dominated by *Lactobacillus*, *Prevotella*, or *Sneathia*, whereas in infants delivered by Cesarean section the gut microbiota is most similar to that found on the mother's skin, dominated by *Staphylococcus*, *Corynebacterium*, and *Propionibacterium*.[8] During the first 2−3 years of life, human infants modulate their gut microbiota until it reaches a stable adult composition.[4] Then, during the course of life, the microbiota composition remains relatively stable.[9] It has been postulated that forces shaping the microbiome during early childhood may contribute to dysbiosis affecting pathologies later in life, including asthma, inflammatory bowel diseases (IBDs), diabetes, and obesity.[7]

10.3 MICROBIOTA EFFECTS ON IMMUNE DEVELOPMENT

Colonization of the gut microbiota is essentially important to the development and normal function of multiple arms of the immune system. It is believed that the gut microbiota can regulate not only the local intestinal immune responses but may also have a profound influence on systemic immune responses. There is a plethora of emerging data relating to the gut microbiota and immune function, described in depth elsewhere.[10−15] In this section we will provide a few examples highlighting the important roles normal microbiota colonization plays on intact development and function of several cellular representatives of the innate and adaptive immune arms.

10.3.1 Lymphoid Tissue and General Immune Responses

GF animals feature profound deficits in both normal gut architecture and the development of the gut-associated lymphoid tissues.[16,17] GF mice exhibit smaller Payer's patches, lymph nodes, and spleen and lack germinal centers. Intestinal epithelial cells, which line the gut and form a physical barrier between luminal contents and mucosal immune cells, show altered patterns of microvilli formation and decreased rates of cellular turnover,[18] coupled with a decreased or absent expression of epithelial antimicrobial peptides and proteins as compared to colonized controls.[19,20] In GF rodents, the cecum was shown to be enlarged by four to eightfold due to the accumulation of mucus and undigested fibers, and the small intestine is less developed, with a considerably smaller surface area, slower peristalsis, irregular villi and reduced renewal of epithelial cells (reviewed in detail in Ref. 21).

10.3.2 Metabolites

Nutrients and metabolites derived from or modulated by commensal bacteria, including bile acid salts, vitamins, amino acids, and short-chain fatty acids (SCFAs),[22] are critically important for the development, homeostasis, and function of the immune system. For example, SCFAs have been reported to show anti-inflammatory properties. Colonic bacteria produce SCFAs after fermentation of dietary fiber; bacteria of the *Bacteroidetes* phylum produce high levels of acetate and propionate, whereas bacteria of the *Firmicutes* phylum produce high amounts of butyrate.[23] GF mice do not produce SCFAs owing to a lack of enteric microbes.[24] SCFAs induce anti-inflammatory properties in both colonic epithelium and immune cells.[19,25−27] Recently, SCFAs, have been found to bind and activate the G-protein-coupled receptor GPR43 to affect inflammatory responses.[28,29] In agreement with that, GPR43-deficient presented a more severe inflammation in models of colitis as compared to WT controls.[30−34]

10.3.3 Dendritic Cells and Macrophages

Mucosal dendritic cells (DCs) have a critical role in the maintenance of gut homeostasis, immune responses against gut infection, and IBDs by regulation of tolerogenic versus protective immune responses.[35] Interestingly in GF mice, a reduced number of intestinal but not systemic DCs was observed. However, colonization of the animals with *Escherichia coli* induced the recruitment of DCs to the intestines.[36,37] Intestinal macrophages represent the largest population of tissue macrophages in the body.[38] In GF mice, peritoneal macrophage functions such as chemotaxis, phagocytosis, microbicidal activities and activation markers are suggested to be severely compromised.[39−41]

10.3.4 Neutrophils

Most data about neutrophils in GF conditions comes from GF rats that are neutropenic[42] and dysfunctional, including impaired superoxide anion and nitric oxide generation, in addition to decreased phagocytic functions. Conventionalization of GF rats could not rescue the normal superoxide anion phenotype,[43] leading to the notion that the lack of microbiota miseducates normal neutrophilic function, an imprinted impairment which is irreversible when colonization is restored during adulthood.

10.3.5 B Cells

DCs induce the activation and differentiation of naive B cells into plasma secreting commensal-specific immunoglobulin A (IgA) in the lamina propria (LP).[44,45] Gut-associated B cells are mostly located in the Peyer's patches where they secrete IgA.[46] A decreased level of IgA and reduced number of plasma cells were observed in the intestine of GF mice. The spleens of GF mice contained fewer and smaller germinal centers, and serum natural IgG level was reduced while serum natural IgM level was normal in GF animals[47,48]

10.3.6 Regulatory T Cells

In the gut, regulatory T cells (Treg) were required to prevent the activation of $CD4^+$ T_H cells against commensal bacteria,[49] and were significantly decreased in the colonic LP of GF mice.[50–52] As was mentioned above and will be further described in the next sections, SCFA are important components for immune cell regulation. SCFAs were described playing an important role in determining normal numbers and function of Tregs in regulating intestinal adaptive immune responses.[33] Antigens induced by microbiota were shown to control the specific homing of T cells, particularly Tregs, to the large intestine.[53,54] Likewise, Tregs were induced by specific populations of commensal bacteria, such as *Clostridium* clusters IV and XIVa.[52] Specifically, 17 strains of human-derived *Clostridia* were able to produce SCFA and other metabolites that induced accumulation of Tregs in the gut. Furthermore, Foxp3 + regulatory T cells contributed to diversification of gut microbiota, particularly of species belonging to the Firmicute family.[32,55] Therefore, Tregs are believed to be essential for the prevention of the development of inappropriate auto-inflammation, a function dependent on normal microbiota colonization.

10.3.7 Antimicrobial Peptides

Antimicrobial peptides, innate immune effectors produced by intestinal epithelial cells, play an important role in host protection from enteric pathogens and in the containment and composition regulation of the intestinal microbiota.[56] Studies in neonatal and GF mice had shown that some of these peptides, including lysozyme and α-defensins, are constitutively produced in the absence of bacterial colonization. Others, such as angiogenins and Reg3g, are induced in response to bacterial colonization (reviewed in Ref. 57). Reg3g is essential for spatial separation of commensal bacteria from the epithelial surface. In Reg3g-deficient mice, the microbiota was found in close contact with the epithelium, resulting in increased expression of inflammatory genes.[58,59] The induction of these epithelial antimicrobials was an outcome of direct signaling of bacterial products in the lumen of the GI tract through TLRs and the myeloid differentiation primary response 88 (MyD88) pathway, a signaling adaptor for multiple TLRs.[60] Consistent with this notion, the gram-negative commensal *Bacteroides thetaiotaomicron* induced the expression of Reg3g by Paneth cells.[60] Production of Reg3g was impaired in mice that lack MyD88, resulting in the increased susceptibility of mice to infection by enteric pathogens.[61–63]

10.3.8 T_H17 Cells

IL-17–producing T_H17 cells are presented in high numbers in the LP of the intestine. They play a role in host defense but when unregulated may contribute to the development of autoimmunity and auto-inflammation by producing the pro-inflammatory cytokines IL-17 and IL-22. Because the number of intestinal T_H17 cells is greatly reduced in antibiotic-treated or GF mice, microbiota seems to have an important role in T_H17 cell development (reviewed inRef. 64). As will be described in the next sections, specific members of the microbiota such as segmented filamentous bacteria (SFB), were found to promote T_H17 cell development in mice.[65–67]

10.3.9 Intestinal CD4+ and CD8+ T Cells

The gut microbiota plays an important role in the development of both mucosal and systemic CD4+ T cells. A marked decrease in the number of LP CD4+ cells was observed in in GF mice. In addition, there was a reduced number and decreased cytotoxicity of intestinal CD8+ T cells in GF mice (reviewed inRef. 21). GF mice were also observed to have a Th1/Th2 imbalance as their immune response is biased toward the Th2 response (reviewed inRef. 46), suggesting that a normally colonized microbiota is essential for normal development and function of the adaptive immune arm.

10.3.10 Natural Killer T Cells

Natural killer T cells (NKT cells) are a diverse group of T cells, which are defined by their ability to recognize self- and nonself-derived lipids in the context of CD1d.[68,69] It was initially thought that generation, maturation, and peripheral accumulation of NKT cells is comparable between GF mice and colonized controls.[70] However, it was later shown that NKT cells isolated from GF mice had a less mature phenotype and were less responsive to activation with α-galactosylceramide. Colonization of GF mice to *Sphingomonas* bacteria, which express iNKT cell antigens, reversed phenotypic maturity of iNKT cells, while colonization with *Escherichia coli*, did not affect the phenotype of iNKT cells.[71] Furthermore, iNKT cells accumulated in the colonic LP and lung of GF mice, resulting in increased IBD disease severity in oxazolone-induced colitis as compared to SPF mice. Colonization of neonatal, but not adult, GF mice with a SPF microbiota protected the animals from iNKT accumulation and colitis pathology.[72]

In addition to microbiota effects on intestinal iNKT cells, CD1d and NKT cells were reciprocally shown to alter intestinal microbiota composition.[73] GF CD1d-deficient mice showed enhanced *Pseudomonas aeruginosa*, *E. coli*, *Staphylococcus aureus*, or *Lactobacillus gasseri* colonization of the small intestine, probably due to a defect in CD1d-mediated release of antimicrobial peptides from small intestinal Paneth cells.[74] CD1d deficiency was associated with intestinal dysbiosis[74,75]

In summary, the microbiota plays critical roles in the normal development and function of major immune arms. Disruption of normal microbiota composition and function may alter normal immune homeostasis. Reconstitution with a complete complex microbiota can restore some, but not all, microbiota-dependent immune functions. For example, reconstitution with a single species of bacteria, such as SFB or even with the *Bacteroides fragilis*, can restore many aspects of immune function that are disturbed in GF mice.[26,65,66] More examples of bacteria or bacterial families that are associated with the differentiation of specific adaptive immune subsets will be discussed further in this chapter.

10.4 MICROBIOTA MODULATION

A state of dysbiotic microbiota may potentially contribute to emergence of immune-mediated disease. In this section we will discuss the ways in which the microbiota composition can be altered and manipulated to potentially restore healthy immune functions. It is important to mention that some of the mechanisms by which the below interventions alter the microbiota remain elusive and at times nonevidence-based, thus more research is needed to validate these methods and decipher their full function and safety profiles.

10.4.1 Antibiotics

Antibiotics are widely used in controlling pathogenic infection. However, antibiotics can have an adverse effect on gut commensal microbial communities by reducing their abundance and diversity.[76,77] Over the past several decades an increasing concern has been raised about the spread of antibiotic resistance among pathogens, as well as growing concern that antibiotic use may disrupt the normal host—microbe interactions that contribute to human health.[78] In addition to their clinical usages, antibiotics are widely used as a research tool in the study of the microbiota, in aiming to assess the contribution of bacterial populations to a given phenotype or disease. Patterns of antibiotic-induced changes in bacterial families could be important indicators of general community disturbances, as antibiotics target different microbial communities depending on of their mechanisms of activity, doses, and durations. For example, 16S rRNA gene sequence analysis of the entire gut microbiota community revealed that the administration of ciprofloxacin (targeting gram negative bacteria) to humans affected the majority of bacterial taxa in the gut, resulting in decreased richness and diversity. In contrast, oral administration of vancomycin (affecting gram positive bacteria) to mice did not decrease the abundance of most mucosal-present bacteria.[77] After antibiotic administration, recovery depends on the type of antibiotic used, its dose, and the duration of administration.[77] Antibiotic alterations of the gut microbiota do not only eliminate bacterial communities, but also, indirectly, provide a vacant niche for other, more resistant microbial strains. As such, antibiotic administration has been linked to susceptibility to resistant potentially pathogenic commensal bacteria (hence termed pathobionts), viral and fungal infections. For example, neomycin administration increased susceptibility of mice to influenza infection in the lungs,[79] suggesting that commensal bacteria may normally provide protection against viral infections. Another example is the emergence of *Clostridium difficile*, mainly in hospitalized patients who are chronically treated with antibiotics that are susceptible to recurrent life-threatening infections by these bacteria.[80] In some cases, the disturbances in gut microbiota composition secondary to antibiotic use remain irreversible following cessation of antibiotic use.[81] This is potentially concerning because loss of specific commensal bacteria may chronically impact host health following antibiotic treatment.

10.4.2 Diet and Prebiotics

Diet can induce compositional changes in the microbiota, potentially as a mechanism by which the gut microbes adapt to changing nutrition as a means of modifying resource supply. In turn, diet plays a major role in shaping gut community structure and function.[82] This approach, employing nutritional strategies to promote the growth of bacteria that are considered beneficial to human health, is termed prebiotics.[83] One example of prebiotics involves a group of carbohydrates that cannot be degraded by the host but can promote the growth and activity of supposedly beneficial bacteria within the GI tract. Nondigestible carbohydrates (fiber), including starch, are the main nutrient source for some colonic bacteria.[84] Bacteria ferment fiber to produce SCFAs,[85] mainly acetate, propionate, and butyrate.[86] SCFAs benefit the host by providing energy and triggering hormonal and immune-related pathways.[87] High fiber diets and prebiotics such as inulin are known to stimulate the growth of beneficial bacteria such as *Bifidobacterium*, and to reduce appetite and the risk of obesity.[88,89] However, specific ways in which these compounds affect microbial community composition or function remain elusive.[90]

10.4.3 Probiotics

Probiotics are microbes that confer host advantages in maintaining microbiota homeostasis. *Lactobacillus* and *Bifidobacteria* species represent the microbes most commonly considered as probiotics conferring health benefits, however *Bifidobacterium*, *Escherichia coli*, *Streptococcus spp.*, *Enterococcus spp.*, and *Saccharomyces boulardii*[91] also were suggested to possess beneficial activity. These bacteria may compete against pathogens by either physically taking over their binding niche or by altering the microenvironment to be incompatible for pathogens growth requirements such as by lowering pH, and secreting toxic bacteriocins and chemicals.[92–94] Many probiotic bacteria are present in fermented foods and believed to be beneficial to human health, including dairy products such as yogurt that contain milk fermented with *L. bulgaricus* and *S. thermophiles*, as well as nondairy fermented foods such as sauerkraut and pickles (reviewed in Ref. 95). As will be described in the sections below, probiotics have been used to attempt to treat immune diseases, however, their efficacy remain inconclusive.

10.4.4 Fecal Microbiota Transplantation

Fecal microbiota transplantation (FMT) was first described in the "Zhou Hou Bei Ji Fang," medical manual for emergencies, written in fourth century China by Ge Hong, a herbal medicine master and alchemist, who successfully saved lives from food poisoning and diarrhea by oral administration of fecal suspension.[96] The therapeutic potential was accepted by modern medicine in the early 1900s, followed by case reports showing significant cure rates for gut-related infections and inflammation.[97–100] The rationale of FMT is that the normal microbiota in the gut protects the GI mucosa against microbial pathogens through "colonization resistance," the ability of the healthy gut microbiota to inhibit colonization and overgrowth by invading microorganisms. This is also known as "barrier effect" which is defined as the spatial and environmental competition, and by fermenting and secreting unused energy substrates, such as butyrate, to train the immune system and prevent growth of harmful, pathogenic bacteria.[97] It is established that perturbation of the gut microbiota, or "dysbiosis" disrupts colonization resistance, altering the microbiota composition, thereby affecting immune responses.

One of the most studied examples today in which FMT has been proven to benefit patients, is *Clostridium difficile* infection. FMT to treat *Clostridium difficile* has been described for over 500 patients in the literature, with efficacy rates of >90%.[101] The use of FMT will be described in the next sections as it was attempted to restore healthy microbiota functions that were lost in some immune-mediated diseases.

10.5 MICROBIOTA INVOLVEMENT IN PREVALENCE AND PROGRESSION IMMUNE-RELATED DISEASE

Immune-mediated disorders are a group of tissue-specific or systemic conditions that share common inflammatory perturbations. These disorders involve excessive, uncontrolled, and improper immune responses and are usually accompanied by dysregulation of the body's normal cytokine milieu. Approximately 5–7% of the population in developed countries is believed to suffer immune-mediated disorders. These "multi-factorial" diseases are caused by combinations of genetic and environmental factors.[102] The incidence of immune-mediated disorders has increased dramatically over the past few decades, therefore environmental factors that may rapidly develop, are suspected as being central mediators of these diseases. For example, the "hygiene hypothesis" proposes that enhanced personal hygiene in modern individuals resulted in reduced opportunities for microbial exposure during childhood, leading to immune system dysregulation and potentially to immune-mediated disease.[103,104] Examples by which compositional and functional alterations of the commensal microbiota (termed dysbiosis) may contribute to immune pathology are provided in this section.[105,106]

10.5.1 Rheumatoid Arthritis (RA)

Rheumatoid arthritis (RA) is an autoimmune inflammatory disease characterized by chronic synovitis, bone and cartilage destruction, and functional impairment and disability of joints. The etiopathogenesis of RA is not clearly understood at present. However, the development of RA appears to be influenced by both genetic and internal/external environmental factors.[107]

10.5.1.1 Lessons from Mouse Models on Microbiota Involvement in RA

More than three decades ago, animal models suggested that a link exists between the risk for inflammatory arthritis and the presence of certain bacterial commensal genera. Rat GF models of adjuvant-induced and streptococcal-induced arthritis showed increased vulnerability to arthritis compared to colonized controls.[108,109] In contrast, a GF environment was shown to be protective against the development of arthritis in the spontaneous spondyloarthropathy model of HLA-B27 transgenic rats,[110] an observation possibly explained by misfolded HLA-B27 in lipopolysaccharide-stimulated macrophages inducing a robust surge of pro-inflammatory cytokines IL-23 and IL-17.[111] Microbial involvement was also suggested from a work demonstrating that induction of chronic arthritis in a rat model induces an enhanced disease severity when the rat is inoculated with *Lactobacillus* strains but not with *fermentum*. The different outcome was suggested to arise from differences in peptidoglycan structure between the two bacterial strains.[112] Moreover, in two mouse models of RA, IL-1 receptor antagonist knockout (IL-1RA$^{-/-}$) and the K/BxN mice, GF conditions protected mice from clinical signs of the disease. Inoculating these mice with *Lactobacillus* or SFB was sufficient for the development of autoimmunity and inflammatory arthritis, via induction of a robust Th17 response.[113,114] Altogether, these studies reveal a role for the microbiota in various RA animal models, suggesting that a mechanistic relationship exists between microbes, mucosal immunity, and joint inflammation.

In contrast, it is not clear whether dysbiosis influences human RA. A study using a low-throughput 16S hybridization technique (only eight probes were included) was used to evaluate the fecal microbiota of patients with newly diagnosed RA. RA patients showed overall lower levels of *Bifidobacteria* and higher abundance of the *Bacteroides-Porphyromonas-Prevotella* group as compared with patients suffering fromfibromyalgia.[115] A second study investigated the composition of fecal *Lactobacillus* communities in newly diagnosed RA patients, as a follow up of a previous mouse study.[112] Using specific *Lactobacillus* primers, the authors discovered that *Lactobacillus* featured a higher strain diversity at the genus level in early RA,[116] including increased levels of *Lactobacillus salivarius*, *Lactobacillus iners*, and *Lactobacillus ruminis* in the RA group as compared to controls, and the presence of *Lactobacillus mucosae* that was unique to RA patients. Thereby, a potential relationship between *Lactobacillus* communities and the development and progression of RA was suggested. A recent human study using 16S rRNA pyrosequencing compared gut microbiota composition of recent onset RA, as compared to untreated RA, unrelated arthritis, and healthy controls.[117] The bacterial species *Prevotella copri* was found to be dramatically more abundant in early onset RA patients, as compared to all control groups. Moreover, the presence of *P. copri* corresponded to a reduction in the abundance of other potentially beneficial bacterial groups. This expansion in *Prevotella* correlated to a pro-inflammatory tendency in a mouse model of gut inflammation, in which antibiotic treated wild-type mice colonized with *P. copri* featured a more severe disease than controls.[117]

10.5.1.2 Probiotics and FMT

Attempted use of probiotics as a possible microbiota-targeting treatment for animal models of RA (collagen-induced arthritis) showed that *Lactobacillus casei* reduced pro-inflammatory cytokine levels, increased IL-10, and improved arthritis scores as compared with control rats.[118,119] There is a lack of evidence of the efficacy of probiotics in human arthritis. Despite the recent animal and human evidence possibly implicating the intestinal microbiota in RA development, it remains uncertain whether gut dysbiosis represent a pivotal factor or rather a secondary effect of local and systemic inflammation. Further work is required to better understand the enzymatic and metabolic effects underlying the changes in gut bacterial communities in RA patients. The potential to manipulate the microbiota, by probiotics and FMT, is now being investigated in this disorder.

10.5.2 Multiple Sclerosis
10.5.2.1 Lessons from Mouse Models on Microbiota Involvement in Multiple Sclerosis

Multiple sclerosis (MS) is a T helper cell (CD4 T cell)-mediated autoimmune disease that is characterized by chronic inflammation involving the central nervous system (CNS).[120] Experimental autoimmune encephalomyelitis (EAE) is an animal model that reproduces many of the features of MS.[121] EAE be can induced by immunization with CNS antigens, such as glycoprotein (MOG), or proteolipid protein, in the presence of bacterial adjuvants. The immunization leads to activation of pathogenic myelin-reactive T- cells that then attack self-antigen present in the CNS and peripheral nervous system similarly to the human disease.

The first links between microbiota disturbances and MS were established by observations done using the EAE model. In an article by Yokote et al. the authors showed that antibiotic administration to mice before EAE induction ameliorated disease severity,[122] accompanied by reduced levels of pro-inflammatory cytokines secreted from draining lymph node cells and a reduction in mesenteric Th17 cells. Another work suggested that this effect[123] may be mediated by microbiota depletion-induced skewing of CD4+ CD25+ regulatory T cell function. Antibiotic administration also increased a CD5 positive B-cell regulatory subset that potentially can ameliorate EAE.[124]

More evidences for the importance of microbiota functions in EAE models were achieved by the use of GF mice, shown to develop significantly reduced EAE symptoms and pathology and expressed lower levels of inflammatory cytokines as compared with colonized mice.[125] These effects were associated with increased numbers of

CD4 + CD25 + regulatory T cells and reduced Th1/Th17 pro-inflammatory responses in the CNS. Moreover, the authors suggested that DCs from GF animals do not prime MOG-specific T cell activation as efficiently as DCs from colonized animals, which might be the cause of reduced T cell pathogenicity and reduced EAE severity in these animals. Furthermore, inoculation of GF mice with SFB, a strain of bacteria that induces Th17 cell differentiation in the gut, enhanced EAE severity in GF mice, thereby linking the presence of a gut microbiota to EAE pathology. Moreover,[126] mice bearing a transgenic T-cell for MOG peptide were protected from spontaneous EAE development if grown under GF condition, but not if inoculated with microbiota.

10.5.2.2 Probiotics

As it became clear that gut microbiota might play a regulatory role in initiation and progression of EAE, various groups attempted to manipulate the microbiota by administration of probiotics. Lavasani et al.[127] showed in mice that therapeutic treatment with a probiotic mixture of three lactobacilli strains successfully reversed clinically established EAE. A synergistic effect of these strains induced systemic IL-10 release and led to an increased number of functional regulatory T cells in intestinal lymph nodes and in the periphery and CNS of diseased animals. Oral immunization with an attenuated *Salmonella typhimurium* expressing the colonization factor antigen I (CFA/I) fimbriae of enterotoxigenic *E. coli* is used as an experimental vaccine for enterotoxigenic *Escherichia coli* to confer protection against it. Unexpectedly, this vaccination conferred prophylactic[128] and therapeutic[129,130] protection against EAE. The mechanisms proposed for this effect include deviation of pathogenic T cells into Th2 cells and induction of CD4 + CD25 + Foxp3 + regulatory T cells that were able to adoptively transfer to ameliorate EAE. Oral immunization with an attenuated *Salmonella typhimurium* bearing a different subunit of (CFA/I) fimbriae, (CFA/I$_{IC}$) induced increased IL-13 and IFNγ but diminished TGF-β production by regulatory T cells.

Phosphorylated dihydroceramides (PE DHC) is a uniquely structured-lipid derived from the common human oral bacterium *Porphyromonas gingivalis*. Administration of PE DHC to mice induced with EAE, significantly enhanced EAE, but not in Toll-like receptor 2 (TLR2)-deficient mice. In addition, PE DHC-treated EAE inflicted mice showed a decreased percentage of spinal cord Foxp3+ T cells, suggesting that these bacterial lipids may regulate innate and adaptive immune responses to increase immune responses in EAE.[131]

Bacteroides species are gram-negative bacteria that are composed of approximately 25% of the microbiota in both humans and other mammals. Studies using mice grown in GF environment showed that monocolonization with *Bacteroides fragilis* was sufficient to stimulate early development of gut associated lymphatic tissue and normal organogenesis of the spleen and thymus.[26] Ochoa-Reparaz et al. [132] investigated the effect of oral antibiotic treatment followed by gut reconstitution with human isolate of *B. fragilis* in the development and protection against EAE. Two *B. fragilis* strains were used: one strain was able to produce the capsular polysaccharide A (PSA), the second was a mutant deficient in its ability to produce PSA. Recolonization of antibiotic-treated mice with PSA-deficient *B. fragilis* restored susceptibility to disease, whereas mice recolonized with the PSA-producing strain of *B. fragilis* remained protected against EAE. Oral administration of PSA conferred both prophylactic and therapeutic protection against EAE that were not subjected to previous treatment with antibiotics. Protection against disease was associated with a significant accumulation of CD103+ DCs and FoxP3+ regulatory T cells in the cervical LN. In addition, CD103+ DCs induced the conversion of naïve into IL-10-producing CD4+ T cells. Thus, this work suggested a role for commensal bacterial antigens in inducing anti-inflammatory responses, thereby improving immune homeostasis.

10.5.2.3 Diet

As discussed above, nutrition can serve as a way by which the microbiota can be manipulated to regulate the course or severity of microbiota-related disorders. There are emerging evidences that dietary factors may contribute to EAE susceptibility through their effects on the gut microbiota. Gut microbiota can respond to factors introduced by dietary substances either directly or via the production of metabolites. One example of dietary factors that can modulate EAE is vitamin A, which was shown to induce regulatory T cells in the intestinal mucosa,[133] while vitamin D3 dietary supplements protected mice from EAE.[134] Another such example is ligands of the aryl hydrocarbon receptor (Ahr) that are widely present in cruciferous vegetables. AhR was shown to be required for the postnatal expansion of intestinal

RORγt + innate lymphoid cells and the formation of intestinal lymphoid follicles, thereby being important in maintaining the intestinal architecture as well as homeostasis.[135] Likewise, mice fed a high fat[136] or high salt[137,138] diet, featured increased Th17 cells, leading to a more severe EAE. Reinforcing these diet-related modulatory functions seen in EAE animal models, epidemiological studies linked dietary vitamin D consumption with the risk of MS.[139] Enhanced MS incidence was also associated with the intake of three or more servings per day of whole milk during adolescence, whereas certain polyunsaturated fatty acids as well as plant fibers may decrease the risk for development of MS.[140] Whether these effects would be seen in larger cohorts, and whether they involve modulation of the gut microbiome merits further studies.

10.5.2.4 Human Studies

FMT has recently been attempted in MS patients. In the first attempt,[141] three patients underwent daily FMT for 1−2 weeks for reasons related to constipation. Surprisingly, progressive improvement in neurological symptoms was noted, with all three patients regaining the ability to walk. Two of the patients with prior indwelling urinary catheters experienced restoration of intact urinary function. In one of the three patients, follow-up MRI 15 years after FMT showed a halting of disease progression.

Other works suggested pathogen infections as means of modulating MS progress. For example, the prevalence of MS was suggested to inversely correlate with the level of sanitation,[142] being extremely rare in countries with a prevalence of *T. trichiura* infection of more than 10%, while being much more prevalent in regions with lower prevalence of parasitic infection.[143] While this observation is entirely correlative, patients with MS who become infected with helminths have a strikingly diminished rate of disease progression, and develop circulating myelin specific regulatory T cells that release IL-10 and TGF-β in response to activation by myelin basic protein.[144] Helminthic infection also induced a population of IL-10-secreting regulatory B cells in these patients.[145] Treatment of helminthic infection was associated with rapid MS exacerbation.[146] Overall, these preliminary results suggest that microbial stimulation may modify MS progression and disease severity. The utility, safety, and persistence of these effects merit further studies.

10.5.3 Systemic Lupus Erythematosus

Systemic lupus erythematosus (SLE) is an autoimmune disorder characterized by the generation of autoantibodies, recruitment of autoreactive or inflammatory T cells, and abnormal production of pro-inflammatory cytokines.[147,148] The disease is characterized by severe and persistent inflammation that leads to tissue damage in multiple organs, including kidneys, lungs, joints, heart, skin, and brain. Disease arises when abnormally functioning B lymphocytes produce autoantibodies against DNA and nuclear proteins, resulting in immune complexes that cause damage to the tissue. While the triggers of SLE are not known, it is widely accepted that it is a consequence of a complex interaction between genetic and environmental factors.[148]

10.5.3.1 Lessons from Mouse Models of Microbiota Involvement in Systemic Lupus Erythematosus

A number of animal models have been used for the study of SLE onset and progression, including the New Zealand black (NZB) mice strain that develops spontaneous disease, and the MRL-lpr mice strain, which is homozygous for the mutation Fas[lpr], and features systemic autoimmunity, lymphadenopathy, and glomerulonephritis.[149] Both animal models have clinical features similar to lupus-associated manifestations in humans.

As early as in the 1960s and 1970s, GF NZB mice exhibited lower levels of serum IgG, and significant decreases in the incidence and severity of renal disease as compared to colonized mice.[150,151] GF MRL-lpr did not show differences in lympho-proliferation, or histologic analysis of the kidneys or autoantibody levels. However, if these GF mice were fed with a diet strictly deficient in bacterial antigens, they exhibited lower severity of nephritis.[152] Therefore, there are conflicting evidences in regard to GF conditions affecting SLE symptoms in mouse models of the disease, and the roles of live versus microbial-related antigens in these models.

Others examined the microbiota composition in the MRL-lpr mouse.[153] Since in mice, as in humans, females are more susceptible to disease,[148] the authors compared the gut microbiota of female MRL-lpr versus control mice, and found them to be vastly distinct from each other. The gut microbiota of lupus-prone MRL-lpr mice was characterized by a reduction in the *Lactobacillaceae* family and a concurrent increase in the *Lachnospiraceae* family, which accounted together for more than 65% of all bacteria in the distal gut. While interesting, these associations do not prove microbial causality in the pathogenesis of SLE and merit further studies.

10.5.3.2 Human Studies

An Ion Torrent PGM sequencing Platform was recently used to characterize SLE patients' microbiota composition as compared to controls.[77] A significant 2.5-fold-reduction was noted in the *Firmicutes/Bacteroidetes* ratio in SLE inflicted individuals as compared to healthy controls. A metabolomics study observed the metabolite profile of the microbiota of SLE patients,[154] as analyzed by a combination of mass spectrometry with liquid chromatography and capillary electrophoresis separation, to be distinct from that of control groups. In this study, microbiota compositions of SLE patients and controls remained similar to each other, suggesting that changes induced by SLE are more apparent at the functional rather than the compositional level. Further studies will be needed to delineate whether these metabolic changes are involved with the pathogenesis of SLE manifestations, or alternatively they are merely a reflection of disease occurrence and severity.

10.5.4 Chronic Urticaria

Chronic urticarial (CU) is a common skin disease characterized by widespread, transient skin lesions occurring daily or almost daily for at least 6 weeks. Masked or overt bacterial, viral, fungal, and protozoan agents have been reported as possible initiating factors for CU. No etiologic factor has been found in most patients, which makes chronic idiopathic urticaria a major problem for physicians and patients alike. *Helicobacter pylori* is a spiral-shaped microaerophilic gram-negative bacterium that colonizes the gastric mucosa and induces a strong inflammatory response with the release of various bacterial and host-dependent cytotoxic substances.[155] Some studies have found an etiopathogenetic link between *H. pylori* infection and CU following observations that *H. pylori* eradication induced skin improvement.[156,157] Other studies, however, disagree with these findings and have found that *H. pylori* prevalence does not differ from that of control groups.[158,159] Thus, the role of *H. pylori* infection as a possible causative agent in CU is still controversial and probably significantly, though weakly, associated with the risk of disease.[160]

10.5.5 Inflammatory Bowel Disease

IBD comprises a group of chronic systemic inflammatory disorders that include Crohn's disease (CD), ulcerative colitis (UC), and indeterminate colitis. IBD manifests as an incurable immune-mediated disease with typical onset during young adulthood and a lifelong course characterized by periods of remission and relapse. CD can involve any part of the GI tract but most commonly the ileum and proximal colon, while UC is most often localized to the descending colon. Worldwide, there is a trend toward increased incidence of both UC and CD,[161] with incidents reaching 120–200/100000 (UC) and 50–200/100000 (CD) in developed regions.[162] Etiology of the disease is complex. Higher risk of IBD development in siblings of an affected individual and significant cooccurrence within families (especially in early-onset disease) supports a role for host genetics in the etiology of the disease.[163,164] Genome-wide association studies have identified 163 distinct loci that confer risk of or protection from the development of CD and UC with a substantial portion of these loci (110 of 163) being common to both diseases.[165] The role of genetics in the development of these diseases appears greater for CD than UC, with roughly 2-fold greater variance explained by associated loci.[166] However, the fact that IBD-associated genetic variants are present in many individuals who do not develop disease,[167] suggests that genetics may not fully explain the etiology of the disease. Several-fold increase in IBD incidence in the developed world during the last six decades[162] and an increase in the disease risk upon migrants[167] suggest an important role for environmental factors in disease pathogenesis. Furthermore, genetic and chemically-induced animal models of IBD showed that most IBD symptoms were attenuated or abrogated by antibiotics and GF conditions and restored or exacerbated by subsequent colonization.[110,168–170] As such, the use of antibiotics in management of IBD in patients was suggested to attenuate some aspects of the disease.[171] The role of microbiota in IBD is extensively studied. Next generation sequencing studies analyzing microbiota composition (based on 16S rRNA phylogenetics) of IBD patients identified enrichment for the *Enterobacteriaceae* and depletion of Clades IV and XIVa Clostridia and decrease in overall community diversity during disease-associated inflammation.[166,172,173] Several studies indicate that these microbial shifts occur prior to, or in conjunction with, the onset of inflammation and clinical phenotypes.[166,167] Metagenomic studies of clinical samples from IBD patients identified reduction in overall gene diversity, enrichment in microbial pathways for oxidative stress tolerance, immune evasion, and host metabolite uptake, with corresponding depletions in SCFA biosynthesis and typical gut carbohydrate metabolism and amino acid biosynthetic processes.[174,175] Intriguingly, similar microbial metabolic shifts have been observed in other inflammatory conditions such as type 2 diabetes,[175] suggesting a common gut microbial response to chronic inflammation and immune activation. Metabolomics studies showed amino acid levels, SCFAs, and additional tricarboxylic acid cycle products to be altered in stool samples of IBD patients.[176] A metagenomic-metaproteomic study dissecting stool samples from monozygotic twin pairs concordant or discordant for IBD identified depletion of most typical carbohydrate utilization and amino acid metabolism pathways in correspondence with overall reduced microbial diversity.[177] While such studies document microbiota changes in IBD, by design they cannot show whether these changes play a causative role in the development of the disorder or are merely an indicator of disease activity. Possible causality[25,32,33,178–180] was suggested by Kenya Honda and colleagues, who characterized 17 strains of *Clostridia* from a healthy human fecal sample to significantly increase the numbers and suppressive function of colonic regulatory T cells in colonized mice, thereby attenuating symptoms of experimental allergic diarrhea and colitis. In another work, administration of SCFAs, which are produced by colonic bacteria after fermentation of dietary fiber, improved disease indices. The lack of SCFAs receptor, *Gpr43*, in mice induced with chronic model of DSS-induced colitis, showed greater morbidity, reduced colon length, and increased colon histology score.[25]

Recently, a metagenome-based microbiome comparison between naïve CD patients with and without antibiotic exposure demonstrated that antibiotic use increased the microbial dysbiosis associated with CD,[166] suggesting that, in contrast to previous belief, the microbial network appears more dysbiotic in the context of antibiotic exposure.

In contrast to *Clostridium difficile* infection[181] FMT in IBD showed mixed results[97,182] indicating that microbiota roles in IBD are more complex and heterogeneous than previously anticipated.[166] Nevertheless "untargeted" probiotic treatment suggested a significant yet small beneficial effect in IBD,[183,184] implying that microbial community modulation has the potential to improve IBD outcome.

Integration of next generation sequencing-based approaches, coupled with more mechanistic animal model studies, and personally tailored probiotic strategies may improve our understanding of microbial contribution to IBD and enable the development of more effective microbiota-targeted interventions.

10.6 SUMMARY AND CONCLUSIONS

Interactions between the gut microbiota and the innate and adaptive mucosal immune arms are essential to both intact immune function and normal composition and function of the gut microbiota. This delicate balance between the host and its microbes, best exemplified in the GI tract, enables the mucosal immune system to tolerate the large microbial burden that exists just one epithelial layer from the mostly sterile inner host, while allowing s potent interaction against both pathogens and commensals when they breach mucosal surfaces. Many of the mechanisms by which host immune cells and microbiota interact in health and disease remain elusive. Equally elusive are the effects the microbiota may have on systemic immunity, which merit further studies.

Several challenges need to be met in order to better understand the contribution of microbiota alterations to immune-related disease. It is becoming clear that alterations in microbiota composition may appear years before clinical manifestations develop and diagnosis is made. As such, studying these effects necessitates a comprehensive profiling and prospective follow-up of large cohorts of human participants. Moreover, it is becoming clearer that dissecting the microbiota at the compositional level may be insufficient in characterizing how it affects and is affected by host and environmental alterations contributing to disease pathogenesis. Thus, more comprehensive microbiota characterization in the form of metagenomics, metatranscriptomics, metabolomics, and metaproteomics will allow the integration of functional analysis to compositional data, thus improving our ability to "connect the dots" between microbiota alterations and host immune consequences. Overall, improved understanding of the interaction between the microbiota and the various cells and arms of the immune systems will enable us to better understand, at the molecular level, how genomics and environmental factors integrate to drive healthy immunity or the propensity towards common "multifactorial" immune mediated disease (Figure 10.1, Tables 10.1 and 10.2).

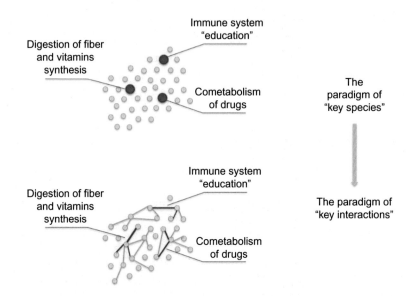

Figure 10.1 Modulation of the complex microbiome

Table 10.1 Human Studies

Disease	Microbiome Composition	FMT	Antibiotics	Probiotics
Rheumatoid arthritis (RA)	Lower levels of *Bifidobacteria* and higher abundance of the *Bacteroides- Porphyromonas- Prevotella*.[115] Higher strain diversity of Lactobacillus in early RA[116] Higher abundance of *Prevotella copri*.[117]			
Multiple sclerosis (MS)		FMT improved clinical symptoms in 3 patients.[141]		
Inflammatory bowel disease (IBD)	Enriched for *Enterobacteriaceae* and depleted of Clades IV and XIVa *Clostridia* during disease-associated inflammation [166,172,173]	FMT in IBD showed mixed results. [97,182,166]	Antibiotic use increased the microbial dysbiosis associated with CD.[166]	Probiotic treatment suggested a significant beneficial effect in IBD.[183,184]

(Continued)

Table 10.1 (Continued)

Disease	Microbiome Composition	FMT	Antibiotics	Probiotics
	Metagenomic studies of clinical sample from IBD patients identified reduction in overall gene diversity, enrichment in microbial pathways for oxidative stress tolerance, immune evasion, and host metabolite uptake, with corresponding depletions in short-chain fatty acid (SCFA) biosynthesis and gut carbohydrate metabolism and amino acid biosynthetic processes.[174,175] Reduced microbial diversity.[177]			
Chronic urticarial (CU)		Contradicting observations regarding An etiopathogenesis link between *H. pylori* infection and CU.[156–160]		

Table 10.2 Animal Studies

Disease	Model	Alterations in microbiome composition	Effect of germ free conditions	Administration of probiotics and effects old diet	Antibiotic Treatment
Rheumatoid arthritis (RA)	Rat RA		Increased vulnerability [108, 109, 113, 114]	*Lactobacillus* strains enhanced RA [112].	
			Protective against disease [110].	*Lactobacillus casei* improved arthritis scores as compared with controls [118, 119].	
Multiple sclerosis (MS)	Mouse EAE		Develop reduced EAE symptoms and pathology [125].	SFB enhanced EAE severity in GF mice [126]. A mixture of three lactobacilli strains reversed clinically established EAE [127]. Oral immunization with an attenuated *Salmonella typhimurium* conferred protection [127–130].	Ameliorated EAE severity [122].

(Continued)

Table 10.2 (Continued)					
Disease	**Model**	**Alterations in microbiome composition**	**Effect of germ free conditions**	**Administration of probiotics and effects old diet**	**Antibiotic Treatment**
				Oral administration of PSA conferred prophylactic and therapeutic protection [132].	
				Vitamin A and vitamin D3 dietary supplements protected mice from EAE [134].	
				Mice fed a high fat [136] or high salt [137, 138] diet, featured a more severe EAE.	
				Polyunsaturated fatty acids as well as plant fibers may decrease the risk for development of MS [140].	
Systemic lupus erythematosus (SLE)	NZB mice		Decreases in incidence and severity of renal disease [150, 151]. No change, unless fed with a diet deficient in bacterial antigens [152].		
	MRL-lpr	Reduction in the *Lactobacillaceae* family and an increase in the *Lachnospiraceae* family [153]			
Inflammatory bowel disease (IBD)		IBD symptoms were attenuated or abrogated by antibiotics and GF conditions and restored or exacerbated by subsequent colonization [110, 168–170] Possible causality [25, 32, 33, 178–180] was suggested by		The lack of SCFAs receptor, *Gpr43*, in mice induced with chronic model of DSS-induced colitis, showed greater morbidity, reduced colon length, and increased colon histology score [25].	

(Continued)

Table 10.2 (Continued)

Disease	Model	Alterations in microbiome composition	Effect of germ free conditions	Administration of probiotics and effects old diet	Antibiotic Treatment
		Kenya Honda and colleagues, that characterized 17 strains of *Clostridia* from a healthy human fecal sample to significantly increase the numbers and suppressive function of colonic regulatory T cells in colonized mice.			

ACKNOWLEDGEMENTS

We thank the members of the Elinav laboratory for their inputs and suggestions. We apologize to all the authors whose work was not cited in this review due to space limitations. E.E. is supported by Yael and Rami Ungar, Israel; Leona M. and Harry B. Helmsley Charitable Trust; the Gurwin Family Fund for Scientific Research; Crown Endowment Fund for Immunological Research; estate of Jack Gitlitz; estate of Lydia Hershkovich; the Benoziyo Endowment Fund for the Advancement of Science; Adelis Foundation; John L. and Vera Schwartz, Pacific Palisades; Alan Markovitz, Canada; Cynthia Adelson, Canada; CNRS (Centre National de la Recherche Scientifique); estate of Samuel and Alwyn J. Weber; Mr and Mrs Donald L. Schwarz, Sherman Oaks; grants funded by the European Research Council; the German-Israel Binational foundation; the Israel Science Foundation; the Minerva Foundation; the Rising Tide foundation; and the Alon Foundation scholar award. E.E. is the incumbent of the Rina Gudinski Career Development Chair.

REFERENCES

1. Backhed F, Ley RE, Sonnenburg JL, Peterson DA, Gordon JI. Host-bacterial mutualism in the human intestine. *Science* 2005;**307**(5717):1915–20 [PMID:15790844 http://dx.doi.org/10.1126/science.1104816].

2. Brown EM, Sadarangani M, Finlay BB. The role of the immune system in governing host-microbe interactions in the intestine. *Nat Immunol* 2013;**14**(7):660–7.

3. Woese CR, Fox GE. Phylogenetic structure of the prokaryotic domain: the primary kingdoms. *Proc Natl Acad Sci USA* 1977;**74**(11):5088–90 [PMID: 270744 PMCID: 432104 DOI: http://www.ncbi.nlm.nih.gov/pubmed/270744].

4. Yatsunenko T, Rey FE, Manary MJ, Trehan I, Dominguez-Bello MG, Contreras M, et al. Human gut microbiome viewed across age and geography. *Nature* 2012;**486**(7402):222–7 [PMID:22699611 PMCID: 3376388 http://dx.doi.org/10.1038/nature11053].

5. Jiménez E, Marín ML, Martín R, Odriozola JM, Olivares M, Xaus J, et al. Is meconium from healthy newborns actually sterile? *Res Microbiol* 2008;**159**(3):187−93.

6. Moles L, Gomez M, Heilig H, Bustos G, Fuentes S, de Vos W, et al. Bacterial diversity in meconium of preterm neonates and evolution of their fecal microbiota during the first month of life. *PLoS One* 2013;**8**(6):e66986.

7. Bravo JA, Julio-Pieper M, Forsythe P, Kunze W, Dinan TG, Bienenstock J, et al. Communication between gastrointestinal bacteria and the nervous system. *Curr Opin Pharmacol* 2012;**12**(6):667−72 [PMID:23041079 http://dx.doi.org/10.1016/j.coph.2012.09.010].

8. Dominguez-Bello MG, Costello EK, Contreras M, Magris M, Hidalgo G, Fierer N, et al. Delivery mode shapes the acquisition and structure of the initial microbiota across multiple body habitats in newborns. *Proc Natl Acad Sci USA* 2010;**107**(26):11971−5.

9. David LA, Materna AC, Friedman J, Campos-Baptista MI, Blackburn MC, Perrotta A, et al. Host lifestyle affects human microbiota on daily timescales. *Genome Biol* 2014;**15**(7):R89 [PMID: 25146375 PMCID: 4405912 http://dx.doi.org/10.1186/gb-2014-15-7-r89].

10. de Zoete MR, Palm NW, Zhu S, Flavell RA. Inflammasomes. *Cold Spring Harb Perspect Biol* 2014;**6**(12):a016287 [PMID:25324215 http://dx.doi.org/10.1101/cshperspect.a016287].

11. Ivanov II K, Atarashi N, Manel EL, Brodie T, Shima U, Karaoz D, et al. Induction of intestinal Th17 cells by segmented filamentous bacteria. *Cell* 2009;**139**(3):485−98 [PMID:19836068 PMCID: 2796826 http://dx.doi.org/10.1016/j.cell.2009.09.033].

12. Lavelle EC, Murphy C, O'Neill LA, Creagh EM. The role of TLRs, NLRs, and RLRs in mucosal innate immunity and homeostasis. *Mucosal Immunol* 2010;**3**(1):17−28 [PMID: 19890268 PMCID: 3428627 http://dx.doi.org/10.1038/mi.2009.124].

13. Palm NW, de Zoete MR, Flavell RA. Immune-microbiota interactions in health and disease. *Clin Immunol* 2015;**159**(4):122−7 [PMID:26141651 http://dx.doi.org/10.1016/j.clim.2015.05.014].

14. Spor A, Koren O, Ley R. Unravelling the effects of the environment and host genotype on the gut microbiome. *Nat Rev Microbiol* 2011;**9**(4):279−90 [PMID: 21407244 http://dx.doi.org/10.1038/nrmicro2540].

15. Belkaid Y, Segre JA. Dialogue between skin microbiota and immunity. *Science* 2014;**346** (6212):954−9 [PMID: 25414304 http://dx.doi.org/10.1126/science.1260144].

16. Macpherson AJ, Harris NL. Interactions between commensal intestinal bacteria and the immune system. *Nat Rev Immunol* 2004;**4**(6):478−85 [PMID:15173836 http://dx.doi.org/10.1038/nri1373].

17. Falk PG, Hooper LV, Midtvedt T, Gordon JI. Creating and maintaining the gastrointestinal ecosystem: what we know and need to know from gnotobiology. *Microbiol Mol Biol Rev* 1998;**62**(4):1157−70 [PMID: 9841668 PMCID: 98942 DOI: http://www.ncbi.nlm.nih.gov/pubmed/9841668].

18. Abrams GD, Bauer H, Sprinz H. Influence of the normal flora on mucosal morphology and cellular renewal in the ileum. A comparison of germ-free and conventional mice. *Lab Invest* 1963;**12**:355−64 [PMID:14010768 DOI: http://www.ncbi.nlm.nih.gov/pubmed/14010768].

19. Round JL, Mazmanian SK. The gut microbiota shapes intestinal immune responses during health and disease. *Nat Rev Immunol* 2009;**9**(5):313−23 [PMID:19343057 PMCID: 4095778 http://dx.doi.org/10.1038/nri2515].

20. Bouskra D, Brezillon C, Berard M, Werts C, Varona R, Boneca IG, et al. Lymphoid tissue genesis induced by commensals through NOD1 regulates intestinal homeostasis. *Nature* 2008;**456**(7221):507−10 [PMID:18987631 http://dx.doi.org/10.1038/nature07450].

21. Al-Asmakh M, Zadjali F. Use of germ-free animal models in microbiota-related research. *J Microbiol Biotechnol* 2015. [PMID:26032361 DOI: http://www.ncbi.nlm.nih.gov/pubmed/26032361].

22. Brestoff JR, Artis D. Commensal bacteria at the interface of host metabolism and the immune system. *Nat Immunol* 2013;**14**(7):676−84 [PMID:23778795 PMCID: 4013146 http://dx.doi.org/10.1038/ni.2640].

23. Macfarlane S, Macfarlane GT. Regulation of short-chain fatty acid production. *Proc Nutr Soc* 2003;**62**(1):67–72 [PMID:12740060 http://dx.doi.org/10.1079/PNS2002207].

24. Hoverstad T, Midtvedt T. Short-chain fatty acids in germfree mice and rats. *J Nutr* 1986;**116** (9):1772–6 [PMID:3761032 DOI: http://www.ncbi.nlm.nih.gov/pubmed/3761032].

25. Maslowski KM, Vieira AT, Ng A, Kranich J, Sierro F, Yu D, et al. Regulation of inflammatory responses by gut microbiota and chemoattractant receptor GPR43. *Nature* 2009;**461** (7268):1282–6 [PMID:19865172 PMCID: 3256734 http://dx.doi.org/10.1038/nature08530].

26. Mazmanian SK, Liu CH, Tzianabos AO, Kasper DL. An immunomodulatory molecule of symbiotic bacteria directs maturation of the host immune system. *Cell* 2005;**122**(1):107–18 [PMID:16009137 http://dx.doi.org/10.1016/j.cell.2005.05.007].

27. Segain JP, Raingeard de la Bletiere D, Bourreille A, Leray V, Gervois N, Rosales C, et al. Butyrate inhibits inflammatory responses through NF-kappaB inhibition: implications for Crohn's disease. *Gut* 2000;**47**(3):397–403 [PMID:10940278 PMCID: 1728045 DOI: http://www.ncbi.nlm.nih.gov/pubmed/10940278].

28. Le Poul E, Loison C, Struyf S, Springael JY, Lannoy V, Decobecq ME, et al. Functional characterization of human receptors for short chain fatty acids and their role in polymorphonuclear cell activation. *J Biol Chem* 2003;**278**(28):25481–9 [PMID:12711604 http://dx.doi.org/10.1074/jbc.M301403200].

29. Brown AJ, Goldsworthy SM, Barnes AA, Eilert MM, Tcheang L, Daniels D, et al. The Orphan G protein-coupled receptors GPR41 and GPR43 are activated by propionate and other short chain carboxylic acids. *J Biol Chem* 2003;**278**(13):11312–19 [PMID:12496283 http://dx.doi.org/10.1074/jbc.M211609200].

30. Cipriani S, Mencarelli A, Chini MG, Distrutti E, Renga B, Bifulco G, et al. The bile acid receptor GPBAR-1 (TGR5) modulates integrity of intestinal barrier and immune response to experimental colitis. *PLoS One* 2011;**6**(10):e25637 [PMID:22046243 PMCID: 3203117 http://dx.doi.org/10.1371/journal.pone.0025637].

31. Obata Y, Furusawa Y, Endo TA, Sharif J, Takahashi D, Atarashi K, et al. The epigenetic regulator Uhrf1 facilitates the proliferation and maturation of colonic regulatory T cells. *Nat Immunol* 2014;**15**(6):571–9 [PMID:24777532 http://dx.doi.org/10.1038/ni.2886].

32. Narushima S, Sugiura Y, Oshima K, Atarashi K, Hattori M, Suematsu M, et al. Characterization of the 17 strains of regulatory T cell-inducing human-derived Clostridia. *Gut Microbes* 2014;**5** (3):333–9 [PMID:24642476 PMCID: 4153770 http://dx.doi.org/10.4161/gmic.28572].

33. Smith PM, Howitt MR, Panikov N, Michaud M, Gallini CA, Bohlooly YM, et al. The microbial metabolites, short-chain fatty acids, regulate colonic Treg cell homeostasis. *Science* 2013;**341** (6145):569–73 [PMID:23828891 PMCID: 3807819 http://dx.doi.org/10.1126/science.1241165].

34. Kamada N, Seo SU, Chen GY, Nunez G. Role of the gut microbiota in immunity and inflammatory disease. *Nat Rev Immunol* 2013;**13**(5):321–35 [PMID:23618829 http://dx.doi.org/10.1038/nri3430].

35. Steinman RM, Hawiger D, Nussenzweig MC. Tolerogenic dendritic cells. *Annu Rev Immunol* 2003;**21**:685–711 [PMID:12615891 http://dx.doi.org/10.1146/annurev.immunol.21.120601.141040].

36. Haverson K, Rehakova Z, Sinkora J, Sver L, Bailey M. Immune development in jejunal mucosa after colonization with selected commensal gut bacteria: a study in germ-free pigs. *Vet Immunol Immunopathol* 2007;**119**(3–4):243–53 [PMID:17643495 http://dx.doi.org/10.1016/j.vetimm.2007.05.022].

37. Williams AM, Probert CS, Stepankova R, Tlaskalova-Hogenova H, Phillips A, Bland PW. Effects of microflora on the neonatal development of gut mucosal T cells and myeloid cells in the mouse. *Immunology* 2006;**119**(4):470–8 [PMID:16995882 PMCID: 2265821 http://dx.doi.org/10.1111/j.1365-2567.2006.02458.x].

38. Lee SH, Starkey PM, Gordon S. Quantitative analysis of total macrophage content in adult mouse tissues. Immunochemical studies with monoclonal antibody F4/80. *J Exp Med* 1985;**161**(3):475–89 [PMID:3973536 PMCID: 2187577 DOI: http://www.ncbi.nlm.nih.gov/pubmed/3973536].

39. Mikkelsen HB, Garbarsch C, Tranum-Jensen J, Thuneberg L. Macrophages in the small intestinal muscularis externa of embryos, newborn and adult germ-free mice. *J Mol Histol* 2004;**35**(4):377−87 [PMID:15503811 DOI: http://www.ncbi.nlm.nih.gov/pubmed/15503811].

40. Mitsuyama M, Ohara R, Amako K, Nomoto K, Yokokura T, Nomoto K. Ontogeny of macrophage function to release superoxide anion in conventional and germfree mice. *Infect Immun* 1986;**52**(1):236−9 [PMID:3007361 PMCID: 262225 DOI: http://www.ncbi.nlm.nih.gov/pubmed/3007361].

41. Morland B, Midtvedt T. Phagocytosis, peritoneal influx, and enzyme activities in peritoneal macrophages from germfree, conventional, and ex-germfree mice. *Infect Immun* 1984;**44**(3):750−2 [PMID:6233226 PMCID: 263691 DOI: http://www.ncbi.nlm.nih.gov/pubmed/6233226].

42. Ohkubo T, Tsuda M, Tamura M, Yamamura M. Impaired superoxide production in peripheral blood neutrophils of germ-free rats. *Scand J Immunol* 1990;**32**(6):727−9 [PMID:1702900 DOI: http://www.ncbi.nlm.nih.gov/pubmed/1702900].

43. Ohkubo T, Tsuda M, Suzuki S, El Borai N, Yamamura M. Peripheral blood neutrophils of germ-free rats modified by in vivo granulocyte-colony-stimulating factor and exposure to natural environment. *Scand J Immunol* 1999;**49**(1):73−7 [PMID:10023860 DOI: http://www.ncbi.nlm.nih.gov/pubmed/10023860].

44. Hooper LV, Littman DR, Macpherson AJ. Interactions between the microbiota and the immune system. *Science* 2012;**336**(6086):1268−73 [PMID:22674334 PMCID: 4420145 http://dx.doi.org/10.1126/science.1223490].

45. Mowat AM. Anatomical basis of tolerance and immunity to intestinal antigens. *Nat Rev Immunol* 2003;**3**(4):331−41 [PMID:12669023 http://dx.doi.org/10.1038/nri1057].

46. Wu HJ, Wu E. The role of gut microbiota in immune homeostasis and autoimmunity. *Gut Microbes* 2012;**3**(1):4−14 [PMID:22356853 PMCID: 3337124 http://dx.doi.org/10.4161/gmic.19320].

47. Pereira P, Forni L, Larsson EL, Cooper M, Heusser C, Coutinho A. Autonomous activation of B and T cells in antigen-free mice. *Eur J Immunol* 1986;**16**(6):685−8 [PMID:2941305 http://dx.doi.org/10.1002/eji.1830160616].

48. Hooijkaas H, Benner R, Pleasants JR, Wostmann BS. Isotypes and specificities of immunoglobulins produced by germ-free mice fed chemically defined ultrafiltered "antigen-free" diet. *Eur J Immunol* 1984;**14**(12):1127−30 [PMID:6083871 http://dx.doi.org/10.1002/eji.1830141212].

49. Powrie F, Leach MW, Mauze S, Caddle LB, Coffman RL. Phenotypically distinct subsets of CD4+ T cells induce or protect from chronic intestinal inflammation in C. B-17 scid mice. *Int Immunol* 1993;**5**(11):1461−71 [PMID: 7903159 DOI: http://www.ncbi.nlm.nih.gov/pubmed/7903159].

50. Weiss JM, Bilate AM, Gobert M, Ding Y, Curotto de Lafaille MA, Parkhurst CN, et al. Neuropilin 1 is expressed on thymus-derived natural regulatory T cells, but not mucosa-generated induced Foxp3+ T reg cells. *J Exp Med* 2012;**209**(10):1723−42 S1721 [PMID:22966001 PMCID: 3457733 http://dx.doi.org/10.1084/jem.20120914].

51. Geuking MB, Cahenzli J, Lawson MA, Ng DC, Slack E, Hapfelmeier S, et al. Intestinal bacterial colonization induces mutualistic regulatory T cell responses. *Immunity* 2011;**34**(5):794−806 [PMID:21596591 http://dx.doi.org/10.1016/j.immuni.2011.03.021].

52. Atarashi K, Tanoue T, Shima T, Imaoka A, Kuwahara T, Momose Y, et al. Induction of colonic regulatory T cells by indigenous Clostridium species. *Science* 2011;**331**(6015):337−41 [PMID:21205640 PMCID: 3969237 http://dx.doi.org/10.1126/science.1198469].

53. Kim SV, Xiang WV, Kwak C, Yang Y, Lin XW, Ota M, et al. GPR15-mediated homing controls immune homeostasis in the large intestine mucosa. *Science* 2013;**340**(6139):1456−9 [PMID:23661644 PMCID: 3762262 http://dx.doi.org/10.1126/science.1237013].

54. Diehl GE, Longman RS, Zhang JX, Breart B, Galan C, Cuesta A, et al. Microbiota restricts trafficking of bacteria to mesenteric lymph nodes by CX(3)CR1(hi) cells. *Nature* 2013;**494** (7435):116−20 [PMID:23334413 PMCID: 3711636 http://dx.doi.org/10.1038/nature11809].

55. Kawamoto S, Maruya M, Kato LM, Suda W, Atarashi K, Doi Y, et al. Foxp3(+) T cells regulate immunoglobulin a selection and facilitate diversification of bacterial species responsible for immune homeostasis. *Immunity* 2014;**41**(1):152−65 [PMID:25017466 http://dx.doi.org/10.1016/j.immuni.2014.05.016].

56. Bevins CL, Salzman NH. Paneth cells, antimicrobial peptides and maintenance of intestinal homeostasis. *Nat Rev Microbiol* 2011;**9**(5):356−68 [PMID:21423246 http://dx.doi.org/10.1038/nrmicro2546].

57. Salzman NH. The role of the microbiome in immune cell development. *Ann Allergy Asthma Immunol* 2014;**113**(6):593−8 [PMID:25466801 http://dx.doi.org/10.1016/j.anai.2014.08.020].

58. Loonen LM, Stolte EH, Jaklofsky MT, Meijerink M, Dekker J, van Baarlen P, et al. REG3gamma-deficient mice have altered mucus distribution and increased mucosal inflammatory responses to the microbiota and enteric pathogens in the ileum. *Mucosal Immunol* 2014;**7**(4):939−47 [PMID:24345802 http://dx.doi.org/10.1038/mi.2013.109].

59. Vaishnava S, Yamamoto M, Severson KM, Ruhn KA, Yu X, Koren O, et al. The antibacterial lectin RegIIIgamma promotes the spatial segregation of microbiota and host in the intestine. *Science* 2011;**334**(6053):255−8 [PMID:21998396 PMCID: 3321924 http://dx.doi.org/10.1126/science.1209791].

60. Cash HL, Whitham CV, Behrendt CL, Hooper LV. Symbiotic bacteria direct expression of an intestinal bactericidal lectin. *Science* 2006;**313**(5790):1126−30 [PMID:16931762 PMCID: 2716667 http://dx.doi.org/10.1126/science.1127119].

61. van Ampting MT, Loonen LM, Schonewille AJ, Konings I, Vink C, Iovanna J, et al. Intestinally secreted C-type lectin Reg3b attenuates salmonellosis but not listeriosis in mice. *Infect Immun* 2012;**80**(3):1115−20 [PMID:22252863 PMCID: 3294648 http://dx.doi.org/10.1128/IAI.06165-11].

62. Abreu MT. Toll-like receptor signalling in the intestinal epithelium: how bacterial recognition shapes intestinal function. *Nat Rev Immunol* 2010;**10**(2):131−44 [PMID:20098461 http://dx.doi.org/10.1038/nri2707].

63. Dessein R, Gironella M, Vignal C, Peyrin-Biroulet L, Sokol H, Secher T, et al. Toll-like receptor 2 is critical for induction of Reg3 beta expression and intestinal clearance of Yersinia pseudotuberculosis. *Gut* 2009;**58**(6):771−6 [PMID:19174417 http://dx.doi.org/10.1136/gut.2008.168443].

64. Min YW, Rhee PL. The role of microbiota on the gut immunology. *Clin Ther* 2015;**37** (5):968−75 [PMID:25846321 http://dx.doi.org/10.1016/j.clinthera.2015.03.009].

65. Farkas AM, Panea C, Goto Y, Nakato G, Galan-Diez M, Narushima S, et al. Induction of Th17 cells by segmented filamentous bacteria in the murine intestine. *J Immunol Methods* 2015;**421**:104−11 [PMID:25858227 http://dx.doi.org/10.1016/j.jim.2015.03.020].

66. Gaboriau-Routhiau V, Rakotobe S, Lecuyer E, Mulder I, Lan A, Bridonneau C, et al. The key role of segmented filamentous bacteria in the coordinated maturation of gut helper T cell responses. *Immunity* 2009;**31**(4):677−89 [PMID:19833089 http://dx.doi.org/10.1016/j.immuni.2009.08.020].

67. Ivanov II, Frutos Rde L, Manel N, Yoshinaga K, Rifkin DB, Sartor RB, et al. Specific microbiota direct the differentiation of IL-17-producing T-helper cells in the mucosa of the small intestine. *Cell Host Microbe* 2008;**4**(4):337−49 [PMID:18854238 PMCID: 2597589 http://dx.doi.org/10.1016/j.chom.2008.09.009].

68. Zeissig S, Blumberg RS. Commensal microbial regulation of natural killer T cells at the frontiers of the mucosal immune system. *FEBS Lett* 2014;**588**(22):4188−94 [PMID:24983499 http://dx.doi.org/10.1016/j.febslet.2014.06.042].

69. Brennan PJ, Brigl M, Brenner MB. Invariant natural killer T cells: an innate activation scheme linked to diverse effector functions. *Nat Rev Immunol* 2013;**13**(2):101−17 [PMID:23334244 http://dx.doi.org/10.1038/nri3369].

70. Park SH, Benlagha K, Lee D, Balish E, Bendelac A. Unaltered phenotype, tissue distribution and function of Valpha14(+) NKT cells in germ-free mice. *Eur J Immunol* 2000;**30**(2):620−5 [PMID:10671219 http://dx.doi.org/10.1002/1521-4141(200002)30:2 < 620::AID-IMMU620 > 3.0. CO;2-4].

71. Wingender G, Stepniak D, Krebs P, Lin L, McBride S, Wei B, et al. Intestinal microbes affect phenotypes and functions of invariant natural killer T cells in mice. *Gastroenterology* 2012;**143**(2):418−28 [PMID:22522092 PMCID: 3404247 http://dx.doi.org/10.1053/j.gastro.2012.04.017].

72. Olszak T, An D, Zeissig S, Vera MP, Richter J, Franke A, et al. Microbial exposure during early life has persistent effects on natural killer T cell function. *Science* 2012;**336**(6080):489−93 [PMID:22442383 PMCID: 3437652 http://dx.doi.org/10.1126/science.1219328].

73. Salzman NH, Hung K, Haribhai D, Chu H, Karlsson-Sjoberg J, Amir E, et al. Enteric defensins are essential regulators of intestinal microbial ecology. *Nat Immunol* 2010;**11** (1):76−83 [PMID:19855381 PMCID: 2795796 http://dx.doi.org/10.1038/ni.1825].

74. Nieuwenhuis EE, Matsumoto T, Lindenbergh D, Willemsen R, Kaser A, Simons-Oosterhuis Y, et al. Cd1d-dependent regulation of bacterial colonization in the intestine of mice. *J Clin Invest* 2009;**119**(5):1241−50 [PMID:19349688 PMCID: 2673876 http://dx.doi.org/10.1172/JCI36509].

75. Dowds CM, Blumberg RS, Zeissig S. Control of intestinal homeostasis through crosstalk between natural killer T cells and the intestinal microbiota. *Clin Immunol* 2015. [PMID:25988859 http://dx.doi.org/10.1016/j.clim.2015.05.008].

76. Dethlefsen L, Huse S, Sogin ML, Relman DA. The pervasive effects of an antibiotic on the human gut microbiota, as revealed by deep 16S rRNA sequencing. *PLoS Biol* 2008;**6**(11): e280 [PMID:19018661 PMCID: 2586385 http://dx.doi.org/10.1371/journal.pbio.0060280].

77. Hevia A, Milani C, Lopez P, Cuervo A, Arboleya S, Duranti S, et al. Intestinal dysbiosis associated with systemic lupus erythematosus. *mBio* 2014;**5**(5). e01548-01514 [PMID:25271284 PMCID: 4196225 http://dx.doi.org/10.1128/mBio.01548-14].

78. Goossens H, Ferech M, Vander Stichele R, Elseviers M, Group EP. Outpatient antibiotic use in Europe and association with resistance: a cross-national database study. *Lancet* 2005;**365** (9459):579−87.

79. Ichinohe T, Pang IK, Kumamoto Y, Peaper DR, Ho JH, Murray TS, et al. Microbiota regulates immune defense against respiratory tract influenza A virus infection. *Proc Natl Acad Sci USA* 2011;**108**(13):5354−9 [PMID:21402903 PMCID: 3069176 http://dx.doi.org/10.1073/pnas.1019378108].

80. Sharma SK, Nakajima K, Shukla PJ. Clostridium difficile infection. *N Engl J Med* 2015;**373** (3):287 [PMID:26176399 http://dx.doi.org/10.1056/NEJMc1506004#SA3].

81. Kremery Jr. V, Matejicka F, Pichnova E, Jurga L, Sulcova M, Kunova A, et al. Documented fungal infections after prophylaxis or therapy with wide spectrum antibiotics: relationship between certain fungal pathogens and particular antimicrobials? *J Chemother* 1999;**11**(5):385−90 [PMID:10632385 http://dx.doi.org/10.1179/joc.1999.11.5.385].

82. Walker AW, Ince J, Duncan SH, Webster LM, Holtrop G, Ze X, et al. Dominant and diet-responsive groups of bacteria within the human colonic microbiota. *ISME J* 2011;**5**(2):220−30 [PMID:20686513 PMCID: 3105703 http://dx.doi.org/10.1038/ismej.2010.118].

83. Gibson GR, Roberfroid MB. Dietary modulation of the human colonic microbiota: introducing the concept of prebiotics. *J Nutr* 1995;**125**(6):1401−12 [PMID:7782892 DOI: http://www.ncbi.nlm.nih.gov/pubmed/7782892].

84. Flint HJ, Scott KP, Duncan SH, Louis P, Forano E. Microbial degradation of complex carbohydrates in the gut. *Gut Microbes* 2012;**3**(4):289–306 [PMID:22572875 PMCID: 3463488 http://dx.doi.org/10.4161/gmic.19897].

85. Wong JM, de Souza R, Kendall CW, Emam A, Jenkins DJ. Colonic health: fermentation and short chain fatty acids. *J Clin Gastroenterol* 2006;**40**(3):235–43 [PMID:16633129 DOI: http://www.ncbi.nlm.nih.gov/pubmed/16633129].

86. Cummings JH, Hill MJ, Bone ES, Branch WJ, Jenkins DJ. The effect of meat protein and dietary fiber on colonic function and metabolism. II. Bacterial metabolites in feces and urine. *Am J Clin Nutr* 1979;**32**(10):2094–101 [PMID:484528 DOI: http://www.ncbi.nlm.nih.gov/pubmed/484528].

87. Sleeth ML, Thompson EL, Ford HE, Zac-Varghese SE, Frost G. Free fatty acid receptor 2 and nutrient sensing: a proposed role for fibre, fermentable carbohydrates and short-chain fatty acids in appetite regulation. *Nutr Res Rev* 2010;**23**(1):135–45 [PMID:20482937 http://dx.doi.org/10.1017/S0954422410000089].

88. Maskarinec G, Takata Y, Pagano I, Carlin L, Goodman MT, Le Marchand L, et al. Trends and dietary determinants of overweight and obesity in a multiethnic population. *Obesity* 2006;**14**(4):717–26 [PMID:16741275 http://dx.doi.org/10.1038/oby.2006.82].

89. Ludwig DS, Pereira MA, Kroenke CH, Hilner JE, Van Horn L, Slattery ML, et al. Dietary fiber, weight gain, and cardiovascular disease risk factors in young adults. *JAMA* 1999;**282** (16):1539–46 [PMID:10546693 DOI: http://www.ncbi.nlm.nih.gov/pubmed/10546693].

90. Zhang H, Sun J, Jin D. Manipulation of microbiome, a promising therapy for inflammatory bowel diseases. *J Clin Cell Immunol* 2014;**5**:234.

91. Martin R, Miquel S, Ulmer J, Kechaou N, Langella P, Bermudez-Humaran LG. Role of commensal and probiotic bacteria in human health: a focus on inflammatory bowel disease. *Microb Cell Fact* 2013;**12**:71 [PMID:23876056 PMCID: 3726476 http://dx.doi.org/10.1186/1475-2859-12-71].

92. Veerappan GR, Betteridge J, Young PE. Probiotics for the treatment of inflammatory bowel disease. *Curr Gastroenterol Rep* 2012;**14**(4):324–33 [PMID:22581276 http://dx.doi.org/10.1007/s11894-012-0265-5].

93. Vanderpool C, Yan F, Polk DB. Mechanisms of probiotic action: implications for therapeutic applications in inflammatory bowel diseases. *Inflamm Bowel Dis* 2008;**14**(11):1585–96 [PMID:18623173 http://dx.doi.org/10.1002/ibd.20525].

94. Salminen S, Salminen E. Lactulose, lactic acid bacteria, intestinal microecology and mucosal protection. *Scand J Gastroenterol Suppl* 1997;**222**:45–8 [PMID:9145446 DOI: http://www.ncbi.nlm.nih.gov/pubmed/9145446].

95. Rauch M, Lynch SV. The potential for probiotic manipulation of the gastrointestinal microbiome. *Curr Opin Biotechnol* 2012;**23**(2):192–201 [PMID:22137452 http://dx.doi.org/10.1016/j.copbio.2011.11.004].

96. Zhang F, Luo W, Shi Y, Fan Z, Ji G. Should we standardize the 1700-year-old fecal microbiota transplantation? *Am J Gastroenterol* 2012;**107**(11):1755 author reply 1755–1756 [PMID:23160295 http://dx.doi.org/10.1038/ajg.2012.251].

97. Borody TJ, Brandt LJ, Paramsothy S. Therapeutic faecal microbiota transplantation: current status and future developments. *Curr Opin Gastroenterol* 2014;**30**(1):97–105 [PMID:24257037 PMCID: 3868025 http://dx.doi.org/10.1097/MOG.0000000000000027].

98. Schwan A, Sjolin S, Trottestam U, Aronsson B. Relapsing Clostridium difficile enterocolitis cured by rectal infusion of normal faeces. *Scand J Infect Dis* 1984;**16**(2):211–15 [PMID:6740251 DOI: http://www.ncbi.nlm.nih.gov/pubmed/6740251].

99. Eiseman B, Silen W, Bascom GS, Kauvar AJ. Fecal enema as an adjunct in the treatment of pseudomembranous enterocolitis. *Surgery* 1958;**44**(5):854–9 [PMID:13592638 DOI: http://www.ncbi.nlm.nih.gov/pubmed/13592638].

100. van Nood E, Speelman P, Nieuwdorp M, Keller J. Fecal microbiota transplantation: facts and controversies. *Curr Opin Gastroenterol* 2014;**30**(1):34–9 [PMID:24241245 http://dx.doi. org/10.1097/MOG.0000000000000024].

101. Mullish BH, Marchesi JR, Thursz MR, Williams HR. Microbiome manipulation with faecal microbiome transplantation as a therapeutic strategy in Clostridium difficile infection. *QJM* 2015;**108**(5):355–9 [PMID:25193538 PMCID: 4410624 http://dx.doi.org/10.1093/ qjmed/hcu182].

102. Davidson A, Diamond B. Autoimmune diseases. *N Engl J Med* 2001;**345**(5):340–50 [PMID:11484692 http://dx.doi.org/10.1056/NEJM200108023450506].

103. Strachan DP. Family size, infection and atopy: the first decade of the "hygiene hypothesis". *Thorax* 2000;**55**(Suppl. 1):S2–10 [PMID:10943631 PMCID: 1765943 DOI: http://www.ncbi. nlm.nih.gov/pubmed/10943631].

104. Strachan DP. Hay fever, hygiene, and household size. *BMJ* 1989;**299**(6710):1259–60 [PMID:2513902 PMCID: 1838109 doi: http://www.ncbi.nlm.nih.gov/pubmed/2513902].

105. Noverr MC, Huffnagle GB. Does the microbiota regulate immune responses outside the gut? *Trends Microbiol* 2004;**12**(12):562–8 [PMID:15539116 http://dx.doi.org/10.1016/j. tim.2004.10.008].

106. Rook GA, Martinelli R, Brunet LR. Innate immune responses to mycobacteria and the downregulation of atopic responses. *Curr Opin Allergy Clin Immunol* 2003;**3**(5):337–42 [PMID:14501431 http://dx.doi.org/10.1097/01.all.0000092602.76804.ad].

107. Edwards CJ. Commensal gut bacteria and the etiopathogenesis of rheumatoid arthritis. *J Rheumatol* 2008;**35**(8):1477–9.

108. Kohashi O, Kuwata J, Umehara K, Uemura F, Takahashi T, Ozawa A. Susceptibility to adjuvant-induced arthritis among germfree, specific-pathogen-free, and conventional rats. *Infect Immun* 1979;**26**(3):791–4.

109. Van den Broek M, Van Bruggen M, Koopman J, Hazenberg M, Van Den Berg W. Gut flora induces and maintains resistance against streptococcal cell wall-induced arthritis in F344 rats. *Clin Exp Immunol* 1992;**88**(2):313.

110. Taurog JD, Richardson JA, Croft JT, Simmons WA, Zhou M, Fernandez-Sueiro JL, et al. The germfree state prevents development of gut and joint inflammatory disease in HLA-B27 transgenic rats. *J Exp Med* 1994;**180**(6):2359–64 [PMID:7964509 PMCID: 2191772 DOI: http://www.ncbi.nlm.nih.gov/pubmed/7964509].

111. DeLay ML, Turner MJ, Klenk EI, Smith JA, Sowders DP, Colbert RA. HLA - B27 misfolding and the unfolded protein response augment interleukin-23 production and are associated with Th17 activation in transgenic rats. *Arthritis Rheum* 2009;**60**(9):2633–43.

112. Šimelyte E, Rimpiläinen M, Lehtonen L, Zhang X, Toivanen P. Bacterial cell wall-induced arthritis: chemical composition and tissue distribution of four lactobacillus strains. *Infect Immun* 2000;**68**(6):3535–40.

113. Abdollahi-Roodsaz S, Joosten LA, Koenders MI, Devesa I, Roelofs MF, Radstake TR, et al. Stimulation of TLR2 and TLR4 differentially skews the balance of T cells in a mouse model of arthritis. *J Clin Invest* 2008;**118**(1):205.

114. Wu H-J, Ivanov II, Darce J, Hattori K, Shima T, Umesaki Y, et al. Gut-residing segmented filamentous bacteria drive autoimmune arthritis via T helper 17 cells. *Immunity* 2010;**32** (6):815–27.

115. Vaahtovuo J, Munukka E, Korkeamäki M, Luukkainen R, Toivanen P. Fecal microbiota in early rheumatoid arthritis. *J Rheumatol* 2008;**35**(8):1500.

116. Liu X, Zou Q, Zeng B, Fang Y, Wei H. Analysis of fecal lactobacillus community structure in patients with early rheumatoid arthritis. *Curr Microbiol* 2013;**67**(2):170–6.

117. Scher JU, Sczesnak A, Longman RS, Segata N, Ubeda C, Bielski C, et al. Expansion of intestinal Prevotella copri correlates with enhanced susceptibility to arthritis. *Elife* 2013;2:e01202.

118. Amdekar S, Singh V, Singh R, Sharma P, Keshav P, Kumar A. Lactobacillus casei reduces the inflammatory joint damage associated with collagen-induced arthritis (CIA) by reducing the pro-inflammatory cytokines. *J Clin Immunol* 2011;31(2):147−54.

119. So J-S, Kwon H-K, Lee C-G, Yi H-J, Park J-A, Lim S-Y, et al. Lactobacillus casei suppresses experimental arthritis by down-regulating T helper 1 effector functions. *Mol Immunol* 2008;45(9):2690−9.

120. Steinman L. A molecular trio in relapse and remission in multiple sclerosis. *Nat Rev Immunol* 2009;9(6):440−7 [PMID:19444308 http://dx.doi.org/10.1038/nri2548].

121. Stromnes IM, Goverman JM. Active induction of experimental allergic encephalomyelitis. *Nat Protoc* 2006;1(4):1810−19 [PMID:17487163 http://dx.doi.org/10.1038/nprot.2006.285].

122. Yokote H, Miyake S, Croxford JL, Oki S, Mizusawa H, Yamamura T. NKT cell-dependent amelioration of a mouse model of multiple sclerosis by altering gut flora. *Am J Pathol* 2008;173(6):1714−23 [PMID:18974295 PMCID: 2626383 http://dx.doi.org/10.2353/ajpath.2008.080622].

123. Ochoa-Reparaz J, Mielcarz DW, Ditrio LE, Burroughs AR, Foureau DM, Haque-Begum S, et al. Role of gut commensal microflora in the development of experimental autoimmune encephalomyelitis. *J Immunol* 2009;183(10):6041−50 [PMID:19841183 http://dx.doi.org/10.4049/jimmunol.0900747].

124. Ochoa-Reparaz J, Mielcarz DW, Haque-Begum S, Kasper LH. Induction of a regulatory B cell population in experimental allergic encephalomyelitis by alteration of the gut commensal microflora. *Gut Microbes* 2010;1(2):103−8 [PMID:21326918 PMCID: 3023588 http://dx.doi.org/10.4161/gmic.1.2.11515].

125. Lee YK, Menezes JS, Umesaki Y, Mazmanian SK. Proinflammatory T-cell responses to gut microbiota promote experimental autoimmune encephalomyelitis. *Proc Natl Acad Sci USA* 2011;108(Suppl. 1):4615−22 [PMID:20660719 PMCID: 3063590 http://dx.doi.org/10.1073/pnas.1000082107].

126. Berer K, Mues M, Koutrolos M, Rasbi ZA, Boziki M, Johner C, et al. Commensal microbiota and myelin autoantigen cooperate to trigger autoimmune demyelination. *Nature* 2011;479(7374):538−41 [PMID:22031325 http://dx.doi.org/10.1038/nature10554].

127. Lavasani S, Dzhambazov B, Nouri M, Fak F, Buske S, Molin G, et al. A novel probiotic mixture exerts a therapeutic effect on experimental autoimmune encephalomyelitis mediated by IL-10 producing regulatory T cells. *PloS one* 2010;5(2):e9009 [PMID:20126401 PMCID: 2814855 http://dx.doi.org/10.1371/journal.pone.0009009].

128. Jun S, Gilmore W, Callis G, Rynda A, Haddad A, Pascual DW. A live diarrheal vaccine imprints a Th2 cell bias and acts as an anti-inflammatory vaccine. *J Immunol* 2005;175 (10):6733−40 [PMID:16272329 DOI: http://www.ncbi.nlm.nih.gov/pubmed/16272329].

129. Ochoa-Reparaz J, Riccardi C, Rynda A, Jun S, Callis G, Pascual DW. Regulatory T cell vaccination without autoantigen protects against experimental autoimmune encephalomyelitis. *J Immunol* 2007;178(3):1791−9 [PMID:17237429 DOI: http://www.ncbi.nlm.nih.gov/pubmed/17237429].

130. Ochoa-Reparaz J, Rynda A, Ascon MA, Yang X, Kochetkova I, Riccardi C, et al. IL-13 production by regulatory T cells protects against experimental autoimmune encephalomyelitis independently of autoantigen. *J Immunol* 2008;181(2):954−68 [PMID:18606647 PMCID: 2599928 DOI: http://www.ncbi.nlm.nih.gov/pubmed/18606647].

131. Nichols FC, Housley WJ, O'Conor CA, Manning T, Wu S, Clark RB. Unique lipids from a common human bacterium represent a new class of Toll-like receptor 2 ligands capable of enhancing autoimmunity. *Am J Pathol* 2009;175(6):2430−8 [PMID:19850890 PMCID: 2789629 http://dx.doi.org/10.2353/ajpath.2009.090544].

132. Ochoa-Reparaz J, Mielcarz DW, Ditrio LE, Burroughs AR, Begum-Haque S, Dasgupta S, et al. Central nervous system demyelinating disease protection by the human commensal Bacteroides fragilis depends on polysaccharide A expression. *J Immunol* 2010;**185** (7):4101–8 [PMID:20817872 http://dx.doi.org/10.4049/jimmunol.1001443].

133. Sun CM, Hall JA, Blank RB, Bouladoux N, Oukka M, Mora JR, et al. Small intestine lamina propria dendritic cells promote de novo generation of Foxp3 T reg cells via retinoic acid. *J Exp Med* 2007;**204**(8):1775–85 [PMID:17620362 PMCID: 2118682 http://dx.doi.org/ 10.1084/jem.20070602].

134. Lemire JM, Archer DC. 1,25-dihydroxyvitamin D3 prevents the in vivo induction of murine experimental autoimmune encephalomyelitis. *J Clin Invest* 1991;**87**(3):1103–7 [PMID:1705564 PMCID: 329907 http://dx.doi.org/10.1172/JCI115072].

135. Kiss EA, Vonarbourg C, Kopfmann S, Hobeika E, Finke D, Esser C, et al. Natural aryl hydrocarbon receptor ligands control organogenesis of intestinal lymphoid follicles. *Science* 2011;**334**(6062):1561–5 [PMID:22033518 http://dx.doi.org/10.1126/science.1214914].

136. Timmermans S, Bogie JF, Vanmierlo T, Lutjohann D, Stinissen P, Hellings N, et al. High fat diet exacerbates neuroinflammation in an animal model of multiple sclerosis by activation of the renin angiotensin system. *J Neuroimmune Pharmacol* 2014;**9**(2):209–17 [PMID:24068577 http://dx.doi.org/10.1007/s11481-013-9502-4].

137. Kleinewietfeld M, Manzel A, Titze J, Kvakan H, Yosef N, Linker RA, et al. Sodium chloride drives autoimmune disease by the induction of pathogenic TH17 cells. *Nature* 2013;**496** (7446):518–22 [PMID:23467095 PMCID: 3746493 http://dx.doi.org/10.1038/nature11868].

138. Wu C, Yosef N, Thalhamer T, Zhu C, Xiao S, Kishi Y, et al. Induction of pathogenic TH17 cells by inducible salt-sensing kinase SGK1. *Nature* 2013;**496**(7446):513–17 [PMID:23467085 PMCID: 3637879 http://dx.doi.org/10.1038/nature11984].

139. Munger KL, Chitnis T, Frazier AL, Giovannucci E, Spiegelman D, Ascherio A. Dietary intake of vitamin D during adolescence and risk of multiple sclerosis. *J Neurol* 2011;**258** (3):479–85 [PMID:20945071 PMCID: 3077931 http://dx.doi.org/10.1007/s00415-010-5783-1].

140. Manzel A, Muller DN, Hafler DA, Erdman SE, Linker RA, Kleinewietfeld M. Role of "Western diet" in inflammatory autoimmune diseases. *Curr Allergy Asthma Rep* 2014;**14** (1):404 [PMID:24338487 PMCID: 4034518 http://dx.doi.org/10.1007/s11882-013-0404-6].

141. Borody TJ, Leis S, Campbell J, et al. Fecal microbiota transplantation (FMT) in multiple sclerosis (MS). *Am J Gastroenterol* 2011;**106**:S352.

142. Leibowitz U, Antonovsky A, Medalie JM, Smith HA, Halpern L, Alter M. Epidemiological study of multiple sclerosis in Israel. II. Multiple sclerosis and level of sanitation. *J Neurol Neurosurg Psychiatry* 1966;**29**(1):60–8 [PMID:5910580 PMCID: 495985 DOI: http://www.ncbi.nlm.nih.gov/pubmed/5910580].

143. Fleming JO, Cook TD. Multiple sclerosis and the hygiene hypothesis. *Neurology* 2006;**67** (11):2085–6 [PMID:17159130 http://dx.doi.org/10.1212/01.wnl.0000247663.40297.2d].

144. Correale J, Farez M. Association between parasite infection and immune responses in multiple sclerosis. *Ann Neurol* 2007;**61**(2):97–108 [PMID:17230481 http://dx.doi.org/10.1002/ ana.21067].

145. Correale J, Farez M, Razzitte G. Helminth infections associated with multiple sclerosis induce regulatory B cells. *Ann Neurol* 2008;**64**(2):187–99 [PMID:18655096 http://dx.doi.org/ 10.1002/ana.21438].

146. Correale J, Farez MF. The impact of parasite infections on the course of multiple sclerosis. *J Neuroimmunol* 2011;**233**(1–2):6–11 [PMID:21277637 http://dx.doi.org/10.1016/j. jneuroim.2011.01.002].

147. Ohl K, Tenbrock K. Inflammatory cytokines in systemic lupus erythematosus. *J Biomed Biotechnol* 2011;**2011**:432595 [PMID:22028588 PMCID: 3196871 http://dx.doi.org/10.1155/ 2011/432595].

148. Tsokos GC. Systemic lupus erythematosus. *N Engl J Med* 2011;**365**(22):2110−21 [PMID:22129255 http://dx.doi.org/10.1056/NEJMra1100359].

149. Andrews BS, Eisenberg RA, Theofilopoulos AN, Izui S, Wilson CB, McConahey PJ, et al. Spontaneous murine lupus-like syndromes. Clinical and immunopathological manifestations in several strains. *J Exp Med* 1978;**148**(5):1198−215 [PMID:309911 PMCID: 2185049 DOI: http://www.ncbi.nlm.nih.gov/pubmed/309911].

150. East J, Prosser PR, Holborow EJ, Jaquet H. Autoimmune reactions and virus-like particles in germ-free NZB mice. *Lancet* 1967;**1**(7493):755−7 [PMID:4164124 DOI: http://www.ncbi.nlm.nih.gov/pubmed/4164124].

151. Unni KK, Holley KE, McDuffie FC, Titus JL. Comparative study of NZB mice under germfree and conventional conditions. *J Rheumatol* 1975;**2**(1):36−44 [PMID: 1185733 DOI: http://www.ncbi.nlm.nih.gov/pubmed/1185733].

152. Maldonado MA, Kakkanaiah V, MacDonald GC, Chen F, Reap EA, Balish E, et al. The role of environmental antigens in the spontaneous development of autoimmunity in MRL-lpr mice. *J Immunol* 1999;**162**(11):6322−30 [PMID:10352243 DOI: http://www.ncbi.nlm.nih.gov/pubmed/10352243].

153. Zhang H, Liao X, Sparks JB, Luo XM. Dynamics of gut microbiota in autoimmune lupus. *Appl Environ Microbiol* 2014;**80**(24):7551−60 [PMID:25261516 PMCID: 4249226 http://dx.doi.org/10.1128/AEM.02676-14].

154. Rojo D, Hevia A, Bargiela R, Lopez P, Cuervo A, Gonzalez S, et al. Ranking the impact of human health disorders on gut metabolism: systemic lupus erythematosus and obesity as study cases. *Sci Rep* 2015;**5**:8310 [PMID:25655524 PMCID: 4319156 http://dx.doi.org/10.1038/srep08310].

155. Tüzün Y, Keskin S, Kote E. The role of Helicobacter pylori infection in skin diseases: facts and controversies. *Clin Dermatol* 2010;**28**(5):478−82.

156. Chiu Y-C, Tai W-C, Chuah S-K, Hsu P-I, Wu D-C, Wu K-L, et al. The clinical correlations of Helicobacter pylori virulence factors and chronic spontaneous urticaria. *Gastroenterol Res Pract* 2013;**2013**.

157. Yadav MK, Rishi JP, Nijawan S. Chronic urticaria and Helicobacter pylori. *Indian J Med Sci* 2008;**62**(4):157.

158. Abdou AG, Elshayeb EI, Farag AG, Elnaidany NF. Helicobacter pylori infection in patients with chronic urticaria: correlation with pathologic findings in gastric biopsies. *Int J Dermatol* 2009;**48**(5):464−9 [DOI: http://onlinelibrary.wiley.com/doi/10.1111/j.1365-4632.2009.04042.x/abstract].

159. Moreira A, Rodrigues J, Delgado L, Fonseca J, Vaz M. Is Helicobacter pylori infection associated with chronic idiopathic urticaria? *Allergol Immunopathol (Madr)* 2003;**31**(4):209−14.

160. Gu H, Li L, Gu M, Zhang G. Association between Helicobacter pylori infection and chronic urticaria: a meta-analysis. *Gastroenterol Res Pract* 2015;**2015**:486974.

161. Molodecky NA, Soon IS, Rabi DM, Ghali WA, Ferris M, Chernoff G, et al. Increasing incidence and prevalence of the inflammatory bowel diseases with time, based on systematic review. *Gastroenterology* 2012;**142**(1):46−54 e42; quiz e30 [PMID:22001864 http://dx.doi.org/10.1053/j.gastro.2011.10.001].

162. Cosnes J, Gower-Rousseau C, Seksik P, Cortot A. Epidemiology and natural history of inflammatory bowel diseases. *Gastroenterology* 2011;**140**(6):1785−94 [PMID:21530745 http://dx.doi.org/10.1053/j.gastro.2011.01.055].

163. Van Limbergen J, Radford-Smith G, Satsangi J. Advances in IBD genetics. Nature reviews. *Gastroenterol Hepatol* 2014;**11**(6):372−85 [PMID:24614343 http://dx.doi.org/10.1038/nrgastro.2014.27].

164. Van Limbergen J, Russell RK, Drummond HE, Aldhous MC, Round NK, Nimmo ER, et al. Definition of phenotypic characteristics of childhood-onset inflammatory bowel disease. *Gastroenterology* 2008;**135**(4):1114–22 [PMID:18725221 http://dx.doi.org/10.1053/j.gastro.2008.06.081].

165. Jostins L, Ripke S, Weersma RK, Duerr RH, McGovern DP, Hui KY, et al. Host-microbe interactions have shaped the genetic architecture of inflammatory bowel disease. *Nature* 2012;**491**(7422):119–24 [PMID:23128233 PMCID: 3491803 http://dx.doi.org/10.1038/nature11582].

166. Gevers D, Kugathasan S, Denson LA, Vazquez-Baeza Y, Van Treuren W, Ren B, et al. The treatment-naive microbiome in new-onset Crohn's disease. *Cell Host Microbe* 2014;**15**(3):382–92 [PMID:24629344 PMCID: 4059512 http://dx.doi.org/10.1016/j.chom.2014.02.005].

167. Huttenhower C, Kostic AD, Xavier RJ. Inflammatory bowel disease as a model for translating the microbiome. *Immunity* 2014;**40**(6):843–54 [PMID:24950204 PMCID: 4135443 http://dx.doi.org/10.1016/j.immuni.2014.05.013].

168. Rakoff-Nahoum S, Paglino J, Eslami-Varzaneh F, Edberg S, Medzhitov R. Recognition of commensal microflora by toll-like receptors is required for intestinal homeostasis. *Cell* 2004;**118**(2):229–41 [PMID:15260992 http://dx.doi.org/10.1016/j.cell.2004.07.002].

169. Rath HC, Schultz M, Freitag R, Dieleman LA, Li F, Linde HJ, et al. Different subsets of enteric bacteria induce and perpetuate experimental colitis in rats and mice. *Infect Immun* 2001;**69**(4):2277–85 [PMID:11254584 PMCID: 98156 http://dx.doi.org/10.1128/IAI.69.4.2277-2285.2001].

170. Sadlack B, Merz H, Schorle H, Schimpl A, Feller AC, Horak I. Ulcerative colitis-like disease in mice with a disrupted interleukin-2 gene. *Cell* 1993;**75**(2):253–61 [PMID:8402910 DOI: http://www.ncbi.nlm.nih.gov/pubmed/8402910].

171. Bernstein LH, Frank MS, Brandt LJ, Boley SJ. Healing of perineal Crohn's disease with metronidazole. *Gastroenterology* 1980;**79**(2):357–65 [PMID: 7399243 DOI: http://www.ncbi.nlm.nih.gov/pubmed/7399243].

172. Michail S, Durbin M, Turner D, Griffiths AM, Mack DR, Hyams J, et al. Alterations in the gut microbiome of children with severe ulcerative colitis. *Inflamm Bowel Dis* 2012;**18**(10):1799–808 [PMID:22170749 PMCID: 3319508 http://dx.doi.org/10.1002/ibd.22860].

173. Willing B, Halfvarson J, Dicksved J, Rosenquist M, Jarnerot G, Engstrand L, et al. Twin studies reveal specific imbalances in the mucosa-associated microbiota of patients with ileal Crohn's disease. *Inflamm Bowel Dis* 2009;**15**(5):653–60 [PMID:19023901 http://dx.doi.org/10.1002/ibd.20783].

174. Morgan XC, Tickle TL, Sokol H, Gevers D, Devaney KL, Ward DV, et al. Dysfunction of the intestinal microbiome in inflammatory bowel disease and treatment. *Genome Biol* 2012;**13**(9):R79 [PMID:23013615 PMCID: 3506950 http://dx.doi.org/10.1186/gb-2012-13-9-r79].

175. Qin J, Li R, Raes J, Arumugam M, Burgdorf KS, Manichanh C, et al. A human gut microbial gene catalogue established by metagenomic sequencing. *Nature* 2010;**464**(7285):59–65 [PMID:20203603 PMCID: 3779803 http://dx.doi.org/10.1038/nature08821].

176. Ooi M, Nishiumi S, Yoshie T, Shiomi Y, Kohashi M, Fukunaga K, et al. GC/MS-based profiling of amino acids and TCA cycle-related molecules in ulcerative colitis. *Inflamm Res* 2011;**60**(9):831–40 [PMID:21523508 http://dx.doi.org/10.1007/s00011-011-0340-7].

177. Erickson AR, Cantarel BL, Lamendella R, Darzi Y, Mongodin EF, Pan C, et al. Integrated metagenomics/metaproteomics reveals human host-microbiota signatures of Crohn's disease. *PLoS One* 2012;**7**(11):e49138 [PMID:23209564 PMCID: 3509130 http://dx.doi.org/10.1371/journal.pone.0049138].

178. Atarashi K, Tanoue T, Oshima K, Suda W, Nagano Y, Nishikawa H, et al. Treg induction by a rationally selected mixture of Clostridia strains from the human microbiota. *Nature* 2013;**500**(7461):232–6 [PMID:23842501 http://dx.doi.org/10.1038/nature12331].

179. Furusawa Y, Obata Y, Fukuda S, Endo TA, Nakato G, Takahashi D, et al. Commensal microbe-derived butyrate induces the differentiation of colonic regulatory T cells. *Nature* 2013;**504**(7480):446–50 [PMID:24226770 http://dx.doi.org/10.1038/nature12721].

180. Arpaia N, Campbell C, Fan X, Dikiy S, van der Veeken J, deRoos P, et al. Metabolites produced by commensal bacteria promote peripheral regulatory T-cell generation. *Nature* 2013;**504**(7480):451–5 [PMID:24226773 PMCID: 3869884 http://dx.doi.org/10.1038/nature12726].

181. Borody TJ, Khoruts A. Fecal microbiota transplantation and emerging applications. Nature reviews. *Gastroenterol Hepatol* 2012;**9**(2):88–96 [PMID:22183182 http://dx.doi.org/10.1038/nrgastro.2011.244].

182. Aroniadis OC, Brandt LJ. Fecal microbiota transplantation: past, present and future. *Curr Opin Gastroenterol* 2013;**29**(1):79–84 [PMID:23041678 http://dx.doi.org/10.1097/MOG.0b013e32835a4b3e].

183. Leone V, Chang EB, Devkota S. Diet, microbes, and host genetics: the perfect storm in inflammatory bowel diseases. *J Gastroenterol* 2013;**48**(3):315–21 [PMID:23475322 PMCID: 3698420 http://dx.doi.org/10.1007/s00535-013-0777-2].

184. Whelan K, Quigley EM. Probiotics in the management of irritable bowel syndrome and inflammatory bowel disease. *Curr Opin Gastroenterol* 2013;**29**(2):184–9 [PMID:23286925 http://dx.doi.org/10.1097/MOG.0b013e32835d7bba].

CHAPTER 11

Natural Products: Immuno-Rebalancing Therapeutic Approaches

Eduardo Penton-Arias[1] and David D. Haines[2]

[1]Latin American School of Medicine (ELAM) and Biomedical Research Direction of Center for Genetic Engineering and Biotechnology (CIGB), Havana, Cuba [2]University of Connecticut, Faculty of Pharmacy, Department of Pharmacology Health Science Center, University of Debrecen, Hungary

11.1 INTRODUCTION

Plants have evolved to express bioactive compounds as adaptive features allowing a particular plant to survive under conditions of environmental stress. Indeed, plants expressing compounds that are beneficial for animal health have gained evolutionary advantages by virtue of the improved capacity for survival that they confer on animals that eat them and spread their seeds. This cooperative relationship is called xenohormesis. A conceptually simple example is the enhanced colonization of territory by plants bearing fruits containing vitamin C, a potent water-soluble antioxidant. Animals consuming such fruits are more resilient than those that do not, and increase in population size. These plant species benefit by the far-ranging deposition of their seeds in animal droppings. Here the unifying principle linking the cooperative success of a particular plant and animal species is the cytoprotective effects of vitamin C. The "donor" of a beneficial compound can be a plant, as illustrated above, but also many other living organisms. These may be aquatic, commensal, poisonous, edible, archaic, extremophils, among others, with features substantially different from the "recipient" organism expected to benefit from them.

From the early days of medicinal preparations up to now, remedies have originated from nature by empiric trial and error. Up to 64% of all drugs and approximately half of those approved by the US Food and Drug Administration (FDA) were initially components found in or obtained from natural products or inspired on them.[1,2] According to a recent World Health Organization (WHO) study, about 80% of

Immune Rebalancing. DOI: http://dx.doi.org/10.1016/B978-0-12-803302-9.00011-7

the world's population relies on traditional medicine.[3] In many cases, the production of natural compounds shifted from complex crude mixtures or partially processed natural materials to better defined extracted ingredients, and eventually they have been obtained by synthetic or semisynthetic procedures. Only recently are drugs starting to be developed by truly "rational design" driven by the structure of the target biological molecule they must reach, interact with, and modify.[4] This is the case, for example, of Imatinib (Glivec, Novartis), a tyrosine kinase inhibitor currently used for chronic myeloid leukemia. It was selected by high throughput screening from a large amount of variants, guided by the drug target molecule structure.[5,6]

Nevertheless, it is predicted that the conventional and traditional ethnomedical natural sources will be used for a long time to come in the search for new drugs by pharmacologists and the pharma industry. Increasingly sophisticated high throughput screening tools and systems[7,8] and the extraction and chemical characterization of isolated components from natural products, will continue to promote the production of synthetic drug analogues and their derivatives. These will be further characterized by their linkage to specific pharmacologic mechanisms of action. However, important patent issues on natural products, not discussed in this context, must be considered to promote the interest and provide incentives to the pharma industry and the academic research systems. These topics are crucial aspects for the development of new safe and effective drugs and treatments derived from natural products and proven on solid and reliable scientific grounds.

For most of the last century, chemical synthesis was considered the paradigm of drug production because of the completely reliable chemical structures obtained and the strict control of the processes, among others. However, the impact on the environment, the increasing prevalence of noncommunicable chronic diseases, and other general drawbacks allegedly linked to chemical pollutants, have started to erode this position. Large population sectors are now seeking food and drug products of natural origin, because of the widespread belief that "natural" is synonymous to beneficial and healthy. Computer-aided procedures of combinatorial chemistry have been introduced into the pharma industry and real or virtual "libraries" of hundreds of thousands of related structures and their screening algorithms have been developed.[9] However, the replacement of natural products as a privileged source—probably the first source—of new drugs is not foreseen.[2]

Natural medicines are typically taken orally and considered safe foods with medicinal use (nutraceuticals), although they are not always safe or nourishing. Toxic episodes have been reported at times and the consistency, quality control, and toxicological evaluation of their formulations are either not done or difficult to assure. This is due to the variability of the environmental, farming, harvesting, processing, and preservation conditions, as well as the genetic diversity of the drug source and of the patients.

It thus becomes clear that the limits between foods, drugs, and toxic agents are fading, and it is often a matter of dose, concentration, interactions, and acute, cumulative, or remote effects, that classify different products into one or another category. In fact, dietary foods may also have pharmacologic, pathogenic, or toxic effects depending on their type, amount, and intake frequency, or the length of the study period considered and the presence of mutual interactions. Increasing attention is now being paid to the cumulative and remote effects on health of substances to which the body is frequently exposed by different routes, regardless of their origin and intended use.[10,11]

Many physicians are still reluctant in prescribing ill-defined mixtures of ingredients that they cannot manage and dose with precision. In any case, whatever the source and the route a medicinal preparation has followed to become a therapeutic option, its pharmacological properties must have been scientifically demonstrated and the risk/benefit ratio must be favourable. Today's rough extracts may, in a not too distant future, evolve into well-defined synthetic or partially synthetic drugs that are chemically, biologically, pharmacologically, and clinically well characterized. Their natural origin will then be forgotten, as has occurred with aspirin, initially derived from the cortex of a certain type of willow and synthetically produced for a long time.

11.2 MODULATION OF IMMUNE RESPONSES FOR DISEASE PREVENTION AND TREATMENT

Natural products are included among immune response-inducing drugs that can keep or restore health by recruiting soluble immune effectors (antibodies [Ab], cytokines, chemokines) and/or immune effector cells (activated immunocompetent cells and their precursors). The procedures may be active immunotherapies that recruit or stimulate the immune system of the recipient for disease prevention or treatment, for example, conventional preventive vaccines. However, more recently, the concept of therapeutic vaccines was introduced, intended for treatment instead of prevention. Then a vaccine as Sipuleucel-T, the first dendritic cell-based therapeutic vaccine for prostate cancer,[12] was approved by FDA in 2010. Alternatively, passive immunotherapies are based on the adoptive transfer of soluble or viable immune effectors. Among them, those found in preparations of whole sera, polyclonal or monoclonal antibodies (mAbs), immune cells, bone marrow, and transfusions of whole blood or its fractions. These effectors may be prepared through biotech means, or taken from other subjects or animal species, or from the same subject before disease onset or after some specific ex vivo treatments.

Cancer has been the most characteristic—and possibly the most productive—goal of immunotherapies, aimed at eliciting the immune system to respond against tumor cells, although their application is only at the early stages when compared to chemo- or radiotherapies. Cell-based adoptive immunotherapies use allogenic or autologous immune cells targeted to recognize and destroy tumor cells. Cells are isolated, enriched, and/or activated or modified ex vivo and then injected into the body.

mAbs have been available for passive immunotherapies since the in vitro production of specific immunoglobulins by hybridoma (immortalized plasma cell) cultures became possible during the late 1970s. They are now the most developed and promising tools for this purpose. mAbs may identify their targets and exert their own effects, including immunosuppression (for example, anti-T cell CD3 or anti-IL-2 receptor). They can also act as targeted carriers of toxins or cell poisons, radioactive particles, or others, delivered to the site of action, which is marked by the epitope recognized by the mAb. Immunotherapies are carried out by immunosuppressors, stimulants, or adjuvants, known as a whole as immunomodulators. Their actions are mediated by cyto/lympho/chemokines, macrophages, dendritic (DC) or natural killer (NK) cells, cytotoxic T lymphocytes (CTL), among others. Immunomodulators may also include immunoenhancers, such as the TLR-9 linked CpG motifs,[13] and adjuvants (substances or cells that boost immune response), such as BCG, interleukin (IL)-2 and interferon (IFN)-alpha.

Natural or recombinant biomolecules may be directly used in immunotherapies, but natural products often work by promoting or interfering (suppressing) their endogenous production or by modifying their activity in some way. Suppressive immunotherapies prevent responses of the immune system that are inconvenient under certain conditions, for example, graft rejection, autoimmunity or sensitivity to allergens. Immunotherapies are normally less risky than other treatments and natural products are frequently proposed as immunomodulators. However, their formal introduction may be at best subjected to clinical trials (CT), since natural products are often neglected or simply not supported by the mainstream pharma industry. For example, for recurrent prostate cancers that increase prostate specific antigen (PSA), pomegranate extract preparations have shown significant improvement in several CTs, while others are in progress.[14] Chinese herbal therapies, muscadine grape skin extract, and a brassica vegetable diet (eg, broccoli), among others, are also undergoing formal CTs.[14] Their mechanism of action, at a preclinical level, focuses on the inhibition of nuclear factor-κB and the Akt signaling pathway.[6]

11.3 TRADITIONAL MEDICINAL PREPARATIONS HAVE IMMUNOACTIVE PROPERTIES

Classical herbal remedies having valuable assets but affected by many of the above mentioned concerns include epigallocatechin-3-gallate (EGCG)[15] from green tea (*Camellia sinensis*), ginger root (*Zingiber officinale*) extracts and Tanshione (TSN) from *Salvia miltiorrhiza* (Chinese Danshen). These principles show immunosuppressive effects; however, ginseng (*Panax genus*, from Korea/China/Japan), a drug candidate with growing expectations,[16] and milk thistle (*Silybum marianum*)[17] produce nonspecific immunostimulant proliferation effects on lymphocytes. Curcumin from turmeric (*Curcuma longa*)[18] seems to have prospects in multiple sclerosis (MS) treatment, due to its immunosuppressive pro-inflammatory cyto and chemokine downregulation properties. Curcumin also inactivates the NF-κB transcription factor, a master regulator of inflammation and oxidative stress.[19,20]

Resveratrol, a promising phenolic component of grape juice and red wine, inhibits phosphodiesterases by increasing the cytosolic second messenger cAMP, with positive outcomes for carbohydrate, lipid, and mitochondrial metabolisms in the elderly.[21,22] Indeed, polyphenolic flavonoids of plant origin, which are highly contained in food, have been constantly described as inhibitors of intracellular phosphorylation pathways. They also function as immunomodulators for inflammatory and cellular autoimmunity processes. Among them, catechins such as EGCG, for example, inhibit DCs derived from monocytes and quercetins have been shown to improve rat experimental autoimmune myocarditis (EAM). This is achieved by conveniently shifting pro-inflammatory (TNFα and IL-17) and/or anti-inflammatory (IL-10) cytokine production.[23]

Immunoactive natural products also include terpenoids, such as those contained in turmeric and *Gingko biloba* and alkaloids, as those obtained from vinca rosea (*Catharantus roseus*), that aside from their main antimitotic action are strongly immunosuppressive. Polysaccharides from herbal and microbial sources are generally considered immunostimulants,[24] and garlic (*Allium sativum*)[25] is not clearly classified, but both have proven anti-inflammatory properties. The traditional Chinese herbal remedy Berberine (BBR)[26] from *Coptis chinensis* and *Hydrastis canadensis* has hypoglycemic/lipemic and antioxidant/inflammatory activities, proven in experimental and clinical studies. BBR inhibits NADPH oxidase, a potential target for diabetes, since its activation has been associated with diabetes onset,[27] and reduces TNFα and IL-6 that are important mediators of insulin resistance.[28] NF-κB, IL-1β, matrix metalloprotease 9 (MMP9), cyclooxygenase-2 (COX-2) are downregulated by BBR, increasing the anti-inflammatory/pro-inflammatory cytokine ratio. Many other natural products are claimed to have immunological properties but their active components may be unknown and/or the supporting evidence is weak.

11.4 NATURAL PRODUCTS CAN INFLUENCE AND MODIFY INTERSYSTEM INTERACTIONS AND INFECTION RESISTANCE

Drugs showing immunopharmacological activities, including natural products, set up a complex interplay with their biological target receptors within the immune system to reestablish a new balance between regulatory events (immunomodulation). A flowing intersystem crosstalk, typically between the immune, nervous, and endocrine systems, takes place through cellular and soluble immune effectors to maintain homeostasis.[29] It is therefore foreseeable that cytokine receptors in neurological and endocrine structures may provide new immunotherapeutic targets.[30] Endotoxins and hormonal effects must be taken into account and kept under control in order to validate experimental results supporting mechanisms of action of components under test from poorly purified natural preparations.

New immunotherapeutic concepts require the identification, purification, and formulation of the pharmacologically active ingredients from natural extracts under high quality control and purity standards. Defining and characterizing the chemical structure of extracted active compound(s) from natural products is crucial for their partial or complete chemical synthesis. Our growing knowledge on gene regulation (genotypic and pregenomic), expression products (as ligands or target receptors), and on immunity modulation at the molecular level, helps to disclose the mechanisms of action of natural products. These avenues would increase our insight on how natural products affect immunity and lead to the development of synthetic analogues.

Immunoactive natural products can also increase the ability of the immune system to prevent, fight or collaborate with more specific therapies for infections and immunodeficient conditions. BCG, for example, has been shown to induce robust T helper (Th)1 immune response, effective as an adjuvant anticancer therapy, especially for bladder carcinoma,[31] although it could be relatively ineffective in developing host resistance against *Mycobacterium tuberculosis* infection. Immunomodulation is becoming a complementary or alternative therapeutic modality for infections based on the belief that host's susceptibility can be as important as, or more so, than the microorganism itself for the infection to take place.[32]

The development of infections depends on the interaction of the host's susceptibility with the characteristics of the microorganism, and if it occurs, the balance disrupted by the infection may be restored by modulating the destabilized immune system of the host. Natural polysaccharides such as β-glucans or lentinan and polysaccharide-K from *Coriolus versicolor*, have immunomodulator properties[33] and are referred to as immunosaccharides. Some of them deserve a close follow up, out of this context, since they may qualify as prebiotics, that is, substances that interact with the gut microbiome to confer specific benefits to the health and well-being of the host.

11.5 IMMUNOSUPPRESSION IS NOT THE ABROGATION BUT THE REBALANCING OF IMMUNE FUNCTIONS

The most challenging clinical conditions for immunoactive natural products are those where immunosuppression is presumably required, such as graft rejection, autoimmune diseases, and allergy treatments. Many of the most important immunosuppressive drugs (ISD) are derived from natural products (NISD) and used to prevent or fight organ graft rejection and treat rheumatoid arthritis, psoriasis, and other human autoimmune diseases (HAD). Most NISD in use come from fungi or bacteria, where they presumably represent a selective bioadaptive response for survival and operate by interfering with leukocyte proliferation or activation.

One of the first NISD described was cyclosporine A (CsA, from the *Beauveria nivea* fungus), an eleven amino acid-long cyclic peptide that includes a D amino acid residue, synthesized without ribosomal intervention and used to suppress the immune response after organ transplants. More recent examples include the macrolides (antibiotic family) tacrolimus (FK-506, from *Streptomyces tsukubaensis*) and sirolimus (rapamicin), an antifungal antibiotic from *Streptomyces higroscopicus*, and others.

A group of NISD bind to immunophylins, their cytosolic target proteins, which are enzymes that catalyze *cis—trans* transposition and their complexes hinder the activity of interleukin 2 (IL-2), which is an essential cytokine for T-cell growth and differentiation. For example, CsA binds to cyclophylin, thus inhibiting the Ca^{2+} dependent enzyme calcineurin, a protein phosphatase responsible for IL-2 transcription, stimulated by calmodulin, a Ca^{2+} signal transduction modulator. Tacrolimus and sirolimus bind to the mTOR complex, a protein kinase regulating IL-2 transcription and biosynthesis (see Table 11.1).

NISD may, however, develop severe side effects, especially due to their liver, kidney, and/or bone marrow toxicity, indicating that they should be used under strictly controlled conditions after carefully analyzing the risk—benefit ratio of each patient. Therefore, the search for new and safer NISD is now a challenge for immunopharmacological research, although those of plant origin seem to be less reactogenic and deserve further attention. Table 11.1 summarizes selected ISD that have been more actively investigated for their immunosuppressant activity.

Table 11.1 Main Natural Medicinal Principles with Immunosuppressive/Rebalancing Effects

Organism, Family and Active Principle(s) if Known	Mechanism(s) of Action	Clinical uses or Clinical Trials (CT)	Refs
Plants			
Camellia sinensis (green tea). Theaceae. Epigallocatechin-3-gallate (EGCG) polyphenols	Reduces autoimmune symptoms in a rat model of human rheumatoid arthritis (RA) and a murine model of Sjögren's syndrome. Inhibits human monocyte-derived DC and T cell responses. EGCG improve EAE symptoms	Anti-inflammatory, analgesic, cardiotonic, CNS-stimulant, digestive, diuretic	34, 35, 15
Salvia miltiorrhiza (Danshen). Labiatae. Tanshione IIA (TSN) and salvianolic acid	Inhibits IL-12 and IFN-γ production, modulating TH1-cytokines. TSN reduces inflammatory cytokines (IL-2, IL-4, IFNγ and TNFα) and amino-transferases in mice, increasing IL-10 anti-inflammatory cytokine (CTK)	Hepatitis, heart, CNS and liver diseases. Shown to be useful in CT for acute pancreatitis	36, 37, 38, 39
Curcuma longa (Turmeric) Zingiberace, (rhizome's yellow pigment). Polyphenolic curcumin (CCM)	Anti-oxidant/inflammatory, inhibits human DCs and regulates transcription factors, cell cycle proteins and signal transducing kinases. CCM inhibits NF-κB, Th17 cell. Reduces IL-17 and EAE. Modulates B cells	Infections, inflammatory diseases, CT bowel diseases. RA, pancreatitis, uveitis	40, 41, 18, 42
Tripterygium wilfordii Hook F TWHf (Thunder god vine) Celastraceae. **Triptolide** (diterpenoid)	Anti-inflammatory and immunosuppressive in a rat kidney transplant model. Prolonged survival of rats with kidney transplants when combined with prednisone Inhibits Th1/Th17 cells, IL-17, Th2 CTKs + PGE2.	Used for HAD such as lupus erythematosus and RA. Efficacy shown in RA CT	43–45
Glycyrrhiza (liquorice radix) Fabaceae. Flavonoid Diam-monium glycyrrhizinate (DG), glycyrol, glycyrrhizin (GR).	Immunomodulatory. DG inhibits lymphocyte recruitment into liver, T cell proliferation and protects hepatocytes from apoptosis. Prevents LPS-induced pulmonary inflammation and mouse T-cell-mediated hepatitis.	Anti-inflammatory, anti-microbial, hepato/cardio-protective. GR cream effective for psoriasis in CT	46–50
Berberis **sp.** Berberidaceae Berbamine (BM) from *Berberis vulgaris*	Strong anti-inflammatory properties in EAE. BM has inhibitory effects on the delayed type hypersensitivity reaction (DTH), STAT4 and IFNγ production	HAD, prolonged allograft survival in skin-transplanted mice	51

(Continued)

Table 11.1 (Continued)			
Organism, Family and Active Principle(s) if Known	**Mechanism(s) of Action**	**Clinical uses or Clinical Trials (CT)**	**Refs**
Fungi			
Isaria sinclairii. Ascomicota. Myriocin (Fingolimod, FG)	FG was synthetized as sphingosine 1-phosphate receptor modulator; first oral drug for MS approved by US Food and Drug Administration (FDA).	MS treatment in EAE and in humans	52
Beauveria nivea Ascomicota Cyclosporine A (CsA)	CsA binds to cyclophylin inhibiting calcineurin, a protein phosphatase responsible for IL-2 transcription	Immunosuppressive in organ transplants and graft rejection treatments and for some HAD	53
Streptomyces higroscopicus Streptomycetae. Sirolimus	Both bind to the mTOR (mammalian target of rapamycin) complex, a protein kinase regulating IL-2 transcription and biosynthesis. Sirolimus has been shown to extend mouse life-span even when applied late in life.		54
Streptomyces tsukubaensis Streptomycetae. Tacrolimus			55
Algae			
Spirulina platensis (Sp) Cyanobacteria. C-phycocyanin (CPC), phycocyanobilin (PCB)	CPC/PCB are antioxidant/inflammatory, ROS scavenger to control oxidative stress. Decrease NADPH oxidase+cyclooxygenase. Activate Treg. Regulate apoptosis and CTKs	MS and other HAD. Hepato/cardio/nephro and CNS cytoprotector	56−58

11.6 THE OXIDANT VERSUS ANTIOXIDANT ARGUMENT DOES NOT PROVIDE RESPONSES BUT CREATES UNCERTAINTY

Certain natural products, typically known for their systemic anti-inflammatory and ROS (reactive oxygen species) scavenging antioxidant function, have been progressively found to include other pharmacological activities, some of them associated to the same component. The newly revealed properties opened multivalent therapeutic possibilities, based on effects that are integrated and interconnected to those previously known, all of them dependent on more basic underlying biological principles. This wide range of possibilities, however, made these products look like cure-all potions, due in part to the complex composition of their crude extracts that may display multiple synergic or divergent activities. Moreover, some components are able to interact with different target molecules at the same time.

A clear example of this is the C-phycocyanin (CPC) protein and its prosthetic moiety phycocyanobilin (PCB), from the blue green algae/cyanobacteria *Spirulina (Arthrospira) platensis* (Sp). Crude Sp extracts and partially purified CPC/PCB preparations also contain pharmacologically active (probably immunoenhancing) polysaccharides, other proteins, and healthy polyunsaturated lipids. A wide array of small molecules and nutrients (all essential amino acids, vitamins, and minerals) are also contained in Sp and may be responsible for more of its pharmacologic activities.

However, isolated CPC/PCB are also very interactive with multiple biological systems, especially through the inhibitory activity of the membrane NADPH oxidase enzyme complex. This complex can directly kill microorganisms within phagosomes by forming hydrogen peroxide and generating ROS.[59] ROS, however, favors the adhesion of macrophages containing cholesterol to the arterial walls, promoting atherosclerosis, and therefore NADPH oxidase inhibitors and antioxidants could prevent or reverse this process.

Antioxidant preparations with ROS scavenging properties have been prepared, distributed, promoted, and sold, mostly as nutraceuticals, for quite a number of problems in the past three decades. This multiplicity of effects has been investigated and published, but interestingly, contradictory results of proven benefit, no benefit/no harm, or even increased morbidity effects have emerged from animal research and CTs. This confusing setting implies that the current experience in the clinical use of antioxidants is not enough for generalizations or predictions. A watchful position is thus recommended, where any therapeutic proposal must be based on direct, sound, and reliable evidence justifying its intended use and not just on the antioxidant or oxidant condition of a product.

Antioxidants are criticized because of the fact that ROS are not necessarily, and not only, deleterious but also trigger signals for important homeostatic and disease-preventing physiological processes. This includes apoptosis, which is interfered with if ROS are excessively downregulated. We are not, however, against these nutraceuticals, but against the explanation of every action based on their antioxidant background without exploring other alternatives. Mechanisms of action, indications, dosage, and other characteristics linked (or not) to their antioxidant condition must be independently studied. It is easily understood that higher animals have evolved under a permanent selective pressure in favor of those with the genetic advantage of responding to fairly high ROS levels as triggering signals. If the intensity of these warning signals is not enough, the mechanism may not get started. Hence, the oxidant/antioxidant concepts should not be mechanically extrapolated from their primary chemical meaning and introduced within the biomedical context. The antioxidant condition is not a medical indication category and it should not affect the exploration of other related or coinciding properties.

For several years, our group has been exploring the properties, basic biological functions, and pharmacological effects of CPC/PCB, regardless of whether those effects are linked or not to their antioxidant condition. Nevertheless, ROS control is essential, since permanent high levels are deleterious, in the long-term, and a good way of doing this is through a healthy lifestyle with the consumption of plenty of fruits and vegetables. The antioxidant activity of many edible plants is substantially linked to their bioflavonoids content, which can be found in high concentrations, particularly in broccoli, berries, dry seeds, pomegranate, mango, grapes, and green tea, among others. But nature has also controlled ROS throughout evolution, by adaptation and selection of organisms that are better fit to respond to ROS increases by metabolically downregulating their levels. On the other hand, oxidant molecules are not necessarily, and not always, deleterious and some may show therapeutic effects. This is the case of metformin, a longstanding antidiabetic biguanide, also originally a natural product (from *Gallega officinalis*), that has a well-known anti-hyperglycemic action and is now being studied for possible anticancer properties.[60,61]

11.7 NEUROPROTECTION/RESTORATION IS ACHIEVABLE BY NATURAL PRODUCTS

The NISD myriocin, isolated from the fungus *Isaria sinclairii*[62] and proven for MS treatment in a mouse experimental autoimmune encephalomyelitis (EAE) model, served as the pattern for FTY720 (Fingolimod, Gilenya)[63] chemical synthesis. Fingolimod was the first oral drug for MS approved by FDA in 2010 as a sphingosine structural analogue with a sphingosine 1-phosphate receptor modulator function. This suggests that it is essential to focus on well-defined natural extractive components or their synthetic analogues to reach international drug regulation standards.

The immunomodulatory properties of FTY720 come from its capacity to sequester lymphocytes in lymph nodes and hinder their trafficking towards the central nervous system (CNS), thereby preventing them from provoking MS relapses. These immunomodulatory properties were confirmed in autoimmune disease models such as lupus nephritis, adjuvant- and collagen-induced arthritis, EAM, autoimmune diabetes, and especially in the EAE model, showing higher efficacy than beta interferon. Taken orally the drug prevents the development of neurological signs in both monophasic and relapsing remitting (RR) models of MS. The therapeutic administration of FTY720 slows down and weakens the first acute episode of the already established RR EAE, and animals remain at low and stable disease scores.[64]

Within the wide range of natural products, CPC, the main biliprotein of Sp, used as a natural food dye additive, was chosen for this description. Sp has been designated as GRAS ("Generally Recognized As Safe") by the US Food and Drug Administration (FDA).[65] CPC, the main Sp phycobiliprotein, is made up of two subunits (alpha and beta) having a protein backbone to which three linear open-chain prosthetic tetrapyrrole chromophores, known as PCB, are covalently bound. The CPC protein subunits help maintain the stability, integrity, and ionic state of the active functional group PCB. CPC has potent antioxidant and anti-inflammatory activity in a variety of in vitro and in vivo systems and shows strong neuroprotective and neurorestoring properties in animal models for important human diseases.[66–69]

11.8 C-PHYCOCYANIN/PHYCOCYANOBILIN PROPERTIES, MECHANISMS AND PROSPECTS

Upon oral administration, CPC is transformed by proteolysis into PCB-bound peptides and free PCB (in charge of the pharmacological actions of CPC). In addition to its antioxidant and free radical scavenging properties, CPC displays a substantial anti-inflammatory activity by selectively inhibiting the COX-2 enzyme, also essential for prostaglandin biosynthesis.[70,71] Moreover, CPC/PCB have shown cytoprotective effects in diabetic nephropathy[72] and atherosclerosis[73,74] models, and after acute cerebral hypoperfusion experiments in a global ischemia/reperfusion (I/R) model in gerbils[75] and rats.[76] They have also been effective in a focal I/R model in retina and chronic cerebral hypoperfusion models in Wistar rats and on isolated mitochondria

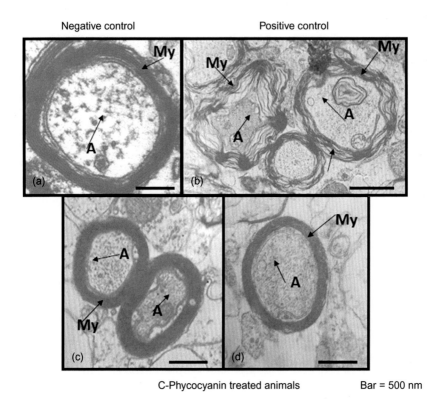

Bar = 500 nm

Figure 11.1 TEM images of myelin in the rat brain. (a) Untreated rats were used as negative control. In the brain, myelin is compact and dense without signs of axonal damage. (b) In the EAE rat brain, myelin is loose, wobbly and unfastened. Most axons show mitochondrial dilation, reflecting axon injury. (C) and (D) EAE rats were treated with C-phycocyanin by oral route. In the brain, myelin is compressed and solid, and no signs of axonal breakdown were observed. Bar = 500 nm. My: myelin; A: axon.

from brains exposed to neurotoxic agents.[77] Neuroprotective effects have been found in acute monophasic and chronic progressive EAE rat and mouse models, preventing cell death. Important immune and inflammatory modifying genes such as IFNγ, IL-6, CD74, Foxp3, TGF-β, CCL12, IL-4, IL-17A, C/EBPβ, CXCL2, ICAM-1, IL-1β, and TNFα were positively modulated by PCB.[78,79]

In the CNS, both CPC and PCB were found to prevent demyelination and/or promote remyelination and to stop or reverse axonal loss[80] in a rat EAE MS model (Fig. 11.1). Activated microglia with high NADPH oxidase and inducible nitric oxide synthase (iNOS) activities can generate cytotoxic oxidant peroxynitrites that mediate neurotoxicity and participate in the pathogenesis of neurodegenerative disorders.[81] Given through the oral route, PCB, as a potent inhibitor of NADPH oxidase, could reach the brain and influence microglial function with a modulatory impact on neuron function to prevent or delay progression in these disorders.[81] The oral route used for CPC/PCB administration, alone or combined with other active ingredients, is a competitive advantage for its application in HAD and CNS disorders such as MS and stroke.[75,79]

However, our most striking finding was that CPC/PCB induces a regulatory T cell (Treg) phenotype in peripheral blood mononuclear cells from MS patients while also expressing their known antioxidant neuroprotective and anti-inflammatory effects.[81] This makes them potential therapeutic candidates for neurodegenerative diseases such as MS[80] and for ischemic ictus.[75] Treg deficiency has been reported in HAD, including MS, indicating that specific Treg activation may be the essential concept involved in the potential therapeutic effect of CPC/PCB in MS and other HAD. Therefore proven active principles, such as IFN, could be complemented by CPC/PCB in synergic combined therapies to enhance their actions, based on immune-rebalancing mechanisms of action.

The oral administration of natural products such as CPC/PCB could influence mucosal immunity, thus reinforcing virus barriers (for example, the human papilloma virus linked to throat and cervical cancer). By linking the effects of CPC/PCB on the immune response to the interaction of endothelial cells with commensal bacteria, the microbiome may also be influenced. This is in line with the role attributed to natural products of approaching different therapeutic trends in immunopharmacology. These trends would also include personalized medicine that matches treatments with patients, and immune reeducation, that ensures tolerance to self and nondangerous antigens. The latter would reduce allergy and autoimmunity hazards.

11.9 CONCLUSIONS

Natural products have made undeniable contributions to the development of the pharma industry and research. Since the start of this century, new procedures for their computer-aided screening and chemical synthesis, as well as their analytical, biological, pharmacological, and clinical characterization, have taken place. Therefore, despite their usefulness, the conventional crude preparations of natural products have been left behind and cannot be considered end points. Instead, purified preparations are obtained; well-defined extracted components are isolated and characterized and semi- or wholly synthetic drug analogues are developed.

Immunoactive properties shown by natural products may be used in immunotherapies both as enhancers and suppressors of the immune response (immunomodulators). However, in spite of the considerable amount of experimental data accumulated from animal and cell models, they seldom reach the clinical trial phase and remain, at best, as nutraceuticals.

This demonstrates that at present natural products are not priorities for the pharma industry beyond the research interest of just a few and patent issues must still be solved to encourage research. The interest of the main companies and research centers on natural products will be mobilized only if very relevant pharmacological properties are identified and synthetic or semisynthetic analogues can be developed.

If the global effect of a product is immunosuppression, instead of the abrogation of immune functions, it will promote a whole rebalancing of the positive and negative regulatory processes and a readjustment of the immunological activities involved. This implies a reaccommodation at a lower level (downregulation) of a repaired and improved response of the entire immune system. A multifactorial approach of this general readaptive response is required to predict outcomes and to correct the problem addressed.

Many pharmacological properties have been described for Sp, CPC, and PCB. Most of them (but not all) are described for all three, meaning that most of the properties observed for Sp would depend ultimately on PCB. Although the well known antioxidant and ROS scavenging capacity of Sp active principals are essential, they cannot solely explain the large array of modified processes that include inflammation, atherosclerosis, immune modulation, cytoprotection, cancer, etc., where other basic mechanisms are therefore involved.

Our group has shown new mechanisms of action of CPC/PCB, such as the activation of Treg, which represents a new therapeutic concept for HAD, as well as the modulation by CPC of the differential expression of genes involved in mechanisms for the regulation of signal transduction, protein transport, synaptic transmission, immune processes, apoptosis, remyelination, and gliogenesis.

REFERENCES

1. Newman DJ, Cragg GM. Natural products as sources of new drugs over the 30 years from 1981 to 2010. *J Nat Prod* 2012;**75**:311−35.

2. Gransalke K. "Mother Nature's Drug Cabinet". Is Mother Nature still the number one source for promising new drugs? *Lab Times Drug Discovery* 2011;**11**:16−19.

3. Traditional medicine strategy launched. (WHO News). 2002;**80**:610.

4. Reynolds CH, Merz KM, Ringe D. *Drug design: structure and ligand-based approaches.* 1st ed. Cambridge, UK: Cambridge University Press; 2010.

5. Druker BJ, Lydon NB. Lessons learned from the development of an Abl tyrosine kinase inhibitor for chronic myelogenous leukemia. *J Clin Invest* 2000;**105**:3−7.

6. Appel S, Rupf A, Weck MM, Schoor O, Brümmendorf TH, Weinschenk T, et al. Effects of Imatinib on monocyte-derived dendritic cells are mediated by inhibition of nuclear factor-κB and Akt signaling pathways. *Clin Cancer Res* 2005;**11**:1928−40.

7. Mishra KP, Ganju L, Sairam M, Banerjee PK, Sawhney RC. A review of high throughput technology for the screening of natural products. *Biomed Pharmacother* 2008;**62**:94−8.

8. Tu Y, Yan B. High-throughput fractionation of natural products for drug discovery. *Methods Mol Biol* 2012;**918**:117−26.

9. Feher M, Schmidt JM. Property distributions: differences between drugs, natural products, and molecules from combinatorial chemistry. *J Chem Inf Comput Sci* 2003;**43**:218−27.

10. World Health Organization (WHO). *Preventing disease through healthy environments.* Geneva, Switzerland: WHO; 2006.

11. Kinney PL. Climate change, air quality, and human health. *Am J Prev Med* 2008;**35**:459−67.

12. Kantoff P. Sipuleucel-T immunotherapy for castration-resistant prostate cancer. *New Engl J Med* 2010;**363**:411−22.

13. Ramirez-Ortiz ZG, Specht CA, Wang JP, Lee CK, Bartholomeu DC, Gazzinelli RT, et al. Toll-like receptor 9-dependent immune activation by unmethylated CpG motifs in *Aspergillus fumigatus* DNA. *Infect Immun* 2008;**76**:2123−9.

14. Di Lorenzo G, Buonerba C, Kantoff PW. Immunotherapy for the treatment of prostate cancer. *Nat Rev Clin Oncol* 2011;**8**:551−61.

15. Yoneyama S, Kawai K, Tsuno NH, Okaji Y, Asakage M, Tsuchiya T, et al. Epigallocatechin gallate affects human dendritic cell differentiation and maturation. *J Allergy Clin Immunol* 2008;**121**:209−14.

16. Baek SH, Bae ON, Park JH. Recent methodology in ginseng analysis. *J Ginseng Res* 2012;**36**:119−34.

17. Wilasrusmee C, Kittur S, Shah G, Siddiqui J, Bruch D, Wilasrusmee S, et al. Immunostimulatory effect of *Silybum marianum* (milk thistle) extract. *Med Sci Monit* 2002;**8**: BR439−43.

18. Jurenka JS. Anti-inflammatory properties of curcumin, a major constituent of *Curcuma longa*: a review of preclinical and clinical research. *Altern Med Rev* 2009;**14**:141−53.

19. Lugrin J, Rosenblatt-Velin N, Parapanov R, Liaudet L. The role of oxidative stress during inflammatory processes. *Biol Chem* 2014;**395**:203−30.

20. Muñoz A, Costa M. Nutritionally mediated oxidative stress and inflammation. *Oxid Med Cell Longev* 2013;**2013**:610950.

21. Tennen RI, Michishita-Kioi E, Chua KF. Finding a target for resveratrol. *Cell* 2012;**148**:387−9.

22. Park S-J, Ahmad F, Philp A, Baar K, Williams T, Luo H, et al. Resveratrol ameliorates aging-related metabolic phenotypes by inhibiting cAMP phosphodiesterases. *Cell* 2012;**148**:421−33.

23. Milenković M, Arsenović-Ranin N, Stojić-Vukanić Z, Bufan B, Vučićević D, Jančić I. Quercetin ameliorates experimental autoimmune myocarditis in rats. *J Pharm Pharm Sci* 2010;**13**:311−19.

24. Schepetkin IA, Quinn MT. Botanical polysaccharides: macrophage immunomodulation and therapeutic potential. *Int Immunopharmacol* 2006;**6**:317−33.

25. Hodge G, Hodge S, Han P. *Allium sativum* (garlic) suppresses leukocyte inflammatory cytokine production in vitro: potential therapeutic use in the treatment of inflammatory bowel disease. *Cytometry* 2002;**48**:209−15.

26. Li Z, Geng Y-N, Jiang J-D, Kong W-J. Antioxidant and anti-inflammatory activities of berberine in the treatment of diabetes mellitus. *Evidence-Based Compl Altern Med* 2014;**2014**:289264.

27. Gray SP, Di Marco E, Okabe J, Szyndralewiez C, Heitz F, Montezano AC, et al. NADPH oxidase 1 plays a key role in diabetes mellitus-accelerated atherosclerosis. *Circulation* 2013;**127**:1888−902.

28. Gratas-Delamarche A, Derbré F, Vincent S, Cillard J. Physical inactivity, insulin resistance, and the oxidative-inflammatory loop. *Free Radical Res* 2014;**48**:93−108.

29. Haddad JJ, Saade NE, Safieh-Garabedian B. Cytokines and neuro-immune-endocrine interactions: a role for the hypothalamic-pituitary-adrenal revolving axis. *J Neuroimmunol* 2002;**133**:1−19.

30. Procaccini C, Pucino V, De Rosa V, Marone G, Matarese G. Neuro-endocrine networks controlling immune system in health and disease. *Front Immunol* 2014;**5**:143.

31. Järvinen R, Kaasinen E, Sankila A, Rintala E. Long-term efficacy of maintenance bacillus Calmette-Guérin versus maintenance mitomycin C instillation therapy in frequently recurrent TaT1 tumours without carcinoma in situ: a subgroup analysis of the prospective, randomised Finn Bladder I study with a 20-year follow-up. *Eur Urol* 2009;**56**:260−5.

32. Pandey R, Sharma S, Khuller GK. Liposome-based antitubercular drug therapy in a guinea pig model of tuberculosis. *Int J Antimicrob Agents* 2004;**23**:414−15.

33. Brown GD, Herre J, Williams DL, Williams JA, Marshall, Gordon S. Dectin-1 mediates the biologic effects of β-glucan. *J Exp Med* 2003;**197**:1119−24.

34. Kawaguchi K, Matsumoto T, Kumazawa Y. Effects of antioxidant polyphenols on TNF-α-related diseases. *Curr Top Med Chem* 2011;**11**:1767−79.

35. Hsu SD, Dickinson DP, Qin H, Borke J, Ogbureke KU, Winger JN, et al. Green tea polyphenols reduce autoimmune symptoms in a murine model for human Sjögren's syndrome and protect human salivary acinar cells from TNF-α-induced cytotoxicity. *Autoimmunity* 2007;**40**:138−47.

36. Ho JH, Hong CY. Salvianolic acids: small compounds with multiple mechanisms for cardiovascular protection. *J Biomed Sci* 2011;**18**:30.

37. Wang X, Wang Y, Jiang M, Zhu Y, Hu L, Fan G, et al. Differential cardioprotective effects of salvianolic acid and tanshinone on acute myocardial infarction are mediated by unique signaling pathways. *J Ethnopharmacol* 2011;**135**:662−71.

38. Peng GL, Zhang XY. Effects of *Salvia miltiorrhiza* on serum levels of inflammatory cytokines in patients with severe acute pancreatitis. *J Chinese Integr Med* 2007;**5**:28−31.

39. Qin XY, Li T, Yan L, Liu QS, Tian Y. Tanshinone IIA protects against immune-mediated liver injury through activation of t-cell subsets and regulation of cytokines. *Immunopharmacol Immunotoxicol* 2010;**32**:51−5.

40. Krasovsky J, Chang DH, Deng G, Yeung S, Lee M, Leung PC, et al. Inhibition of human dendritic cell activation by hydroethanolic but not lipophilic extracts of turmeric (*Curcuma longa*). *Planta Med* 2009;**75**:312−15.

41. Xie L, Li XK, Funeshima-Fuji N, Kimura H, Matsumoto Y, Isaka Y, et al. Amelioration of experimental autoimmune encephalomyelitis by curcumin treatment through inhibition of IL-17 production. *Int Immunopharmacol* 2009;**9**:575−81.

42. Decoté-Ricardo D, Chagas KK, Rocha JD, Redner P, Lopes UG, Cambier JC, et al. Modulation of in vitro murine B-lymphocyte response by curcumin. *Phytomedicine* 2009;**16**:982−8.

43. Wang Y, Mei Y, Feng D, Xu L. Triptolide modulates T-cell inflammatory responses and ameliorates experimental autoimmune encephalomyelitis. *J Neurosci Res* 2008;**86**: 2441−9.

44. Wong KF, Chan JK, Chan KL, Tam P, Yang D, Fan ST, et al. Immunochemical characterization of the functional constituents of *Tripterygium wilfordii* contributing to its anti-inflammatory property. *Clin Exp Pharmacol Physiol* 2008;**35**(1):55−9.

45. Xu W, Lin Z, Yang C, Zhang Y, Wang G, Xu X, et al. Immunosuppressive effects of demethylzeylasteral in a rat kidney transplantation model. *Int Immunopharmacol* 2009;**9**:996−1001.

46. Ni YF, Kuai JK, Lu ZF, Yang GD, Fu HY, Wang J, et al. Glycyrrhizin treatment is associated with attenuation of lipopolysaccharide-induced acute lung injury by inhibiting cyclooxygenase-2 and inducible nitric oxide synthase expression. *J Surg Res* 2011;**165**:29−35.

47. Xie YC, Dong XW, Wu XM, Yan XF, Xie QM. Inhibitory effects of flavonoids extracted from licorice on lipopolysaccharide-induced acute pulmonary inflammation in mice. *Int Immunopharmacol* 2009;**9**:194−200.

48. Cassano N, Mantegazza R, Battaglini S, Apruzzi D, Loconsole F, Vena GA. Adjuvant role of a new emollient cream in patients with palmar and/or plantar psoriasis: a pilot randomized open-label study. *G Ital Dermatol Venereol* 2010;**145**:789−92.

49. Gumpricht E, Dahl R, Devereaux MW, Sokol RJ. Licorice compounds glycyrrhizin and 18β-glycyrrhetinic acid are potent modulators of bile acid-induced cytotoxicity in rat hepatocytes. *J Biol Chem* 2005;**280**:10556−63.

50. Li J, Tu Y, Tong L, Zhang W, Zheng J, Wei Q. Immunosuppressive activity on the murine immune responses of glycyrol from *Glycyrrhiza uralensis* via inhibition of calcineurin activity. *Pharm Biol* 2010;**48**:1177−84.

51. Ren Y, Lu L, Guo TB, Qiu J, Yang Y, Liu A, et al. Novel immunomodulatory properties of berbamine through selective down-regulation of STAT4 and action of IFN-γ in experimental autoimmune encephalomyelitis. *J Immunol* 2008;**181**:1491−8.

52. Adachi K, Kohara T, Nakao N, Arita M, Chiba K, Mishina T, et al. Design, synthesis, and structure−activity relationships of 2-substituted-2-amino-1,3-propanediols: discovery of a novel immunosuppressant, FTY720. *Bioorg Med Chem Lett* 1995;**5**:853−6.

53. Svarstad H, Bugge HC, Dhillion SS. From Norway to Novartis: cyclosporin from *Tolypocladium inflatum* in an open access bioprospecting regime. *Biodiversity Conservation* 2000;**9**:1521−41.

54. Harrison DE, Strong R, Sharp ZD, Nelson J, Astle CM, Flurkey K, et al. Rapamycin fed late in life extends lifespan in genetically heterogeneous mice. *Nature* 2009;**460**:392−5.

55. Abou-Jaoude MM, Naim R, Shaheen J, Naufal N, Abboud S, AlHabash M, et al. Tacrolimus (FK506) vs cyclosporin micro-emulsion (Neoral) as maintenance immunosuppression therapy in kidney transplant recipients. *Transplantation Proc* 2005;**37**:3025−8. Available from: http://dx.doi.org/10.1016/j.transproceed.2005.08.040.

56. McCarty MF, Barroso-Aranda J, Contreras F. Oral phycocyanobilin may diminish the pathogenicity of activated brain microglia in neurodegenerative disorders. *Med Hypotheses* 2010;**74**:601–5.

57 Karnati RR, Kalle MA, Nishant PR, Bhavanasi D, Gorla VR, Pallu R. Alteration of mitochondrial membrane potential by *Spirulina platensis* C-phycocyanin induces apoptosis in the doxorubicin resistant human hepatocellular-carcinoma cell line HepG2. *Biotechnol Appl Biochem* 2007;**47**:159–67.

58. Riss J, Décordé K, Sutra T, Delage M, Baccou JC, Jouy N, et al. Phycobiliprotein C-phycocyanin from *Spirulina platensis* is powerfully responsible for reducing oxidative stress and NADPH oxidase expression induced by an atherogenic diet in hamsters. *J Agric Food Chem* 2007;**55**:7962–7.

59. Castellheim A, Brekke O-L, Espevik T, Harboe M, Mollnes TE. Innate immune responses to danger signals in systemic inflammatory response syndrome and sepsis. *Scand J Immunol* 2009;**69**:479–91.

60. Kasznicki J, Sliwinska A, Drzewoski J. Metformin in cancer prevention and therapy. *Ann Transl Med* 2014;**2**:57.

61. Evans J, Donnelly MM, Emslie-Smith AM, Alessi DR, Morris AD. Metformin and reduced risk of cancer in diabetic patients. *BMJ* 2005;**330**:1304–5.

62. Fujita T, Inoue K, Yamamoto S, Ikumoto T, Sasaki S, Toyama R, et al. Fungal metabolites. Part 11. A potent immunosuppressive activity found in *Isaria sinclairii* metabolite. *J Antibiot* 1994;**47**:208–15.

63. Kataoka H, Sugahara K, Shimano K, Teshima K, Koyama M, Fukunari A, et al. FTY720, sphingosine 1-phosphate receptor modulator, ameliorates experimental autoimmune encephalomyelitis by inhibition of T cell infiltration. *Cell Mol Immunol* 2005;**2**:439–48.

64. Foster CA, Howard LM, Schweitzer A, Persohn E, Hiestand PC, Balatoni B, et al. Brain penetration of the oral immunomodulatory drug FTY720 and its phosphorylation in the CNS during experimental autoimmune encephalomyelitis: consequences for mode of action in multiple sclerosis. *J Pharmacol Exp Ther* 2007;**323**:469–75.

65. Eriksen NT. Production of phycocyanin – a pigment with applications in biology, biotechnology, foods and medicine. *Appl Microbiol Biotechnol* 2008;**80**:1–14.

66. Remirez D, Ledón N, González R. Role of histamine in the inhibitory effects of phycocyanin in experimental models of allergic inflammatory response. *Mediators Inflamm* 2002;**11**:81–5.

67. Romay C, Armesto J, Remirez D, González R, Ledon N, García I. Antioxidant and anti-inflammatory properties of C-phycocyanin from blue-green algae. *Inflamm Res* 1998;**47**:36–41.

68. Hwang JH, Chen JC, Chan YC. Effects of C-phycocyanin and *Spirulina* on salicylate-induced tinnitus, expression of NMDA receptor and inflammatory genes. *PLoS One* 2013;**8**: e58215.

69. Leung PO, Lee HH, Kung YC, Tsai MF, Chou TC. Therapeutic effect of C-phycocyanin extracted from blue green algae in a rat model of acute lung injury induced by lipopolysaccharide. *Evid Based Complement Alternat Med* 2013;**2013**:916590.

70. Reddy MC, Subhashini J, Mahipal SV, Bhat VB, Srinivas Reddy P, Kiranmai G, et al. C-Phycocyanin a selective cyclooxygenase-2 inhibitor, induces apoptosis in lipopolysaccharide-stimulated RAW 264.7 macrophages. *Biochem Biophys Res Commun* 2003;**304**:385–92.

71. Reddy CM, Bhat VB, Kiranmai G, Reddy MN, Reddanna P, Madyastha KM. Selective inhibition of cyclooxygenase-2 by C-phycocyanin, a biliprotein from *Spirulina platensis*. *Biochem Biophys Res Commun* 2000;**277**:599–603.

72. Zheng J, Inoguchi T, Sasaki S, Maeda Y, McCarty MF, Fujii M, et al. Phycocyanin and phycocyanobilin from *Spirulina platensis* protect against diabetic nephropathy by inhibiting oxidative stress. *Am J Physiol Regul Integr Comp Physiol* 2013;**304**:R110–20.

73. Li B, Chu XM, Xu YJ, Yang F, Lv CY, Nie SM. CD59 underlines the antiatherosclerotic effects of C-phycocyanin on mice. *Biomed Res Int* 2013;**2013**:729413.

74. Cheong SH, Kim MY, Sok DE, Hwang SY, Kim JH, Kim HR, et al. *Spirulina* prevents atherosclerosis by reducing hypercholesterolemia in rabbits fed a high-cholesterol diet. *J Nutr Sci Vitaminol* 2010;**56**:34–40.

75. Penton-Rol G, Marín-Prida J, Pardo-Andreu G, Martínez-Sánchez G, Acosta-Medina EF, Valdivia-Acosta A, et al. C-Phycocyanin is neuroprotective against global cerebral ischemia/reperfusion injury in gerbils. *Brain Res Bull* 2011;**86**:42–52.

76. Thaakur S, Sravanthi R. Neuroprotective effect of *Spirulina* in cerebral ischemia-reperfusion injury in rats. *J Neural Transm* 2010;**117**(9):1083–91.

77. Marín-Prida J, Penton-Rol G, Rodrigues FP, Alberici LC, Stringhetta K, Leopoldino AM, et al. C-Phycocyanin protects SH-SY5Y cells from oxidative injury, rat retina from transient ischemia and rat brain mitochondria from Ca2 + /phosphate-induced impairment. *Brain Res Bull* 2012;**89**:159–67.

78. Marín-Prida J, Pavón N, Llópiz A, Fernández J, Delgado L, Mendoza Y, et al. Phycocyanobilin promotes PC12 cell survival and modulates immune and inflammatory genes and oxidative stress markers in acute cerebral hypoperfusion in rats. *Toxicol Appl Pharmacol* 2013;**272**:49–60.

79. Boraschi D, Penton-Rol G. Perspectives in immunopharmacology: the future of immunosuppression. *Immunol Lett* 2014;**161**:211–15.

80. Penton-Rol G, Martínez-Sánchez G, Cervantes-Llanos M, Lagumersindez-Denis N, Acosta-Medina EF, Falcón-Cama V, et al. C-Phycocyanin ameliorates experimental autoimmune encephalomyelitis and induces regulatory T cells. *Int Immunopharmacol* 2011;**11**:29–38.

81. McCarty MF. Clinical potential of *Spirulina* as a source of phycocyanobilin. *J Med Food* 2007;**10**:566–70.

CHAPTER *12*

Nanomedicine

Albert Duschl
Department of Molecular Biology, University of Salzburg, Salzburg, Austria

12.1 WHY NANOMATERIALS?

Nanomedicine is a "hot" field. Up to 2004, only 72 scientific articles on "nanomedicine" had been published according to Medline, but during 2005–2015 that number soared to 10.502 (data retrieved July 30, 2015 from www.pubmed.gov). It can be argued, however, that nanoparticles (NPs) have an old history in medicine. Nanosilver used against bacterial infections is a well-known example, but nanosized agents have also been applied for many years to modulate immune responses. Colloidal gold used to treat rheumatoid arthritis[1] and alum used as adjuvant for various vaccines[2] have contained nanomaterials long before that term became familiar, or before the presence of nanosized components has been considered to be relevant. It is thus not quite true that there is no experience on effects of artificial nanomaterials on the human body. Many practical uses of NPs go back a long time, but medical applications are of special relevance, since here the agents are applied to health-compromised persons, they are applied intentionally, often locally, and usually in doses that would never be reached, for example, during unintentional work place exposure.

The use of NPs for modulating immunity seems to be an obvious perspective. Engineered NPs are nonself and they overlap in size with viruses (mostly 10–200 nm size range[3]), so they fall well within the target size range to which immunity is capable to respond, and since at least some types of NPs are toxic, they can be expected to result in danger signals as well (Fig. 12.1).

In addition, some nanomaterials exhibit repetitive patterns originating from the process of synthesis, so even recognition by pattern recognition receptors may be envisioned. The present overview will highlight features

Immune Rebalancing. DOI: http://dx.doi.org/10.1016/B978-0-12-803302-9.00012-9

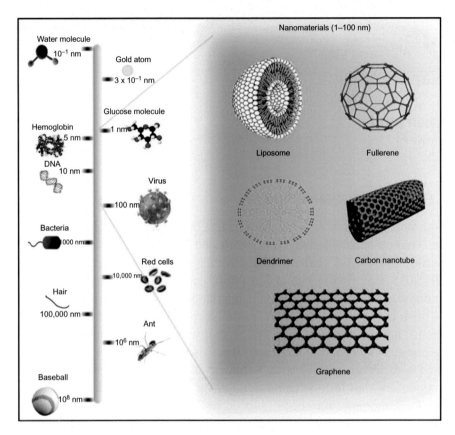

Figure 12.1 Nanoscale sizes compared to other relevant objects. Nanomaterials are in the size range of biological molecules and entities. The biological and the physical world interact on the same scale, which is the basis for many nanospecific effects that can be exploited for medical purposes. Source: Figure reprinted with permission from[130].

of nanomedical agents without restricting itself to the ISO standard, which defines nanoparticles as objects that have in all three dimensions sizes between 1–100 nm (*ISO/TS 27687:2008 Nanotechnologies – Terminology and definitions for nano objects – nanoparticle, nanofibre and nanoplate*). Objects with sizes up to several hundred nm have been described and used as "nanomedical" agents, so in the present review, all materials that have been described as such will be considered as nanomedical agents. Strictly defined, nanopharmaceuticals should not only be in the nanosize range, but should also exploit the particular properties of the nanoscale for the therapeutic effect, so the nanoscale should add functionalities that cannot be obtained by using either the compound chemicals or bulk materials.[4]

Considering investigational and approved nanomedical products, the most prominent area of current use is in the treatment of cancers, where drug targeting is a major issue, but several approved drugs are also aiming at immunity.[5-7] A general overview of interactions between nanomaterials and the immune system has been provided by several recent books.[8-10] Here we will focus on medical applications that aim at modifying immune responses in a preventive or a therapeutic setting. In the context of nanosafety research, some types of NPs have been shown to stimulate the immune system, while others were reported to repress immunity. Confusingly, both claims have been made sometimes for very similar materials, reflecting the by now well recognized problem that many nanotoxicology studies have not provided enough data to rule out problems like contamination with endotoxin or with synthesis chemicals, insufficiently well described materials, particle aging effects, assay interference by particles, or batch-to-batch variation between nominally identical particle preparations.[11] Quality issues in nanosafety testing have recently been extensively described by H. Krug.[12]

12.2 PRODUCTS ON THE MARKET OR IN DEVELOPMENT

As recently reviewed by Weissig et al.,[6] there are currently 43 approved drugs that are publicized as nanopharmaceuticals, excluding components of medical devices, which constitute the majority of nanomedical products on the market.[5] Whether all these formulations really have unique properties due to nanotechnological input is critically discussed by the authors, but if the manufacturers' claims to provide nanomedical therapeutics are taken at face value, 17 of these drugs are used in cancer treatment, with some other drugs aiming to support cancer therapy, for example to suppress emesis associated with chemotherapy. Overall, a wide spectrum of conditions is addressed by approved nanodrugs. Specifically aiming at the immune system are several vaccines, one immunosuppressant, and two drugs for autoimmune conditions, all of which will be discussed below. The numbers, however, make clear that many exciting concepts are still in the pipeline[7] and even more have not yet left the laboratory. It is thus important to take into account concepts that are presently being investigated and to be realistic about the possibilities that nanopharmaceuticals offer for clinical use right now and in the near future. Many different materials are in use, both inorganic and organic (Fig. 12.2).

(a)

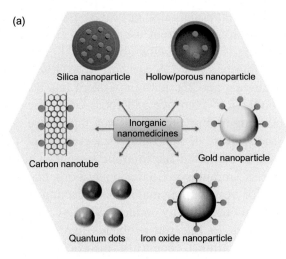

● Chemotherapeutic or diagnosis probe

(b)

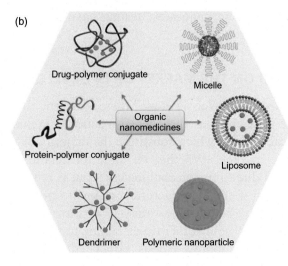

● Chemotherapeutic or diagnosis probe

Figure 12.2 Types of nanoparticles used in medicine. Numerous types of nanoparticles (a: Inorganic, b: Organic) have been used in biomedical experiments and several of them are in clinical use. For the concept of drug delivery, highlighted here, it is interesting to see that that payload can be both on the outside or the inside of the particle. Alternatively, the entire particle may be made up of the payload compound. Source: Figures reprinted with permission from[131].

12.3 SUPPRESSING IMMUNITY: AUTOIMMUNITY AND OTHER CASES

Currently there are two nanopharmaceuticals on the market which target autoimmune diseases. Cimzia® (Certolizumab pegol) is approved in the US (but not in the EU) for the treatment of Crohn's disease and in both the US and the EU for rheumatoid arthritis.[13,14] The agent is a pegylated Fab fragment of a therapeutic antibody against TNFα. In terms of size, Cimzia® is a nanomaterial, but so are essentially all protein drugs. An even more problematic case in terms of being described as a nanopharmaceutical is Copaxone® (Glatiramer acetate), which is a random polymer composed of four amino acids (alanine, glutamic acid, lysine, and tyrosine) which is suggested to resemble sequences in myelin basic protein and is approved for treatment of multiple sclerosis in the US, Europe, and other countries.[15,16] It can be questioned whether these drugs derive an additional property or functionalization from nanoengineering, which in the first case is just pegylation and in the second is not clear at all. These agents were derived based on conventional immunological and pharmaceutical work, so the term "nano" attached to them is at least not a particularly informative label.[6]

Rapamune® is an immunosuppressant that is mainly used to prevent organ rejection following kidney transplants. Its active ingredient is the well-known drug sirolimus (rapamycin, SRL), which is here included in the form of nanocrystals consisting of the pure drug.[17] The nanocrystal form offers a genuine advantage of the nanosize range, addressing the problem of poor solubility of the drug in free form. Normally, the saturation solubility is considered to be a constant that depends on the compound, but for particles below $1-2\,\mu m$ size it becomes also a function of the particle size that increases with decreasing particle size.[18] NPs thus provide higher saturation solubility, which makes more drug molecules available and thus also increases the concentration gradient between gut lumen and blood, increasing the absorption by passive diffusion.[18] Rapamune® is thus a drug that genuinely obtains advantages from being formulated as a nanopharmaceutical. The same principle is used for poorly soluble drugs prescribed for other conditions, including fenofibrate to lower cholesterol levels (Tricor®, Lipanthyl®, Lipidil®) and aprepitant (Emend®) to reduce postoperative nausea and vomiting related to cancer chemotherapy.[6,18,19]

Nanoparticles have been extensively studied with a view towards possible immunotoxicity.[20−23] Several of the principles observed in studying that issue have the potential for clinical use, including stimulation of pattern recognition receptors (for vaccines), modulation of type 1 versus type 2 adaptive immune response (for autoimmunity and allergy) and the release of toxins that may be NP compounds (eg, metal ions), or are "piggybacking" on the NPs, that act as carriers. Suppressing immunity should thus be easy: Cytotoxic NPs may be directed more or less specifically towards immune cells, and functionalized NPs may bind immune mediators like complement factors or antibodies. In principle, such effects could be beneficial in situations where immune reactivity should be reduced or abolished, but lack of selectivity may create problems for clinical use. Nevertheless, it has to be considered that solid tumors show enhanced permeability and retention of NPs due to disruptions of vascular architecture and lymphatic draining.[24] The resulting "EPR effect" (enhanced permeability and retention) applies also to inflamed sites, where the microarchitecture is also compromised.

Nanosized liposomes were applied in many studies, for example to treat neuroinflammation in rabbits,[25] lung injury induced inflammation in pigs,[26] arthritis in rats,[27] and malaria-related inflammation in mice.[28] Several liposome preparations are already in clinical use and liposomes are considered to be especially promising carriers for numerous delivery systems.[29−32] They can be readily produced from biological compounds and have usually good biocompatibility. It has long been known that administered liposomes are rapidly taken up by monocytes and macrophages,[33,34] a fate which can sometimes limit their utility as drugs. However, if mononuclear phagocytic cells are the intended target, liposome properties are naturally advantageous for modulating immunity.[35,36]

Single-walled carbon nanotubes (SWCNT) have been shown to suppress dendritic cell functions[37] and multiwalled carbon nanotubes (MWCNT) suppressed T cell proliferation and function,[38] both in mouse models. The possibility to affect immune cells directly adds an additional impetus to work towards nanotherapeutics, but of course loading them with conventional or NP-specific drugs is readily possible and different versions of nanotubes have been investigated as drug targeting and delivery vehicles.[39−41] Carbon sheets (graphene) are considered to have tremendous potential for many novel applications, but in the form of nanotubes they also have raised serious concerns. Some variants, in particular long MWCNT, resemble asbestos fibers (being long and stiff). Animal studies have shown carcinogenic effects and in consequence, this type of nanomaterial is now categorized as a possible human carcinogen.[42,43] However, it has been suggested that chemical modifications and limited length overcome these problems.[44] In this context—and possibly of special interest to immunologists—is the surprising finding that carbon nanotubes can be degraded by myelo-peroxidase in neutrophils[45] and by peroxidase in eosinophils.[46] The mononuclear phagocytic cells where these agents are most likely to accumulate seem to lack an effective clearance mechanism, but it will be interesting to see whether degradation of CNT by specific cell types can be used for therapeutic purposes.

Immigration of NPs into inflamed sites can also be used to visualize these sites. For example, in mouse models, avidin-nucleic acid nanoassembly (ANANAS) particles were shown to reach inflamed but not healthy bowel tissue, allowing imaging via fluorescent markers[47] and superparamagnetic iron oxide NPs (SPIONS) were used to detect in an arthritis model joint inflammation by Magnetic Resonance Imaging.[48] Importantly, these agents have like many others been shown not to induce adverse reactions. The concept of a "theranostic" is here close to reality, since, for example, a gold NP loaded with a drug still remains a gold NP, which implies that it can be readily visualized by numerous techniques and can be used for photothermal therapy.[1,49] Immunosuppression is based on already existing drugs (that make for nanopharmacuticals ...) rests on core concepts that make for nanopharmaceuticals use of the nanoscale. Fundamental processes are illustrated in Fig. 12.3. Note that the same chains of events could also lead to immune activation or modulation.

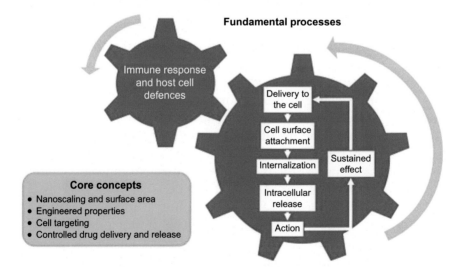

Figure 12.3 Core concepts of nanomedical intervention in immunity. Delivery of a particle to a cell depends on mechanisms of recognition, uptake and processing. Manipulation of cellular functions can result in immune modulation. How sustained this process is will be largely determined by particle properties. Depending on the purpose, different stabilities in the biological system will be desired. Both excretion and dissolution of particles can limit their lifetime in the body. Source: Figure reprinted with permission from[132].

12.4 ACTIVATING IMMUNITY: THE FUTURE OF VACCINES?

It has been mentioned that the size ranges of NPs and viruses overlap. Additional virus-like properties can be present, including repetitive surface patterns, lipid membrane components, and human derived antigens. The most straightforward approach to use these characteristics is to take a virus as a model for NP construction: The results are virus-like particles (VLP).

VLP are, in the chemistry-dominated world of nanotechnology, an example of biotechnology making use of the nanoscale. They correspond to empty viruses with intact protein hull and if desired also membrane envelopes, but they lack genetic material which makes them safe for use in humans. Production is usually by expression of viral proteins in mammalian cells, but avian, insect, plant, yeast, and bacterial cells have also been successfully employed to form VLPs.[50] Alternatively, fully synthetic VLPs have also been produced and the choice of system will depend on the context.[51] Even smaller units made of virus proteins or fragments derived from them have been described as subviral particles.[52] Out of this family of agents, five products are in clinical use for vaccination: Gardasil® and Cervavix® against human papillomavirus,[53,54] Recombivax HB® and Engerix-B against hepatitis B virus[55–57] and, most recently, Hecolin® against hepatitis E virus.[58]

In addition to the already used VLP, other NPs can act as powerful adjuvants and are among the "next generation" compounds that are now developed for vaccination, including emulsions, liposomes alginates, chitosan, and polylactide-coglycolide (PLGA) NPs.[59,60] An attractive feature of nanocarriers is that they can be used as nearly universal platforms that carry not only antigen, but also additional immune modifiers. The addition of ligands for Toll-like receptors (TLRs) is a powerful immune stimulus. Examples of NP/TLR ligand preparations that were used to induce immune responses are ligands for TLR2 (Pam(3)Cys),[61] TLR9 (Poly I: C),[62,63] TLR4 (3-O-desacyl-4′-monophosphoryl lipid A (MPL)),[64] TLR7 (9-benzyl-8-hydroxyadenine),[65] TLR7/8 (resiquimod, R848),[66] and TLR9 (CpG DNA).[66] Considering that other families of pattern recognition receptors, like the NOD-like receptors (NLRs), are also investigated as adjuvants,[67] it can be expected that even more biologicals and their synthetic analogues will be included in particle-based vaccines in the future.

As far as particles go, aluminum hydroxide (Alum) preparations are the paradigmatic adjuvant, used for decades both in animals and humans. It has indeed been reported that the particle nature is an important aspect, leading to direct activation of the NLRP3 inflammasome[68] and characteristics of Alum NPs, like shape and crystallinity, can be used to design adjuvant particles that specifically engage the NLRP3 inflammasome.[69] Activation of NLRP3 has also been reported for other NPs, including SiO_2 and TiO_2 particles.[70] This has been discussed as a safety hazard related to unintentional exposure to NPs; however, the doses needed to stimulate vigorous immune responses are generally quite high. For vaccination, however, high doses are both possible and intended. The highest dose of NP exposure that we can normally encounter would be due to an injection in a diagnostic or therapeutic context. For vaccination, the ability of NPs to stimulate a vigorous immune activation is one of their most interesting features. Nanoparticle features that enable them to be effective vaccines are illustrated in Fig. 12.4.

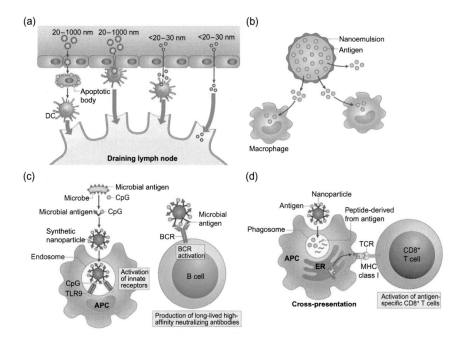

Figure 12.4 Mechanisms involved in immune modulation by nanoparticles. Vigorous immune responses can be stimulated via many different routes. Nanoparticles are able to mimic a wide range of activities known from already existing adjuvants or immune stimulating agents. (a) Delivery of antigens. (b) Depot effect. (c) Repetitive antigen display. (d) Cross-presentation. Source: Figure reprinted with permission from[133].

12.5 CANCER AS AN IMMUNOLOGICAL DISEASE

Cancer is the leading application for approved nanopharmaceuticals. Most products are designed as carriers for drugs,[71,72] but often more special functionalities are in focus, like crossing the blood–brain barrier,[73] enabling visualization techniques,[74,75] or treatments by hyperthermia.[76,77] Tumors, however, strongly interact with the immune system, in ways that are beneficial or detrimental for the patient. While cytotoxic T-cells and natural killer cells destroy tumor cells recognized as compromised self (corresponding to nonself), a lack of danger signals and other costimuli can also induce tolerance and promote tumor survival and growth via wound healing mechanisms.[78–80] Modulating immunity is thus a promising avenue for novel cancer treatments. Both inhibition and activation of certain immune functions can be intended.

Antitumor responses can be promoted by inhibition of immune cells that maintain tumor tolerance, including T_{reg} cells, tumor-associated macrophages and myeloid-derived suppressor cells, a group of cells for which STAT3 was identified as a suitable drug target.[81,82] In vitro studies with PLGA NPs loaded with siRNA showed efficient silencing of STAT3 expression.[83] The advantage of using NPs as a carrier was in this case improved uptake by tumor-tolerized dendritic cells (DCs) and reduced toxicity. Knockdown of STAT3 enabled the DCs to revert to an antitumor mode as shown by TNFα secretion and T-cell priming. In vivo effects of this agent have not yet been reported. Another group has combined siRNA for STAT3 knockdown in PLGA NPs with the chemotherapeutic drug paclitaxel, achieving higher sensitivity of tumor cells compared to free paclitaxel.[84] RNA is a very attractive payload for NPs in tumor therapy, since nonself RNA can stimulate immune reactions by binding to TLRs and siRNA can specifically downregulate gene expression via DNA interference. Improved biodistribution and pharmacokinetics can be achieved by coupling RNA to NPs, but possibly the most essential advantage of using RNA coupled to NPs is a substantially reduced toxicity compared to the free agent, since systemic TLR activation would clearly be detrimental.[85]

As already mentioned, more than one function may be included in NPs design. To mention just one example, in one study gold NPs were loaded with β-cyclodextrin that served to improve water solubility of the anticancer drug, paclitaxel. Biotin was added to target biotin receptors which are overexpressed on the surface of some cancer cells and polyethylene glycol was conjugated to enhance solubility. Rhodamine B was linked for visualization and finally, the gold itself provides options for detection or hyperthermia treatment. The whole NP-based assembly—with 5 functionalizations—was effective for killing cancer cells in vitro.[86] While candidate drugs like this one may appear at first glance to be a bit "over-designed," there is no actual reason why NPs could not carry even more functions. In the context of immune modulation one would like to suggest adding drugs aiming at immunity to the collection. The huge surface area of NPs allows envisioning highly functionalized entities and it may also find a unique role in personalizing medicine.

An alternative to shutting down tumor-protecting immune cells is to activate immunity against the tumor, a strategy that is pursued in the development of cancer vaccines.[87] One strategy is to induce antitumor responses via general immunostimulating signals. This approach is supported by the already mentioned disruptions in tissue microenvironment of tumor sites, which can enable preferential immigration of NPs, and can prolong retention due to disturbed vascularization via the enhanced vascularization and retention effect. An interesting concept is to use gelatin NPs of 100 nm size that accumulate well around the leaky regions of tumor vasculature, but then shrink to 10 nm, which more readily diffuse through the tumor's interstitial space.[88] Another study used direct intratumor injection of nanosized liposomes in a mouse model.[89] The active agents in this case were agonistic antibodies against the costimulatory receptor CD40, which is expressed on the surface of antigen-presenting cells, and CpG-DNA, a ligand for the pro-inflammatory receptor TLR9. Both agents have displayed potent antitumor responses before, but the liposome carriers limited systemic toxicity and led to an accumulation of the drugs in the local tumor tissue and in tumor-draining lymph nodes.[89]

Cancer specific antigens offer the possibility to target specifically tumor cells by harnessing mechanisms of adaptive immunity.[87] NPs are useful for targeting since they accumulate in the lymphatic system in a size dependent manner. A size range of 20−40 nm has been found to be optimal for delivery to DCs in the lymph nodes using poly(ethylene glycol)-stabilized poly(propylene sulfide) NPs,[90] virus-like particles[91] and carboxylated polystyrene micro- and nanospheres.[92] The preferential delivery to DCs and the subsequent vaccine responses are thus independent of the material used and represent a true nanoeffect. Other advantageous properties of NPs that have been reported in studies on cancer vaccine development include simultaneous delivery of antigens and adjuvants to antigen presenting cells,[93] enhanced cross-presentation of antigens,[94,95] and the ability to act as a local antigen depot.[95,96]

12.6 ALLERGY

Another area where NPs have been explored for vaccination is allergy. The only causal therapies (not symptomatic ones) involve immunotherapy with repeated doses of the specific allergen, either as subcutaneous immunotherapy (SCIT), sublingual immunotherapy (SLIT) or—so far experimentally—as oral food allergen immunotherapy (OIT).[97,98] Problems with these therapeutic approaches include the possibility of adverse reactions including anaphylactic shock, long duration of the treatment, and uncertain success. These factors induce many patients to terminate a course of therapy prematurely or decline to enter it at all.

It has been shown that NPs as such can modify ongoing or experimentally induced allergic reactivity, but the data on this topic are confusing, with both reduced and enhanced responses reported. Since different models, different allergens, and different NPs were used it is so far difficult to predict whether a novel NP type would react in one or the other way. One of the major effects that are utilized in experimental studies using actual allergens is the high local concentration that can be achieved (Fig. 12.5). This is an especially important aspect for type 2 adaptive immune responses, which are highly dependent on antigen concentration.

(a)   (b)

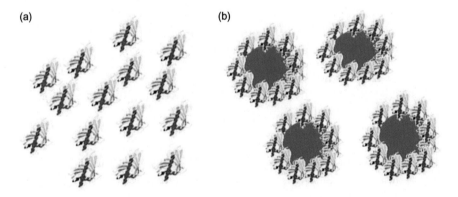

Figure 12.5 Allergen coated to np vs. free allergen. Symbolic representation of an allergen (the major birch pollen allergen Bet v1) in free form (a) and coated to a particle (b). It is possible to achieve a complete single-layer coating, which results in a local concentration of epitopes that could never be achieved by soluble allergen. Source: Data and figure are courtesy of Isabella Radauer-Preiml, University of Salzburg.

Fullerenes were reported to inhibit both IgE induced mediator release from human mast cells and basophils,[99] and to attenuate delayed-type hypersensitivity against methylated BSA in mice.[100] TiO_2 NP suppressed allergic pulmonary inflammation in asthmatic mice.[101] Similar findings were reported for silver NPs[102] and for Fe_2O_3 NPs.[103] On the other hand, SiO_2 impaired lung function of rats in an asthma model,[104] and NPs composed of carbon black,[105] SiO_2,[106] TiO_2,[107] and gold[107] all exacerbated pulmonary inflammation in mouse models of allergic asthma.

Numerous examples for both positive and negative contributions to allergic processes could be mentioned, but even though the actual mechanisms usually remain unclear, it is possible to conclude that NPs as such can have an impact on type 2 adaptive immunity. Using NP properties both as adjuvants that suppress an ongoing type 2 response and as delivery vehicles of allergen immunotherapy has been attempted in many studies.[108,109] The benefit of NPs could be similar as for other vaccinations: (i) they can provide both direct immune activation and a depot effect (acting like a classical adjuvant); (ii) they can be designed in terms of size, shape, surface charge, functionalization, etc., to target specific cells; and (iii) the high surface area potentially accommodates an extremely high local dose of the allergen. The latter effect is especially desired in allergy immunotherapy, where the clinical effect is derived from "overloading" the type 2 branch of the adaptive immune system, resulting in the formation of a tolerogenic response associated with T_{reg} cells. A wide variety of different NP materials have been used for that purpose, as recently reviewed by De Souza Reboucas et al.[109] Here we will focus on clinical studies, which are, up to now, very limited.

Only one agent has been tested in humans so far, a TLR9 antagonist (CYT003-QbG10) loaded into VLP, which showed clinical efficacy in phase IIb studies against allergic rhinoconjunctivitis[110] and against persistent allergic asthma.[111] That this reagent does not contain a specific allergen is not necessarily a disadvantage. Patients are mostly sensitized against different allergens from the same source and often have multiple allergies, so they show IgE dependent responses against allergens from different sources. In addition, there is a strong person-to person variation for reactions against the same allergen, including recognition of different epitopes and vast differences in the severity of symptoms. Under these circumstances, an agent that generally suppresses IgE dependent responses would be very useful. Of note, a second NP-based antiallergic drug has successfully passed a phase IIa study, but in this case for the treatment of horses suffering from recurrent allergic airway obstruction.[112] The therapeutic agent is also a TLR9 agonist, cytosine-phosphate-guanosine-oligodeoxynucleotides (CpG-ODN), in this case loaded onto gelatin NPs.[113] Again, no allergens are contained in the NP preparation and the benefits that various NP/allergen conjugates have shown in animal models still have to be reproduced in clinical studies.

12.7 WHAT ARE WE REALLY USING?

A general issue with all NP drugs is the question what the agent really looks like in the body. The question is addressed by the familiar concept of ADME (absorption, distribution, metabolism, excretion) which applies to all drugs. However, for NPs the situation is more complex than for chemical drugs. NPs are usually described in terms of their monomeric state, but many NPs form more or less loosely bound agglomerates and even quite stable aggregates.[114] This may already occur in storage, but a powerful trigger for agglomeration is often the insertion into liquid medium, in particular if it contains biological substances. Biologicals readily bind to nearly all NPs, forming a corona that is usually dominated by proteins, but can also contain lipids, nucleic acids, amino acids, and other compounds that NPs encounter upon entry into the body.[115] This protein shell may have immediate effects on immunity, in particular if the particle associates with immune proteins. The binding of proteins is not random and depends on the characteristics of the particular NP surface and on the available proteins.[116] Formation of the bioshell changes NP properties like size, surface charge (zeta potential), and in some cases stability—the NP may dissociate. Confusingly, NPs may also reform or grow when they enter a different medium. Overall, one must be aware that the body is usually not exposed to NPs, but rather to bio−nano complexes, which may or may not have the same critical properties as the original particle.[117]

As an example, consider oral uptake: An NP will be first coated by sputum proteins and other mucosal compounds, including the bacterial flora of the oral cavity. When the NP is swallowed it passes through the acid bath of the stomach and then reaches the alkaline environment of the gut lumen, being all the time subjected to the activity of different digestive enzymes. If it is absorbed it may pass through a gut epithelial cell and an endothelial cell, reach the blood and can be taken up by a monocyte, where it travels through endosomal and lysosomal environments, and could then arrive in the cytoplasm where it may find its intended drug target. That is an NP with quite a history. If we consider that we are all the time in reality dealing with a bio—nano complex, it is not easy to predict how this complex is going to look after all these passages. The corona may shield the particle surface and could thus prevent binding to receptors and thus biological responses, but if the right proteins are part of the corona it becomes a means of targeting particles to specific cells (Fig. 12.6).

The protein corona may, however, be useful by reducing the potential for toxicity. Immersion of NPs in serum containing media can reduce the release of toxic metal ions[118] and the production of reactive oxygen species (ROS)[119] on the surface of the NPs, both known mechanisms of nanotoxicity. The self-proteins coating the NPs can also contribute to immune tolerance, since the immune receptors are confronted mainly with self-proteins, which reduces the risk of unplanned immune responses. It has been suggested that protein binding to NPs leads to changes of protein conformation which may result in the exposure of cryptic epitopes in self-proteins.[120] Immune activation has been detected due to partial unfolding of NP-bound fibrinogen,[121] which, as an unfolded protein, constitutes a danger signal and promotes inflammation.[122] Gold nanorods have been shown to unveil

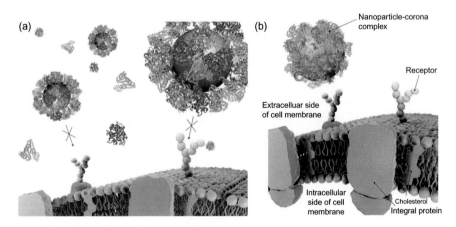

Figure 12.6 The protein corona. Proteins are the predominant components of the nanoparticle corona and can prevent (a) or enable (b) binding to cells. Note that the artist has not depicted nanoparticles lacking a protein shell. That is quite right: That situation does for most particles not exist in biological media. Source: Figure reprinted with permission from[134].

cryptic epitopes of collagen[123] and silicate NPs acted similarly for albumin,[124] but so far there is no indication that binding of self-proteins to NPs would lead to a breakdown of self-tolerance and consequently to the development of autoimmunity. The structural change induced in albumin, for example, could also be achieved by heat denaturation and, if triggered, binding of scavenger receptors. It may thus actually be a normal mechanism to clear particles.[124] That such mechanisms should exist is not surprising, since organisms have been exposed to particles of all sizes throughout evolution.

12.8 REBALANCING EXCITING NEW PROSPECTS AND OVER-OPTIMISTIC HYPE

In the excitement of many new nano-based therapeutic, diagnostic, and theranostic concepts, it is important to retain a careful analysis of the gap between visons and realities. Promising too much may raise false hopes that will be disappointed, leading not only to personal suffering but also to a weaker position for the whole field due to loss of confidence. If agents are not working as well as nice graphics may imply, it should be clearly stated. As a positive example, Rosenberg et al. have reported that the objective response rate in one of their cancer vaccine studies was a sobering 2.6%, out of 440 patients with solid tumors.[125] This is not a unique finding, as oncology has overall one of the lowest success rates for investigational drugs, due to complications like tumor heterogeneity and evolution of malignancy in the process of metastasis.[126] Nanopharmaceuticals have to overcome the same problems. They are no miracle drugs.

One of the important goals for the field as a whole is to improve prediction of possible adverse effects of nanopharmaceuticals, taking into account the complex interactions occurring in the body.[127] Most desired would be prediction on the basis of known structural properties in comparison to data on other, similar materials, which means to apply the principle of quantitative structure−function relationship approaches (QSAR or QSTR) to nanomaterials.[128] In the absence of this, a tiered approach for nanospecific safety effects is desirable. While this is well established in the development of pharmaceutics, the special challenges of NPs will require some adjustments, taking into account issues like assay interference by particles, different approaches to establish a "dose" that is not based on chemical concentration, and the evolution of NP−bio complexes in the human body.

Immune modulation will be an important area for nanomedical research. Autoimmunity is considered to be one of the key areas in the near future.[129] In addition to the obvious importance of getting better therapies for these diseases, this may also help to improve our understanding about interactions between NPs and the immune system. Understanding and controlling the molecular mechanisms involved may lead to progress in other clinical areas as well. It is clear that many exciting new concepts will not be able to get approval for clinical use. Nevertheless, nanomaterials do have unique features and are very promising candidates for new options in immune rebalancing.

12.9 ACKNOWLEDGEMENTS

The author gratefully acknowledges funding received from the European Union (EU) Seventh Framework Programme (FP7/2007–2013) under grant agreement no 263147 (NanoValid—Development of reference methods for hazard identification, risk assessment and LCA of engineered nanomaterials) and the EU FP7 Marie Curie Actions Network for Initial Training NanoTOES (PITN-GA-2010-264506).

REFERENCES

1. Dreaden EC, Alkilany AM, Huang X, Murphy CJ, El-Sayed MA. The golden age: gold nanoparticles for biomedicine. *Chem Soc Rev* 2012;**41**(7):2740–79.

2. Powell BS, Andrianov AK, Fusco PC. Polyionic vaccine adjuvants: another look at aluminum salts and polyelectrolytes. *Clin Exp Vaccine Res* 2015;**4**(1):23–45.

3. Lipscomb MF, Masten BJ. Dendritic cells: immune regulators in health and disease. *Physiol Rev* 2002;**82**(1):97–130.

4. Rivera Gil P, Huhn D, del Mercato LL, Sasse D, Parak WJ. Nanopharmacy: inorganic nanoscale devices as vectors and active compounds. *Pharmacol Res* 2010;**62**(2):115–25.

5. Etheridge ML, Campbell SA, Erdman AG, Haynes CL, Wolf SM, McCullough J. The big picture on nanomedicine: the state of investigational and approved nanomedicine products. *Nanomedicine* 2013;**9**(1):1–14.

6. Weissig V, Pettinger TK, Murdock N. Nanopharmaceuticals (part 1): products on the market. *Int J Nanomedicine* 2014;**9**:4357–73.

7. Weissig V, Guzman-Villanueva D. Nanopharmaceuticals (part 2): products in the pipeline. *Int J Nanomedicine* 2015;**10**.

8. Fadeel B, Shvedova A, Pietroiusti A. *Adverse effects of engineered nanomaterials*. Burlington: Elsevier Science; 2012. 1 online resource (367 s.) p.

9. Dobrovolskaia MA, McNeil SE. *Handbook of immunological properties of engineered nanomaterials*. Singapore: World Scientific Publishing Company; 2012. 1 online resource (721 s.) p.

10. Boraschi D, Duschl A. *Nanoparticles and the immune system safety and effects*. Amsterdam: Academic Press; 2014. XIII, 124 s. p.

11. Oostingh GJ, Casals E, Italiani P, Colognato R, Stritzinger R, Ponti J, et al. Problems and challenges in the development and validation of human cell-based assays to determine nanoparticle-induced immunomodulatory effects. *Part Fibre Toxicol* 2011;**8**(1):8.

12. Krug HF. Nanosafety research – are we on the right track? *Angew Chem Int Ed Engl* 2014;**53**(46):12304–19.

13. Lang L. FDA approves Cimzia to treat Crohn's disease. *Gastroenterology* 2008;**134**(7):1819.

14. Reis RV, Amorim EP, Ledo CA, Pestana RK, Goncalves ZS, Borem A. Selection of putative Terra Maranhao plantain cultivar mutants obtained by gamma radiation. *Genet Mol Res* 2015;**14**(2):4687–95.

15. Scott LJ. Glatiramer acetate: a review of its use in patients with relapsing-remitting multiple sclerosis and in delaying the onset of clinically definite multiple sclerosis. *CNS Drugs* 2013;**27**(11):971–88.

16. McKeage K. Glatiramer acetate 40 mg/mL in relapsing-remitting multiple sclerosis: a review. *CNS Drugs* 2015;**29**(5):425–32.

17. Shen LJ, Wu FL. Nanomedicines in renal transplant rejection – focus on sirolimus. *Int J Nanomedicine* 2007;**2**(1):25–32.

18. Junghanns JU, Muller RH. Nanocrystal technology, drug delivery and clinical applications. *Int J Nanomedicine* 2008;**3**(3):295–309.

19. Hafner A, Lovric J, Lakos GP, Pepic I. Nanotherapeutics in the EU: an overview on current state and future directions. *Int J Nanomedicine* 2014;**9**:1005–23.

20. Jang J, Lim DH, Choi IH. The impact of nanomaterials in immune system. *Immune Netw* 2010;**10**(3):85–91.

21. Fadeel B. Clear and present danger? Engineered nanoparticles and the immune system. *Swiss Med Wkly* 2012;**142**:w13609.

22. Hussain S, Vanoirbeek JA, Hoet PH. Interactions of nanomaterials with the immune system. *Wiley Interdiscip Rev Nanomed Nanobiotechnol* 2012;**4**(2):169–83.

23. Boraschi D, Costantino L, Italiani P. Interaction of nanoparticles with immunocompetent cells: nanosafety considerations. *Nanomedicine (Lond)* 2012;**7**(1):121–31.

24. Maeda H, Wu J, Sawa T, Matsumura Y, Hori K. Tumor vascular permeability and the EPR effect in macromolecular therapeutics: a review. *J Control Release* 2000;**65**(1–2):271–84.

25. Kannan S, Dai H, Navath RS, Balakrishnan B, Jyoti A, Janisse J, et al. Dendrimer-based postnatal therapy for neuroinflammation and cerebral palsy in a rabbit model. *Sci Transl Med* 2012;**4**(130):130ra46.

26. Gaca JG, Palestrant D, Lukes DJ, Olausson M, Parker W, Davis Jr. RD. Prevention of acute lung injury in swine: depletion of pulmonary intravascular macrophages using liposomal clodronate. *J Surg Res* 2003;**112**(1):19–25.

27. Richards PJ, Williams BD, Williams AS. Suppression of chronic streptococcal cell wall-induced arthritis in Lewis rats by liposomal clodronate. *Rheumatology (Oxford)* 2001;**40**(9):978–87.

28. Guo J, Waknine-Grinberg JH, Mitchell AJ, Barenholz Y, Golenser J. Reduction of experimental cerebral malaria and its related proinflammatory responses by the novel liposome-based beta-methasone nanodrug. *BioMed Res Int* 2014;**2014**:292471.

29. Henderson CS, Madison AC, Shah A. Size matters – nanotechnology and therapeutics in rheumatology and immunology. *Curr Rheumatol Rev* 2014;**10**(1):11–21.

30. Sharma AR, Kundu SK, Nam JS, Sharma G, Priya Doss CG, Lee SS, et al. Next generation delivery system for proteins and genes of therapeutic purpose: why and how? *BioMed Res Int* 2014;**2014**:327950.

31. Ozbakir B, Crielaard BJ, Metselaar JM, Storm G, Lammers T. Liposomal corticosteroids for the treatment of inflammatory disorders and cancer. *J Control Release* 2014;**190**:624–36.

32. Zhao G, Rodriguez BL. Molecular targeting of liposomal nanoparticles to tumor microenvironment. *Int J Nanomedicine* 2013;**8**:61–71.

33. Woodle MC, Lasic DD. Sterically stabilized liposomes. *Biochim Biophys Acta* 1992;**1113**(2): 171–99.

34. Van Rooijen N, Sanders A. Liposome mediated depletion of macrophages: mechanism of action, preparation of liposomes and applications. *J Immunol Methods* 1994;**174**(1–2): 83–93.

35. Lee WH, Loo CY, Traini D, Young PM. Nano- and micro-based inhaled drug delivery systems for targeting alveolar macrophages. *Expert Opin Drug Deliv* 2015;**12**(6): 1009–26.

36. Bartneck M, Warzecha KT, Tacke F. Therapeutic targeting of liver inflammation and fibrosis by nanomedicine. *Hepatobiliary Surg Nutr* 2014;**3**(6):364–76.

37. Tkach AV, Shurin GV, Shurin MR, Kisin ER, Murray AR, Young SH, et al. Direct effects of carbon nanotubes on dendritic cells induce immune suppression upon pulmonary exposure. *ACS Nano* 2011;**5**(7):5755–62.

38. Mitchell LA, Gao J, Wal RV, Gigliotti A, Burchiel SW, McDonald JD. Pulmonary and systemic immune response to inhaled multiwalled carbon nanotubes. *Toxicol Sci* 2007;**100**(1): 203–14.

39. Mehra NK, Jain NK. Multifunctional hybrid-carbon nanotubes: new horizon in drug delivery and targeting. *J Drug Target* 2015;1–15.

40. Martincic M, Tobias G. Filled carbon nanotubes in biomedical imaging and drug delivery. *Expert Opin Drug Deliv* 2015;**12**(4):563–81.

41. Lacerda L, Bianco A, Prato M, Kostarelos K. Carbon nanotubes as nanomedicines: from toxicology to pharmacology. *Adv Drug Deliv Rev* 2006;**58**(14):1460–70.

42. Donaldson K, Poland CA, Murphy FA, MacFarlane M, Chernova T, Schinwald A. Pulmonary toxicity of carbon nanotubes and asbestos – similarities and differences. *Adv Drug Deliv Rev* 2013;**65**(15):2078–86.

43. Toyokuni S. Genotoxicity and carcinogenicity risk of carbon nanotubes. *Adv Drug Deliv Rev* 2013;**65**(15):2098–110.

44. Nagda P. Nanomedicine: experts state safety concerns regarding carbon nanotubes have been allayed by chemistry. *Nanomedicine (Lond)* 2013;**8**(3):325–6.

45. Shvedova AA, Kisin ER, Murray AR, Kommineni C, Castranova V, Fadeel B, et al. Increased accumulation of neutrophils and decreased fibrosis in the lung of NADPH oxidase-deficient C57BL/6 mice exposed to carbon nanotubes. *Toxicol Appl Pharmacol* 2008;**231**(2):235–40.

46. Andon FT, Kapralov AA, Yanamala N, Feng W, Baygan A, Chambers BJ, et al. Biodegradation of single-walled carbon nanotubes by eosinophil peroxidase. *Small* 2013;**9** (16):2721–9 2720

47. Buda A, Facchin S, Dassie E, Casarin E, Jepson MA, Neumann H, et al. Detection of a fluorescent-labeled avidin-nucleic acid nanoassembly by confocal laser endomicroscopy in the microvasculature of chronically inflamed intestinal mucosa. *Int J Nanomedicine* 2015;**10**: 399–408.

48. Vermeij EA, Koenders MI, Bennink MB, Crowe LA, Maurizi L, Vallee JP, et al. The in-vivo use of superparamagnetic iron oxide nanoparticles to detect inflammation elicits a cytokine response but does not aggravate experimental arthritis. *PLoS ONE* 2015;**10**(5): e0126687.

49. Mieszawska AJ, Mulder WJ, Fayad ZA, Cormode DP. Multifunctional gold nanoparticles for diagnosis and therapy of disease. *Mol Pharm* 2013;**10**(3):831−47.

50. Naskalska A, Pyrc K. Virus like particles as immunogens and universal nanocarriers. *Pol J Microbiol* 2015;**64**(1):3−13.

51. Boato F, Thomas RM, Ghasparian A, Freund-Renard A, Moehle K, Robinson JA. Synthetic virus-like particles from self-assembling coiled-coil lipopeptides and their use in antigen display to the immune system. *Angew Chem Int Ed Engl* 2007;**46**(47):9015−18.

52. Tan M, Jiang X. Subviral particle as vaccine and vaccine platform. *Curr Opin Virol* 2014; **6**:24−33.

53. Kirnbauer R, Booy F, Cheng N, Lowy DR, Schiller JT. Papillomavirus L1 major capsid protein self-assembles into virus-like particles that are highly immunogenic. *Proc Natl Acad Sci USA* 1992;**89**(24):12180−4.

54. Jagu S, Kwak K, Garcea RL, Roden RB. Vaccination with multimeric L2 fusion protein and L1 VLP or capsomeres to broaden protection against HPV infection. *Vaccine* 2010;**28** (28):4478−86.

55. McAleer WJ, Buynak EB, Maigetter RZ, Wampler DE, Miller WJ, Hilleman MR. Human hepatitis B vaccine from recombinant yeast. *Nature* 1984;**307**(5947):178−80.

56. Safary A, Andre F. Clinical development of a new recombinant DNA hepatitis B vaccine. *Postgrad Med J* 1987;**63**(Suppl. 2):105−7.

57. Adkins JC, Wagstaff AJ. Recombinant hepatitis B vaccine: a review of its immunogenicity and protective efficacy against hepatitis B. *BioDrugs* 1998;**10**(2):137−58.

58. Li S, Zhang J, Xia N. Lessons from hepatitis E vaccine design. *Current Opin Virol* 2015; **11**:130−6.

59. Brito LA, O'Hagan DT. Designing and building the next generation of improved vaccine adjuvants. *J Control Release* 2014;**190**:563−79.

60. Buonaguro L, Tagliamonte M, Visciano ML, Tornesello ML, Buonaguro FM. Developments in virus-like particle-based vaccines for HIV. *Expert Rev Vaccines* 2013;**12**(2): 119−27.

61. Heuking S, Adam-Malpel S, Sublet E, Iannitelli A, Stefano A, Borchard G. Stimulation of human macrophages (THP-1) using Toll-like receptor-2 (TLR-2) agonist decorated nanocarriers. *J Drug Target* 2009;**17**(8):662−70.

62. Luo Z, Wang C, Yi H, Li P, Pan H, Liu L, et al. Nanovaccine loaded with poly I:C and STAT3 siRNA robustly elicits antitumor immune responses through modulating tumor-associated dendritic cells in vivo. *Biomaterials* 2015;**38**:50−60.

63. Hafner AM, Corthesy B, Merkle HP. Particulate formulations for the delivery of poly(I:C) as vaccine adjuvant. *Adv Drug Deliv Rev* 2013;**65**(10):1386−99.

64. Ma T, Wang L, Yang T, Ma G, Wang S. M-cell targeted polymeric lipid nanoparticles containing a Toll-like receptor agonist to boost oral immunity. *Int J Pharm* 2014;**473**(1−2): 296−303.

65. Heuking S, Borchard G. Toll-like receptor-7 agonist decoration enhances the adjuvanticity of chitosan-DNA nanoparticles. *J Pharm Sci* 2012;**101**(3):1166−77.

66. Ilyinskii PO, Roy CJ, O'Neil CP, Browning EA, Pittet LA, Altreuter DH, et al. Adjuvant-carrying synthetic vaccine particles augment the immune response to encapsulated antigen and exhibit strong local immune activation without inducing systemic cytokine release. *Vaccine* 2014;**32**(24):2882−95.

67. Maisonneuve C, Bertholet S, Philpott DJ, De Gregorio E. Unleashing the potential of NOD- and Toll-like agonists as vaccine adjuvants. *Proc Natl Acad Sci USA* 2014;**111**(34):12294−9.

68. Li H, Willingham SB, Ting JP, Re F. Cutting edge: inflammasome activation by alum and alum's adjuvant effect are mediated by NLRP3. *J Immunol* 2008;**181**(1):17−21.

69. Sun B, Ji Z, Liao YP, Wang M, Wang X, Dong J, et al. Engineering an effective immune adjuvant by designed control of shape and crystallinity of aluminum oxyhydroxide nanoparticles. *ACS Nano* 2013;**7**(12):10834−49.

70. Baron L, Gombault A, Fanny M, Villeret B, Savigny F, Guillou N, et al. The NLRP3 inflammasome is activated by nanoparticles through ATP, ADP and adenosine. *Cell Death Disease* 2015;**6**:e1629.

71. Mundra V, Li W, Mahato RI. Nanoparticle-mediated drug delivery for treating melanoma. *Nanomedicine (Lond)* 2015;1−21.

72. Adebowale AS, Choonara YE, Kumar P, du Toit LC, Pillay V. Functionalized nanocarriers for enhanced bioactive delivery to squamous cell carcinomas: targeting approaches and related biopharmaceutical aspects. *Curr Pharm Des* 2015;**21**(22):3167−80.

73. Kim SS, Harford JB, Pirollo KF, Chang EH. Effective treatment of glioblastoma requires crossing the blood-brain barrier and targeting tumors including cancer stem cells: the promise of nanomedicine. *Biochem Biophys Res Commun* 2015.

74. Almer G, Mangge H, Zimmer A, Prassl R. Lipoprotein-related and Apolipoprotein-mediated Delivery Systems for Drug Targeting and Imaging. *Curr Med Chem* 2015.

75. Miller-Kleinhenz JM, Bozeman EN, Yang L. Targeted nanoparticles for image-guided treatment of triple-negative breast cancer: clinical significance and technological advances. *Wiley Interdiscip Rev Nanomed Nanobiotechnol* 2015.

76. Frazier N, Ghandehari H. Hyperthermia approaches for enhanced delivery of nanomedicines to solid tumors. *Biotechnol Bioeng* 2015.

77. Sawdon A, Weydemeyer E, Peng CA. Antitumor therapy using nanomaterial-mediated thermolysis. *J Biomed Nanotechnol* 2014;**10**(9):1894−917.

78. Khatami M. 'Yin and Yang' in inflammation: duality in innate immune cell function and tumorigenesis. *Expert Opin Biol Ther* 2008;**8**(10):1461−72.

79. Ono M. Molecular links between tumor angiogenesis and inflammation: inflammatory stimuli of macrophages and cancer cells as targets for therapeutic strategy. *Cancer Sci* 2008;**99**(8):1501−6.

80. Bodduluru LN, Kasala ER, Madhana RM, Sriram CS. Natural killer cells: the journey from puzzles in biology to treatment of cancer. *Cancer Lett* 2015;**357**(2):454−67.

81. Dauer DJ, Ferraro B, Song L, Yu B, Mora L, Buettner R, et al. Stat3 regulates genes common to both wound healing and cancer. *Oncogene* 2005;**24**(21):3397−408.

82. Kortylewski M, Jove R, Yu H. Targeting STAT3 affects melanoma on multiple fronts. *Cancer Metastasis Rev* 2005;**24**(2):315−27.

83. Alshamsan A, Haddadi A, Hamdy S, Samuel J, El-Kadi AO, Uludag H, et al. STAT3 silencing in dendritic cells by siRNA polyplexes encapsulated in PLGA nanoparticles for the modulation of anticancer immune response. *Mol Pharm* 2010;**7**(5):1643−54.

84. Su WP, Cheng FY, Shieh DB, Yeh CS, Su WC. PLGA nanoparticles codeliver paclitaxel and Stat3 siRNA to overcome cellular resistance in lung cancer cells. *Int J Nanomedicine* 2012;**7**:4269−83.

85. Landesman-Milo D, Peer D. Altering the immune response with lipid-based nanoparticles. *J Control Release* 2012;**161**(2):600−8.

86. Heo DN, Yang DH, Moon HJ, Lee JB, Bae MS, Lee SC, et al. Gold nanoparticles surface-functionalized with paclitaxel drug and biotin receptor as theranostic agents for cancer therapy. *Biomaterials* 2012;**33**(3):856−66.

87. Mehta NK, Moynihan KD, Irvine DJ. Engineering new approaches to cancer vaccines. *Cancer Immunol Res* 2015;**3**(8):836–43.

88. Wong C, Stylianopoulos T, Cui J, Martin J, Chauhan VP, Jiang W, et al. Multistage nanoparticle delivery system for deep penetration into tumor tissue. *Proc Natl Acad Sci USA* 2011;**108**(6):2426–31.

89. Kwong B, Liu H, Irvine DJ. Induction of potent antitumor responses while eliminating systemic side effects via liposome-anchored combinatorial immunotherapy. *Biomaterials* 2011;**32**(22):5134–47.

90. Reddy ST, Rehor A, Schmoekel HG, Hubbell JA, Swartz MA. In vivo targeting of dendritic cells in lymph nodes with poly(propylene sulfide) nanoparticles. *J Control Release* 2006;**112**(1):26–34.

91. Manolova V, Flace A, Bauer M, Schwarz K, Saudan P, Bachmann MF. Nanoparticles target distinct dendritic cell populations according to their size. *Eur J Immunol* 2008;**38**(5):1404–13.

92. Fifis T, Gamvrellis A, Crimeen-Irwin B, Pietersz GA, Li J, Mottram PL, et al. Size-dependent immunogenicity: therapeutic and protective properties of nano-vaccines against tumors. *J Immunol* 2004;**173**(5):3148–54.

93. Kourtis IC, Hirosue S, de Titta A, Kontos S, Stegmann T, Hubbell JA, et al. Peripherally administered nanoparticles target monocytic myeloid cells, secondary lymphoid organs and tumors in mice. *PLoS ONE* 2013;**8**(4):e61646.

94. Moon JJ, Suh H, Bershteyn A, Stephan MT, Liu H, Huang B, et al. Interbilayer-crosslinked multilamellar vesicles as synthetic vaccines for potent humoral and cellular immune responses. *Nat Mater* 2011;**10**(3):243–51.

95. Shen H, Ackerman AL, Cody V, Giodini A, Hinson ER, Cresswell P, et al. Enhanced and prolonged cross-presentation following endosomal escape of exogenous antigens encapsulated in biodegradable nanoparticles. *Immunology* 2006;**117**(1):78–88.

96. Krishnamachari Y, Geary SM, Lemke CD, Salem AK. Nanoparticle delivery systems in cancer vaccines. *Pharm Res* 2011;**28**(2):215–36.

97. Vadlamudi A, Shaker M. New developments in allergen immunotherapy. *Curr Opin Pediatr* 2015.

98. Chelladurai Y, Suarez-Cuervo C, Erekosima N, Kim JM, Ramanathan M, Segal JB, et al. Effectiveness of subcutaneous versus sublingual immunotherapy for the treatment of allergic rhinoconjunctivitis and asthma: a systematic review. *J Allergy Clin Immunol Pract* 2013;**1**(4):361–9.

99. Ryan JJ, Bateman HR, Stover A, Gomez G, Norton SK, Zhao W, et al. Fullerene nanomaterials inhibit the allergic response. *J Immunol* 2007;**179**(1):665–72.

100. Yamashita K, Sakai M, Takemoto N, Tsukimoto M, Uchida K, Yajima H, et al. Attenuation of delayed-type hypersensitivity by fullerene treatment. *Toxicology* 2009;**261**(1–2):19–24.

101. Rossi EM, Pylkkanen L, Koivisto AJ, Nykasenoja H, Wolff H, Savolainen K, et al. Inhalation exposure to nanosized and fine TiO_2 particles inhibits features of allergic asthma in a murine model. *Part Fibre Toxicol* 2010;**7**:35.

102. Jang S, Park JW, Cha HR, Jung SY, Lee JE, Jung SS, et al. Silver nanoparticles modify VEGF signaling pathway and mucus hypersecretion in allergic airway inflammation. *Int J Nanomedicine* 2012;**7**:1329–43.

103. Ban M, Langonne I, Huguet N, Guichard Y, Goutet M. Iron oxide particles modulate the ovalbumin-induced Th2 immune response in mice. *Toxicol Lett* 2013;**216**(1):31–9.

104. Han B, Guo J, Abrahaley T, Qin L, Wang L, Zheng Y, et al. Adverse effect of nano-silicon dioxide on lung function of rats with or without ovalbumin immunization. *PLoS ONE* 2011;**6**(2):e17236.

105. Inoue K, Takano H. Aggravating impact of nanoparticles on immune-mediated pulmonary inflammation. *ScientificWorldJournal* 2011;**11**:382–90.

106. Brandenberger C, Rowley NL, Jackson-Humbles DN, Zhang Q, Bramble LA, Lewandowski RP, et al. Engineered silica nanoparticles act as adjuvants to enhance allergic airway disease in mice. *Part Fibre Toxicol* 2013;**10**:26.

107. Hussain S, Vanoirbeek JA, Luyts K, De Vooght V, Verbeken E, Thomassen LC, et al. Lung exposure to nanoparticles modulates an asthmatic response in a mouse model. *Eur Respir J* 2011;**37**(2):299–309.

108. Broos S, Lundberg K, Akagi T, Kadowaki K, Akashi M, Greiff L, et al. Immunomodulatory nanoparticles as adjuvants and allergen-delivery system to human dendritic cells: implications for specific immunotherapy. *Vaccine* 2010;**28**(31):5075–85.

109. De Souza Reboucas J, Esparza I, Ferrer M, Sanz ML, Irache JM, Gamazo C. Nanoparticulate adjuvants and delivery systems for allergen immunotherapy. *J Biomed Biotechnol* 2012;**2012**:474605.

110. Klimek L, Willers J, Hammann-Haenni A, Pfaar O, Stocker H, Mueller P, et al. Assessment of clinical efficacy of CYT003-QbG10 in patients with allergic rhinoconjunctivitis: a phase IIb study. *Clin Exp Allergy* 2011;**41**(9):1305–12.

111. Beeh KM, Kanniess F, Wagner F, Schilder C, Naudts I, Hammann-Haenni A, et al. The novel TLR-9 agonist QbG10 shows clinical efficacy in persistent allergic asthma. *J Allergy Clin Immunol* 2013;**131**(3):866–74.

112. Klier J, Lehmann B, Fuchs S, Reese S, Hirschmann A, Coester C, et al. Nanoparticulate CpG immunotherapy in RAO-affected horses: phase I and IIa study. *J Vet Intern Med* 2015;**29**(1):286–93.

113. Klier J, Fuchs S, May A, Schillinger U, Plank C, Winter G, et al. A nebulized gelatin nanoparticle-based CpG formulation is effective in immunotherapy of allergic horses. *Pharm Res* 2012;**29**(6):1650–7.

114. Bruinink A, Wang J, Wick P. Effect of particle agglomeration in nanotoxicology. *Arch Toxicol* 2015;**89**(5):659–75.

115. Monopoli MP, Aberg C, Salvati A, Dawson KA. Biomolecular coronas provide the biological identity of nanosized materials. *Nat Nanotechnol* 2012;**7**(12):779–86.

116. Docter D, Westmeier D, Markiewicz M, Stolte S, Knauer SK, Stauber RH. The nanoparticle biomolecule corona: lessons learned – challenge accepted? *Chem Soc Rev* 2015.

117. Pearson RM, Juettner VV, Hong S. Biomolecular corona on nanoparticles: a survey of recent literature and its implications in targeted drug delivery. *Front Chem* 2014;**2**:108.

118. Casals E, Pfaller T, Duschl A, Oostingh GJ, Puntes VF. Hardening of the nanoparticle-protein corona in metal (Au, Ag) and oxide (Fe$_3$O$_4$, CoO, and CeO$_2$) nanoparticles. *Small* 2011;**7**(24):3479–86.

119. Schlinkert P, Casals E, Boyles M, Tischler U, Hornig E, Tran N, et al. The oxidative potential of differently charged silver and gold nanoparticles on three human lung epithelial cell types. *J Nanobiotechnology* 2015;**13**:1.

120. Lynch I, Dawson KA, Linse S. Detecting cryptic epitopes created by nanoparticles. *Sci STKE* 2006;**2006**(327):pe14.

121. Deng ZJ, Liang M, Toth I, Monteiro MJ, Minchin RF. Molecular interaction of poly(acrylic acid) gold nanoparticles with human fibrinogen. *ACS Nano* 2012;**6**(10):8962–9.

122. Deng ZJ, Liang M, Monteiro M, Toth I, Minchin RF. Nanoparticle-induced unfolding of fibrinogen promotes Mac-1 receptor activation and inflammation. *Nat Nanotechnol* 2011;**6** (1):39−44.

123. Lo JH, von Maltzahn G, Douglass J, Park JH, Sailor MJ, Ruoslahti E, et al. Nanoparticle amplification photothermal unveiling of cryptic collagen binding sites. *J Mater Chem B, Mater Biol Med* 2013;**1**(39):5235−40.

124. Mortimer GM, Butcher NJ, Musumeci AW, Deng ZJ, Martin DJ, Minchin RF. Cryptic epitopes of albumin determine mononuclear phagocyte system clearance of nanomaterials. *ACS Nano* 2014;**8**(4):3357−66.

125. Rosenberg SA, Yang JC, Restifo NP. Cancer immunotherapy: moving beyond current vaccines. *Nat Med* 2004;**10**(9):909−15.

126. Kamb A, Wee S, Lengauer C. Why is cancer drug discovery so difficult? *Nat Rev Drug Discov* 2007;**6**(2):115−20.

127. Pelaz B, Charron G, Pfeiffer C, Zhao Y, de la Fuente JM, Liang XJ, et al. Interfacing engineered nanoparticles with biological systems: anticipating adverse nano-bio interactions. *Small* 2013;**9**(9−10):1573−84.

128. Winkler DA, Mombelli E, Pietroiusti A, Tran L, Worth A, Fadeel B, et al. Applying quantitative structure-activity relationship approaches to nanotoxicology: current status and future potential. *Toxicology* 2013;**313**(1):15−23.

129. Clemente-Casares X, Santamaria P. Nanomedicine in autoimmunity. *Immunol Lett* 2014; **158**(1−2):167−74.

130. Ganji DD, Kachapi SHH. Introduction to nanotechnology, nanomechanics, micromechanics, and nanofluid. In: *Application of Nonlinear Systems in Nanomechanics and Nanofluids*, William Andrew; 2015.

131. Tang L, Cheng J. Nonporous silica nanoparticles for nanomedicine application. *Nano Today* 2013;**8**:290−312.

132. Summers H. Nanomedicine—biological warfare at the cellular level. *Front Nanosci* 2013;**5**:1−26.

133. Zhu X, Radovic-Moreno AF, Wu J, Langer R, Shi J. Nanomedicine in the management of microbial infection — Overview and perspectives. *Nano Today* 2014;**9**:478−98.

134. Caracciolo G. Liposome−protein corona in a physiological environment: challenges and opportunities for targeted delivery of nanomedicines. *Nanomedicine* 2015;**11**:543−57.

INDEX

Note: Page numbers followed by "*f*" and "*t*" refer to figures and tables, respectively.

A

Abatacept, 17*t*, 22−23
Abilify, 4*t*
Abiraterone, 106−107
ABIRISK (Anti-Biopharmaceutical
    Immunization: Prediction and Analysis
    of Clinical Relevance to Minimize the
    Risk), 8
Acute diseases versus chronic diseases,
    105−106
Acute myocardial infarction (AMI), 162
Adalimumab (ADA), 4*t*, 22, 45−46
ADME (absorption, distribution, metabolism,
    excretion), 264
Advair/Seretide, 4*t*
Advanced Her-2 positive breast cancer, 109
Advanced nonsmall cell lung carcinoma,
    109−110
Aerobic glycolysis, 135−136
Aflibercept, 109
AJM 300, 50
Alarmins, 16
Alemtuzumab, 72, 74
Allergic diseases, therapeutic approaches in, 85
    allergen-specific immunotherapy (SIT),
        88−89
    general aspects, 85−87
    IgE and FcεRI, targeting, 94−96
    mast cells and eosinophils, targeting, 96−98
    modulation of allergen-specific responses,
        88−92
    Th2 cytokines, targeting, 92−94
Allergy, 262−264
Aluminum hydroxide (Alum) preparations,
    259
Alzheimer's disease (AD), 74−75
AMG 181, 49−50
5-Aminoimidazole-4-carboxamide
    ribonucleotide (AICAR), 41−42
Amyotrophic lateral sclerosis (ALS), 74−75
Anakinra, 17*t*, 23, 154, 154*f*, 160−163
Androgen deprivation therapy (ADT)
    for advanced prostate cancer, 109
Annexin A1, 28−29
Anti-AQP4 Abs, 76

Anti-B-cell therapy, for RA, 17*t*, 23
Antibiotics, 198−199
Antibody to infliximab (ATI), 45
Anticancer drugs for long-term use, 109−110
Anticitrullinated proteins antibodies
    (ACPA), 15
Anticytokine antibodies, 2*t*, 3
Antidrug antibodies (ADA), 8
Antigen presentation pathway, 181
Antigen presenting cells (APCs), 22−23,
    66−67
Anti-IgE mAb, 96
Anti-inflammatory plasma cells, 77
Anti-integrin antibody agents, 47−49
Antimalarials, 17*t*, 21
Antimetabolites, 1, 2*t*
Antimicrobial peptides, 195−196
Anti-TNF agents, 44−47
Anti-TNF therapy, 6
Anti-TNFα biologics, 3
Aprepitant, 255
AQP4-IgG, 77
Aripiprazole, 4*t*
Aryl hydrocarbon receptor (Ahr), 205−206
Aspirin-triggered 15-epi-lipoxin A4 (ATL), 27
Atherosclerosis, 130−131
Atripla, 4*t*
Autoimmune diseases, Systems Medicine
    of, 173
    and emerging technologies, 175−176
        application, in autoimmune research,
        176−182
    Systems Biology and, 175
Avastin, 4*t*
Avidin-nucleic acid nanoassembly (ANANAS)
    particles, 257
Avonex, 4*t*
Azathioprine (AZA), 1, 2*t*, 17*t*, 21, 41, 72, 78

B

Bacteroides fragilis, 197, 205
Bacteroides thetaiotaomicron, 195−196
Bacteroides-Porphyromonas-Prevotella group,
    202
BCG, 235

Beauveria nivea, 236, 237*t*
Behçet's disease, 159–160
Benralizumab, 93, 94*t*
Berberine (BBR), 234
Berberis sp., 237*t*
Bevacizumab, 4*t*, 106–107
BG12, 71–72
Bifidobacterium, 199
Big-data information and computation technology, 182
Bimodality, 107–108
Biological agents, 42–49
  anti-integrin antibody agents, 47–49
  anti-TNF agents, 44–47
Biologics
  as immunomodulatory agents, 1
    from immunosuppression to immune rebalancing, 6–8
    immunosuppressive approaches, 2–5
  in rheumatoid arthritis management, 22
Blood brain barrier (BBB), 66, 70–72, 76
Blood transcriptome studies, 179
Budesonide and formoterol, 4*t*

C

Cabazitaxel, 106–107
Calmodulin, 236
Calprotectin, 51
Calreticulin, 112
Camellia sinensis, 237*t*
Canakinumab Anti-Inflammatory Thrombosis Outcomes Study (CANTOS), 162
Canakinumab, 154*f*, 155, 160
Cancer as an immunological disease, 260–262
Caspase-1, 74–75, 152–153, 163
CCX-282B (Vercirnon), 50
CD8$^+$CD44^{hi} memory T cells, 111–112
CD25, 111–112
CD39, 24–25
CD40, 140–141, 261
CD41 lymphocytes, 178
CD48, 98
CD300a, 98
Celebrex, 4*t*
Celecoxib, 4*t*
Cell adhesions molecules, 42
Cell-based adoptive immunotherapies, 232
Center of Molecular Immunology (CIM), in Cuba, 109–110
  cancer therapy pipeline at, 111–112
Central nervous system (CNS), 63, 65–67, 77, 203
Certolizumab pegol, 46, 255

Cervavix®, 258
Cetuximab, 106–107
Chemo/radiochemotherapy, 107
Chemokine inhibitors, 50–51
Chronic diseases, 105–106
  basic biology of, 105–106
  immune rebalancing, 114–117
  immunotherapy, expanding role of, 110–112
  mathematical modeling, 117
  methodological consequence, 113–114
  pharmacologic consequence, 109–110
  quality of life (QoL), 105–106, 114
  research agenda for age of chronicity, 114–117
  transformation of advanced cancer into, 106–108
    increasing survival, in advanced disease, 106–107
    second tumors, in long-term survivors, 108
    shape of survival curves, 107–108
Chronic inflammation, defined, 115–116
Chronic urticaria (CU), 208, 212*t*
Cimavax, 107
Cimzia®, 255
Classical IL-1 family members, 151–153
Clinically isolated syndrome (CIS), 64
Clostridium difficile, 198–200, 210–211
Colonization factor antigen I (CFA/I), 204
Colonization resistance, 200
Colony-stimulating factor (CSF), 66
Colorectal cancer, advanced, 106–107
Computation technology, 182
Copaxone, 4*t*, 255
Coptis chinensis, 234
Corticosteroids, 1, 2*t*, 7–8
C-phycocyanin (CPC), 237*t*, 239, 241
C-phycocyanin/phycocyanobilin (CPC/PCB), 241–243
C-reactive protein (CRP), 51–52
Crestor, 4*t*
Crohn's disease (CD), 209–210
  immune based therapy for.
    See Inflammatory bowel disease (IBD)
Cryopyrin associated periodic syndromes (CAPS), 157–158
Cryopyrin, 157–158
CTLA-4, 110–111
Curcuma longa, 237*t*
β-Cyclodextrin, 260–261
Cyclophosphamide, 17*t*, 21, 72
Cyclosporine A (CsA), 17*t*, 20–21, 237*t*

Cytokine(s), 16
  immunoregulatory, 42
  inflammatory, 42, 151
  inhibitors, 3
  macrophage activation, 125
  Th2-related, 85–86, 125

D

Damage-associated molecular patterns
    (DAMPs), 125–127, 132
Deficiency of Interleukin-1 Receptor
    Antagonist (DIRA), 155–156
Deficiency of Interleukin-36 Receptor
    Antagonist (DITRA), 156
Delayed tails, 107–108
Dendritic cells (DCs), 152–153, 194
Density survival curves, 108f
Diet and prebiotics, 199
Dimethyl fumarate, 71–72
Disease modifying drugs (DMDs), 69
Disease-modifying antirheumatic drugs
    (DMARDs), 3, 16, 20, 23–24
Disoproxil fumarate, 4t
DNA sequencing techniques, 112, 115–116
Docetaxel, 106–107
Dupilumab, 93, 94t
Dysbiosis, 191–192, 200–201

E

Efavirenz, 4t
Efferocytosis, 26–27
EGF-Vaccine, 109–110
Eicosanoids, 26
Eldelumab, 50
Embryonic stem cells (ESCs), 53
Emergency hematopoiesis, 6–7
Emerging technologies
  application of, in autoimmune research,
      176–182
    big-data information and computation
        technology, 182
    genomics, 177–178
    network biology, 180–182
    proteomics approach, 179–180
    transcriptomic profiling and disease
        stratification, 179
  and precision medicine, 183
  Systems Biology and, 175–176
Emtricitabine, 4t
Enbrel, 3, 4t
Endotoxins, 234–235
Engerix-B, 258
Enterococcus faecium, 192–193

Enzalutamide, 106–107
Eosinophils, 86–87, 92
  targeting, 96–98
Epigallocatechin-3-gallate, 233, 237t
Epigenetic landscape, 136
Epigenetic reprogramming, 136–137
Epigenetics, 177t, 178
Epstein Barr virus (EBV) infection, 64, 163
Ertolizumabpegol, 22
Escalation therapy, 73, 74f
Escherichia coli, 28, 204
Esomeprazole, 4t
Etanercept, 4t, 22
Etrolizumab, 50
Experimental autoimmune encephalomyelitis
    (EAE), 65–67, 203–204, 240–241
Ezetimibe, 4t

F

Factor forkhead box P3 (Foxp3), 24–25
Familial cold auto-inflammatory syndrome
    (FCAS), 157–158
Familial cold urticarial, 157–158
Familial Hibernian fever, 158
Familial Mediterranean fever (FMF),
    156–157
FcεRI, targeting, 94–96
Fecal microbiota transplantation (FMT), 200,
    206
  probiotics and, 202–203
Fingolimod, 71, 74, 240
Firmicute family, 195
Flavonoid Diammonium glycyrrhizinate, 237t
Fluoropyrimidines, 106–107
Fluticasone-salmeterol, 4t
Free fatty acids (FFA), 161–162
FTY720, 240–241
Fullerenes, 263

G

Gardasil®, 258
Gastrointestinal (GI) tract, 191–193
Gelatin NPs, 261, 263–264
Genomics, 177–178, 177t
Germ-free (GF) mice, 191–192, 194
Ginger root extracts, 233
Ginseng, 233
Glatiramer, 4t
Glatiramer acetate (GA), 70
Gleevec, 4t
β-Glucans, 235
Glucocorticoids (GCs), 16–19, 17t
Glycyrol, 237t

Glycyrrhiza, 237*t*
Glycyrrhizin, 237*t*
GM-CSF, 134
Golimumab, 22, 46–47
G-protein-coupled receptor (GPR43), 194
Graft-versus-host disease (GVHD), 7–8
GRAS ("Generally Recognized As Safe"), 241
Gut microbiota, development of, 192–193
GW766994, 98

H
H1 antihistamines (anti-H1R), 96–97
H3K4, trimethylation of, 136–137
Healthy related quality of life (HRQoL), 63
Hecolin®, 258
Helicobacter pylori, 208
Helminthic infection, 206
Hematological disorders, 162–163
Hematopoietic stem cells (HSCs), 53
Herceptin, 4*t*
Hereditary auto-inflammatory diseases,
    155–159
HLA haplotype linkages, 177
Hormone therapy, 109
Human autoimmune diseases (HAD), 236,
    243–244
Humanization, 8
Humira, 3, 4*t*
Hydrastis canadensis, 234
Hygiene hypothesis, 200–201
Hyper IgD syndrome (HIDS), 157
Hypoxia, 137–138
Hypoxia-inducible factor (HIF)
    HIF-1α, 135–138
    HIF-2α, 137–138

I
Imatinib, 109, 229–230
Imatinib mesylate, 4*t*
Immune response-inducing drugs, 231–232
Immunoglobulin A (IgA), 195
Immunoglobulin E (IgE), 85–86
    targeting, 94–96
Immunoglobulins, 78
Immunomodulation with biologics, 1
    from immunosuppression to immune
        rebalancing, 6–8
    from nonspecific to targeted
        immunosuppression, 2–5
Immunomodulators, 124, 232–233
    for inflammatory bowel disease treatment,
        39–42
    methotrexate, 41–42

thiopurines, 41
Immunosaccharides, 235
Immunosuppressant, 253, 255
Immunosuppressive approaches, 1–8
Immunosuppressive drugs (ISD), 236, 237*t*
Immunosuppressive regimens, 1, 2*t*
Induced natural killer T (iNKT) cells, 197
Inducible nitric oxide synthase (iNOS),
    124–125, 242–243
Induction therapy, 74
Inflammasome, 152–153
Inflammation, resolution of, 25–29
Inflammatory bowel disease (IBD), 37,
    209–211, 212*t*
    biological agents, 42–49
        anti-integrin antibody agents, 47–49
        anti-TNF agents, 44–47
    current immune based therapies in, 39, 40*f*,
        40*t*
    immune regulation in, 37–38
    immunomodulators, 39–42
        methotrexate, 41–42
        thiopurines, 41
    innate and adaptive immune system in, 39*f*
    next generation immune based therapies in,
        43*t*, 49–54
        IL-12/23 pathway inhibitor, 52–53
        JAK-stat pathway inhibitor, 51
        laquinimod, 52
        leukocyte trafficking, blockage of, 49–51
        stem cell therapy, 53–54
        TGFβ/SMAD7 pathway inhibitor, 51–52
Inflammatory cytokines, modulating, 151
    biologicals targeting IL-1, 154–155
    blocking IL-1 in disease, 155–163
        acute myocardial infarction (AMI), 162
        hematological disorders, 162–163
        hereditary auto-inflammatory diseases,
            155–159
        metabolic diseases, 161–162
        rheumatic diseases, 160
        systemic inflammatory diseases, 159–160
    classical IL-1 family members, 151–153
    IL-1 receptor signaling, 153–154
Infliximab, 4*t*, 22, 44–45, 158
Innovative Medicine Initiative-Joint
    Undertaking (IMI-JU), 8
Insulin glargine, 4*t*
Interferon (IFN/INF), 179
    IFN-β, 69–70
    IFNγ/INFγ, 91, 93–94, 138–139
Interleukin(s)
    IL-1. *See* Interleukin-1 (IL-1)

IL-12/23 pathway inhibitor, 52–53
IL-13, 93
IL-1 receptor (IL-1R), 153–154
IL-3, 86–87
IL-36Ra, 156
IL-36RN, 156
IL-4, 86, 93, 134
IL-5, 86–87, 92–93, 97–98
IL-6, 23–24, 90–91, 139
Interleukin-1 (IL-1), 27, 151
  biologicals targeting, 154–155
  blocking, in disease, 155–163
    acute myocardial infarction (AMI), 162
    hematological disorders, 162–163
    hereditary auto-inflammatory diseases, 155–159
    metabolic diseases, 161–162
    rheumatic diseases, 160
    systemic inflammatory diseases, 159–160
  IL-1α and IL-1β, 151–153
  receptor signaling, 153–154
Intracellular cell adhesion molecule (ICAM)-1, 42
Ion channel dysfunction, during multiple sclerosis, 69
Ipilimumab, 106–107
Ipilizumab, 6–7
Irinotecan, 106–107
Iron accumulation, during multiple sclerosis, 68
Isaria sinclairii, 237t
Ischemia/reperfusion (I/R) model, 241–242

J

Janus kinase (JAK), 24, 38
  JAK-stat pathway inhibitor, 51
Januvia, 4t
JNJ-27390467, 97

L

Lactobacillus gasseri, 197
Lamina propria (LP), 195
Lantus, 4t
Lapatinib, 106–107
Laquinimod, 52
Leflunomide, 17t, 19–20, 23
Lenalidomide, 4t
Lentinan, 235
Leukocyte trafficking, blockage of, 47, 47f, 49–51
Ligelizumab, 94t, 96
Lipid mediators, 26–28
Liposomes, nanosized, 256

Lipoxin A4 (LXA4), 26–28
Liquid chromatography with tandem mass spectrometry (LC-MS/MS), 26
Lymphoid tissue and general immune responses, 193–194
Lyrica, 4t

M

M1 macrophages, 124–125, 126f, 135–136, 140–141
M1/M2 skewing, 128–132, 130f
M2 macrophages, 124–125, 126f, 127–128, 132–135, 137–139
Mab Thera, 4t
Macrophage activation syndrome (MAS), 163
Macrophage activation
  endogenous factors, 134
  epigenetic reprogramming, 136–137
  local conditions and cell–cell interactions, 137–139
    hypoxia, 137–138
    interaction with MSCs in microenvironment, 138–139
  M1/M2 skewing, 128–132
  metabolic reprogramming, 135–136
  microRNA, 134–135
  modulation of, 121, 132–137, 142f
  polarization/activation, 123–128
  signaling, 132–134
  therapeutic applications based on, 140–141
Macrophage plasticity, 141–142
Magnetic resonance imaging (MRI), 66, 71, 73, 74f, 75f
Major histocompatibility complex (MHC), 1
Maresin 1, 27–28
Mast cells, 86
  targeting, 96–98
M-CSF, 134
Mepolizumab, 92, 94t
6-Mercaptopurine (6MP), 41
Mesenchymal stem cells (MSCs) therapy, 53–54, 137–139
Messenger RNA transcriptome, 178
Metabolic diseases, 161–162
Metabolic reprogramming, 135–136
Metabolic syndrome, 130–131
Metabolomics, 177t, 191–192
Metastatic colorectal cancer, 109
Methotrexate (MTX), 16, 17t, 19–21, 23, 41–42
Mevalonate kinase (MVK), 157

Microbiota, 191
  barrier effect, 200
  development of, 192–193
  effects on immune development, 193–197
    antimicrobial peptides, 195–196
    B cells, 195
    dendritic cells and macrophages, 194
    intestinal CD4 + and CD8 + T cells, 196
    lymphoid tissue and general immune
      responses, 193–194
    metabolites, 194
    natural killer T cells, 197
    neutrophils, 194–195
    regulatory T cells, 195
    T_H17 cells, 196
  modulation, in immune-mediated disorders,
    197–200
    antibiotics, 198–199
    diet and prebiotics, 199
    fecal microbiota transplantation (FMT),
      200
    probiotics, 199–200
  prevalence and progression immune-related
    disease, 200–211
    chronic urticarial (CU), 208
    inflammatory bowel disease (IBD),
      209–211
    multiple sclerosis (MS), 203–206
    rheumatoid arthritis (RA), 201–203
    systemic lupus erythematosus (SLE),
      207–208
Microglia activation, 68
MicroRNA (miRNAs), 179
  and macrophage polarization, 134–135
Mitochondrial injury, during multiple sclerosis,
    68–69
Mitoxantrone, 72
Mongersen, 51–52
Monoclonal antibodies (mAbs), 140–141,
    232–233
Monocyte-derived macrophages, 123–124
Monocytes, 123–124, 128, 152–153
mTORC1/mTORC2, 138
Muckle-Wells syndrome (MWS), 157–158
Mucosal addressin cell adhesion molecule
    (MAdCAM), 42, 47–50, 47f
Mucosal dendritic cells, 194
Multi-factorial diseases, 200–201
Multiple myeloma (MM), 162–163
Multiple sclerosis (MS), 63, 180–181, 212t
  acute disease attacks, treatment of, 77
  clinical features, 64
  current therapy of, 69–70

    alemtuzumab, 72
    cyclophosphamide and mitoxantrone, 72
    dimethyl fumarate, 71–72
    fingolimod, 71
    glatiramer acetate (GA), 70
    interferon-β, 70
    mechanism of action, efficacy, and safety
      concerns, 70–72
    natalizumab, 70–71
    teriflunomide, 71
  disease forms, 64–65
    benign and malign MS, 65
    clinically isolated syndrome (CIS), 64
    primary progressive MS (PP-MS), 65
    relapsing–remitting MS (RR-MS), 65
    secondary progressive MS (SP-MS), 65
  etiology, 63–64
  future therapies for, 78–79
  immunopathogenesis, 66–67
  mechanism underlying progressive forms of,
    67–69
  microbiota involvement, 203–206
    diet, 205–206
    human studies, 206
    mouse models on microbiota involvement,
      203–204
    probiotics, 204–205
  and neurodegenerative diseases, 63, 74–76
  neuromyelitis optica (NMO), long-term
    treatment of, 78
  pathology and neuroradiology, 65–66
  treatment strategies, 72–77
    early treatment, 73
    escalation therapy, 73
    induction therapy, 74
    pathogenesis of NMO, 76–77
Multipotent stromal cells (MSCs), 137–139
Multiwalled carbon nanotubes (MWCNT),
    256–257
Mycobacterium tuberculosis, 6
Mycophenolate mofetil (MMF), 78
MyD88, 132–134, 153–154
  MyD88 pathway, 195–196
Myriocin, 237t, 240

N

NADPH oxidase, 234, 239, 242–243
Nanocarriers, 258
Nanomedicine, 9, 251
  activating immunity, 258–259
  allergy, 262–264
  cancer as an immunological disease,
    260–262

nanoparticles (NPs), 251–253
products on market or in development,
    253–254
reality, 264–266
rebalancing exciting new prospects and
    overoptimistic hype, 266–267
suppressing immunity, 255–257
Nanoparticles (NPs), 251–253, 254*f*, 255–256
immune modulation by, 259*f*
Nanotechnology, 9, 258
Natalizumab, 47–49, 70–71, 74
Natural killer T cells (NKT cells), 197
Natural products
    C-phycocyanin/phycocyanobilin (CPC/
        PCB), 241–243
    disease prevention and treatment,
        modulation of immune responses for,
        231–233
    immunosuppression and rebalancing of
        immune functions, 236–237
    influencing and modifying intersystem
        interactions and infection resistance,
        234–235
    and neuroprotection/restoration, 240–241
    oxidant versus antioxidant argument,
        238–240
    rediscovering, 9
    traditional medicinal preparations, 233–234
Negative feedback control loops, 105–106
Neonatal-onset multisystem inflammatory
    disease (NOMID), 157–158
Network biology, 180–182
Neulasta/Neupogen, 4*t*
Neurodegenerative diseases
    future therapies for, 78–79
    multiple sclerosis and, 63
Neuromyelitis optica (NMO), 74–75
    long-term treatment of, 78
    pathogenesis of, 76–77
Neuromyelitis optica spectrum disorders
    (NMOSD), 75–76
Neuroprotection/restoration, by natural
    products, 240–241
Neutrophils, 152–153, 161–162, 194–195
New Zealand black (NZB) mice, 207
Nexium, 4*t*
Next generation immune based therapies in
    IBD, 43*t*, 49–54
Next generation compounds, 258
Nimotuzumab, 107, 109–110
NISD, 236, 240
Nivolumab, 6–7, 106–107
NK1.1 cells, 111–112

NLRP3, 157–158
NLRP3, activation of, 259
NOD-like receptors (NLRs), 258
Notch signaling, 134
NP/TLR ligand preparations, 258
Nutrition, for regulation of microbiota-related
    disorders, 205–206

O
Obesity, 129–131, 161–162, 191–192
OC000459, 97–98
Omalizumab, 94*t*, 95–96
Omics data types, 177*t*
Oral food allergen immunotherapy
    (OIT), 262
Osteoimmunology, 30–31
Osteoprotegerin (OPG), 30–31
Oxaliplatin, 106–107
Oxidant versus antioxidant, 238–240

P
Pam3CSK4, 91
Paneth cells, 9, 195–196
Panitumumab, 106–107
PAPA syndrome, 158–159
Parkinson's disease (PD), 74–75
Pathguide, 181
Pathogen-associated molecular patterns
    (PAMPs), 125–127, 132
Payer's patches, 193–195
Pegfilgrastim, 4*t*
Pembrolizumab, 106–107
Pembrolizuman, 6–7
Periodic fever, aphthous stomatitis,
    pharyngitis, and adenopathy (PFAPA)
    syndrome, 159–160
Pertuzumab, 106–107, 109
PF00547659, 50
Phosphorylated dihydroceramides (PE DHC),
    204–205
Phycocyanobilin (PCB), 237*t*, 239, 241–244
Piggybacking, 255–256
Plasticity, 124
Polyphenolic curcumin, 237*t*
Polysaccharide-K, 235
Porphyromonas gingivalis, 204–205
Prebiotics, 199
Precision medicine, 9, 183
Pregabalin, 4*t*
Prevnar, 4*t*
Prevotella copri, 202
Primary progressive MS (PP-MS), 65, 68–69
Probability functions, 107–108

Probiotics, 199–200, 204–205
  and fecal microbiota transplantation,
      202–203
Progressive multifocal leukoencephalopathy
      (PML), 48–49, 71
Prostate specific antigen (PSA), 233
Protectin 1 (PD1), 27–28, 110–111, 117
Protein kinase inhibitors
  in rheumatoid arthritis management, 24
Protein-protein interaction (PPI), 180
Proteomics, 174, 177t, 179–180
  database searching, 179–180
  de novo sequencing, 179–180
  laser-capture microdissection, 180
  mass spectrometry, 180
Pseudomonas aeruginosa, 197
PSTPIP1 gene, 158–159

Q
QGE031 (Ligelizumab), 96
Quantitative structure–function relationship
      approaches (QSAR/QSTR)

R
Racotumomab, 109–110
Radium 223, 106–107
Rapamune®, 255
Rapamycin, 255
Reactive oxygen species (ROS), 66–69, 77
Receptor activator of nuclear factor κB ligand
      (RANKL), 30–31
Recombivax HB®, 258
Regorafenib, 109
Regulatory T cells (Tregs), 7–8, 24–25,
      66–67, 91, 111–112, 140–141, 195,
      205–206, 243–244
Relapsing–remitting MS (RR-MS), 65–69
Remicade, 3, 4t
Reslizumab, 92, 94t
Resolvin E1 (RvE1), 27–28
Resveratrol, 233–234
Revlimid, 4t
Rheumatic diseases, 160
Rheumatoid arthritis (RA), 15, 160, 201–203,
      212t
  advance in therapies for, 13
  challenges, 29–31
  loss of immune tolerance as factor for,
      24–25
  management, 16–24
    Anakinra, 23
    anti-B-cell therapy, 23

antimalarials, 21
azathioprine, 21
biologics, 22
cyclophosphamide, 21
cyclosporine A, 20–21
glucocorticoids, 16–19
leflunomide, 19–20
methotrexate, 19
protein kinase inhibitors, 24
sulfasalazine, 20
T-lymphocyte costimulation blocker,
    22–23
Tocilizumab, 23–24
tumor necrosis factor inhibitors, 22
new alternatives for treatment of, 24
resolution of inflammation, 25–29
  annexin A1, 28–29
  lipid mediators, 26–28
Rhodamine B, 260–261
Rilonacept, 155
Rituxan, 3, 4t
Rituximab, 4t, 17t, 23, 78
RNA, 260
ROS (reactive oxygen species), 77, 135–136,
      238–240
Rosuvastatin calcium, 4t

S
Saccharomyces boulardii, 199–200
Salmonella typhimurium, 204
Salvia miltiorrhiza, 237t
Salvianolic acid, 237t
SAPHO syndrome, 159–160
Schnitzler syndrome, 162–163
Second primary neoplasms, 108
Second tumors, in long-term survivors, 108
Secondary amyloidosis, 157–158
Secondary progressive MS (SP-MS), 65
Segmented filamentous bacteria (SFB),
      196–197, 203–204
Self-proteins, 265–266
Short-chain fatty acids (SCFAs), 194–195,
      199, 209–210
Shotgun metagenomic sequencing, 191–192
Single nucleotide polymorphism (SNP),
      177–178, 181
Single-walled carbon nanotubes (SWCNT),
      256–257
Sipuleucel-T, 231–232
SiRNA, for STAT3, 260
Sirolimus, 236, 237t, 255
Sitagliptin, 4t

SOCS family members, 134
Sofosbuvir, 4t
Sovaldi, 3, 4t
Specialized proresolving mediators (SPMs),
    26–28
Sphingomonas bacteria, 197
Spirulina platensis (Sp), 237t
Squamous cell carcinoma of the head and neck
    (SCCHN), 107, 109–110
Staphylococcus aureus, 28, 197
STAT3, 260
Stem cell factor (SCF), 97
Stem cell therapy
    for inflammatory bowel disease, 53–54
Still's disease, 159–160, 163
Streptomyces higroscopicus, 237t
Streptomyces tsukubaensis, 237t
Subcutaneous immunotherapy (SCIT), 262
Sublingual immunotherapy (SLIT), 91, 262
Sulfasalazine (SSZ), 17t, 20
Superparamagnetic iron oxide NPs (SPIONS),
    257
Suppressing immunity, 255–257
Suppressive immunotherapies, 233
Symbicort, 4t
Synovial neovascularization, 20, 23–24
Systemic inflammatory diseases, 159–160
Systemic lupus erythematosus (SLE), 163,
    207–208
Systems Biology
    and emerging technologies, 175–176
    and Systems Medicine, 175
    tools, 173
Systems Medicine of autoimmune diseases.
    See Autoimmune diseases, Systems
    Medicine of
Systems modeling approaches, 182

T
T cell depletion, 7, 69
T regulatory cells. See Regulatory T cells
    (Tregs)
T regulatory epitopes, 8
Tacrolimus, 236, 237t
Tamoxifen, 109
Tanshione (TSN), 233
Tanshione IIA, 237t
Targeted therapies, 106–107, 109, 113–115
T-DM1 drug conjugate, 106–107
Tenofovir, 4t
Teriflunomide, 71
TGFβ/SMAD7 pathway inhibitor, 51–52

Th2 cytokines, targeting, 87, 92–94
Th2 lymphocyte-derived signals, 138–139
Th2-related cytokines, 85–86, 125
Therapeutic plasma exchange (TPE), 77
6-Thioguanine nucleotides (6TGN), 41
Thiopurines, 41, 44–45
Thiopurine-S-methyltransferase (TPMT), 41
Thymidylatesynthetase (TS), 41–42
Timothy grass allergens, 90
Tissue-resident macrophages, 123–124, 129
TLR signaling, 132–134
TLR2/6 agonists, 91
TLR4 ligands, 90–91
TLR9 antagonist, 263–264
T-lymphocyte costimulation blocker, for RA,
    17t, 22–23
TNFRSF1, 158
Tocilizumab, 17t, 23–24
Tofacitinib, 24, 51
Tolerance, restoration of, 7
Toll-like receptors (TLRs), 91, 125–127,
    132–134, 153–154, 195–196, 258
    ligands for, 258
    targeting, 90
    TLR2, 90–91, 204–205
    TLR4, 90–91, 135–136
    TLR5, 92
    TLR6, 91
    TLR7, 91
    TLR8, 90–91
    TLR9, 91, 261, 263–264
Traditional medicine, 229–230
Transcriptomics, 177t
    profiling and disease stratification, 179
Transplantation immunity, 1
Trastuzumab, 4t, 106–107
TRIF, 132–134
Tripterygium wilfordii, 237t
Triptolide, 237t
Truvada, 4t
Tumor antigen-specific mAbs, 140–141
Tumor growth, 6–7, 106–107, 110–111, 115,
    117
Tumor necrosis factor (TNF)
    alpha-inducible protein 3 gene, 177
    anti-TNF treatments, 3
    in rheumatoid arthritis management, 17t, 22
    TNFα, 22
    TNF receptor-1 associated periodic
        syndrome (TRAPS), 158
Tumor progression, 109–110, 113–114,
    137–138

Tumor types, 107−108
Tumor-associated macrophages (TAMs),
        137−138, 140−141
Type 2 diabetes mellitus (T2DM), 161−162
Tyrosine kinase 2 (TYK2), 24

U
Ulcerative colitis (UC), 38, 42, 209−210
    immune based therapy for.
        See Inflammatory bowel disease (IBD)
Ustekinumab, 52−53

V
Vaccines, future of, 258−259
Vaxira, 107

Vedolizumab, 47−50
VEGF/VEGFR signaling pathway, 109
Virus-like particles (VLP), 258, 263−264
Vitamin C, 229

W
Warburg effect, 135−136

X
Xenohormesis, 229
XmAb7195, 94*t*, 96

Z
Zetia/Vytorin, 4*t*